The Society of Fire Protection Engineers Series

Series Editor
Chris Jelenewicz, Society of Fire Protection Engineers
Gaithersburg, MD, USA

The Society of Fire Protection Engineers Series provides rapid dissemination of the most recent and advanced work in fire protection engineering, fire science, and the social/human dimensions of fire.

The Series publishes outstanding, high-level research monographs, professional volumes, contributed collections, and textbooks.

Marcus Runefors • Ragnar Andersson
Mattias Delin • Thomas Gell
Editors

Residential Fire Safety

An Interdisciplinary Approach

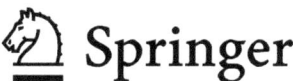

Editors
Marcus Runefors
Division of Fire Safety Engineering
Lund University
Lund, Sweden

Mattias Delin
The Swedish Fire Research Foundation
(Brandforsk)
Stockholm, Sweden

Ragnar Andersson
Risk and Environmental Studies, Centre for
Societal Risk Research
Karlstad University
Karlstad, Sweden

Thomas Gell
The Swedish Fire Research Foundation
(Brandforsk)
Stockholm, Sweden

Division of Fire Safety Engineering
Lund University
Lund, Sweden

ISSN 2731-3638   ISSN 2731-3646 (electronic)
The Society of Fire Protection Engineers Series
ISBN 978-3-031-06324-4   ISBN 978-3-031-06325-1 (eBook)
https://doi.org/10.1007/978-3-031-06325-1

© The Editor(s) (if applicable) and The Author(s), under exclusive license to Springer Nature Switzerland AG 2023
This work is subject to copyright. All rights are solely and exclusively licensed by the Publisher, whether the whole or part of the material is concerned, specifically the rights of translation, reprinting, reuse of illustrations, recitation, broadcasting, reproduction on microfilms or in any other physical way, and transmission or information storage and retrieval, electronic adaptation, computer software, or by similar or dissimilar methodology now known or hereafter developed.
The use of general descriptive names, registered names, trademarks, service marks, etc. in this publication does not imply, even in the absence of a specific statement, that such names are exempt from the relevant protective laws and regulations and therefore free for general use.
The publisher, the authors, and the editors are safe to assume that the advice and information in this book are believed to be true and accurate at the date of publication. Neither the publisher nor the authors or the editors give a warranty, expressed or implied, with respect to the material contained herein or for any errors or omissions that may have been made. The publisher remains neutral with regard to jurisdictional claims in published maps and institutional affiliations.

This Springer imprint is published by the registered company Springer Nature Switzerland AG
The registered company address is: Gewerbestrasse 11, 6330 Cham, Switzerland

Preface

This anthology aims to give a comprehensive overview of deaths and injuries from residential fires and evidence-based approaches to reducing this problem. We believe that the residential area – where most fire-related fatalities and injuries occur – has not received the attention it merits compared to larger-scale fire events. Even if there are many specific papers and reports available on the topic, a comprehensive textbook in the area was still lacking.

Between 2013 and 2018, the Swedish Civil Contingencies Agency, MSB, funded a substantial research effort on residential fires that resulted in new knowledge, not least on deaths and injuries from these fires. The Swedish Fire Research Foundation, Brandforsk, coordinated this work. When looking at the many new research findings, it was natural to come to the conclusion that these, together with results from published international research, deserved to be made more widely available.

Although many of the authors are Swedish, we believe that most of the findings are generically valid and applicable to other Western countries and regions. The connection to previously published scientific papers in the chapters, together with the peer-review process that all chapters have undergone, should guarantee this.

We hope this book will serve as a textbook for education at both universities and fire service schools. It also aims to be an accessible guideline for practitioners from different disciplines – fire, health, social, and policy sciences – as well as for different professional actors affecting the residential fire safety, such as authorities, standardization organizations, and insurance companies.

The interdisciplinary approach, where the authors represent broad expertise from different disciplines such as fire protection engineering, public health science, medicine, psychology, and policy sciences, is believed to be unique. Based on research and practice on the different aspects, the book summarizes the current level of knowledge, and some practical examples, giving guidance concerning preventive efforts and future research. Traditional textbooks on fire protection tend to describe the problem as mainly technical, whereas it rather should be seen as a problem of human vulnerability.

We hope that this book can serve as one small but important step to reduce further the number of individuals injured by fire in the place that should be the safest – their home.

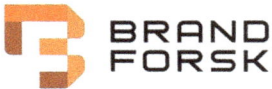

Lund, Sweden	Marcus Runefors
Karlstad, Sweden	Ragnar Andersson
Stockholm, Sweden	Mattias Delin
Stockholm, Sweden	Thomas Gell

Acknowledgments

The initiative for this anthology was taken by the Swedish Fire Research Foundation – Brandforsk – which, together with the Swedish Civil Contingencies Agency (MSB), also funded the editorial work. Brief presentations of these two organizations are given at the end of this section.

As editors, we wish to express our sincere gratitude to all contributors without whose generous efforts this volume would not have been made possible.

The main contributory work was, of course, laid down by all chapter authors, as presented separately. You willingly and generously shared your valuable time and extensive expertise for a good and important cause. Thank you!

We also want to thank our panel of reviewers, as listed below, for careful reading and valuable comments on the chapter manuscripts before publishing:

Ms. Marty Ahrens, National Fire Protection Association, USA
Dr. Michelle Ball, Victoria University, Australia
Prof. Ulf Björnstig, Umeå University, Sweden
Dr. Karen Boyce, Ulster University, United Kingdom
Dr. Juan B. Echeverria, University of Navarra, Spain
Mr. Len Garis, University of the Fraser Valley, Canada
Dr. Dag Glebe, RISE Research Institutes of Sweden, Sweden
Dr. Johanna Gustavsson, Karlstad University, Sweden
Dr. Matt Hinds-Aldrich, American Association of Insurance Services, USA
Dr. Fredrik Huss, Uppsala University, Sweden
Prof. Kenneth Isman, University of Maryland, USA
Dr. Charles Jennings, City University of New York, USA
Dr. Nils Johansson, Lund University, Sweden
Dr. Stephen Kerber, Underwriters Laboratory, USA
Ms. Emelie Lantz, West Blekinge Fire and Rescue Service, Sweden
Prof. Olle Mattsson, Uppsala University, Sweden
Prof. Per Nilsen, Linköping University, Sweden
Prof. Finn Nilson, Karlstad University, Sweden
Dr. Lynn Ranåker, Swedish Civil Contingencies Agency, Sweden

Dr. Linda Ryen, Örebro County Region, Sweden
Mr. Erik Smedberg, Lund University, Sweden
Prof. Anne Steen-Hansen, Norwegian University of Science and Technology, Norway
Dr. Anders Svensson, Linnaeus University, Sweden
Ms. Karolina Storesund, Norwegian University of Science and Technology, Norway
Prof. Björn Sundström, Luleå University, Sweden

A special thanks goes to Kathleen Almand, former Vice President, National Fire Protection Association, for valuable help.

Last but not least, we want to thank Springer Nature and its staff for their very professional interaction during the whole process, from project idea up to technical production and issuing.

> Brandforsk, **the Swedish Fire Research Foundation**, is an independent non-profit organization working, since 1979, to develop and communicate fire safety knowledge to decrease the consequences of fire in the society. The work is funded by a wide variety of supporting organizations in Sweden, making Brandforsk a unique platform for collaboration between public authorities, the private sector, and non-profit organizations. The vision is a fire-safe society built on knowledge. https://www.brandforsk.se/en/
>
> The **Swedish Civil Contingencies Agency** (MSB) is a government agency responsible for issues concerning civil protection, public safety, emergency management, and civil defense. https://www.msb.se/en/

Marcus Runefors
Ragnar Andersson
Mattias Delin
Thomas Gell

Contents

Part I Determinants, Mechanisms and Risk Groups

1. **Fire-Related Mortality from a Global Perspective** 3
   Syed Moniruzzaman

2. **Fire Fatalities and Fatal Fires – Risk Factors and Risk Groups** 13
   Anders Jonsson, Colin McIntyre, and Marcus Runefors

3. **The Residential Fire Injury Pyramid** 29
   Finn Nilson

4. **Fire-Related Injury Mechanisms**............................. 45
   Fredrik Huss

5. **The Evacuation of People with Functional Limitations** 67
   Enrico Ronchi, Erik Smedberg, Gunilla Carlsson,
   and Björn Slaug

6. **Fire Safety Surveillance: Theoretical and Practical Challenges**..... 89
   Colin McIntyre and Anders Jonsson

7. **Implications for Prevention** 111
   Ragnar Andersson and Marcus Runefors

Part II Preventive Measures for Residential Fires

8. **Smoke Alarms and the Human Response**...................... 123
   Michelle Ball and Kara Dadswell

9. **Impact of Interior Doors on Residential Fire Safety** 143
   Victoria N. Hutchison and Simo Hostikka

10	**Prevention of Ignition and Limitation of Fire Development in Furnishing and Home Environment**........................ 159 Anne Steen-Hansen and Karolina Storesund	
11	**Active Fire Protection Systems for Residential Applications**....... 177 Magnus Arvidson	
12	**Residential Fire Rescues: Building a Model of Rescue Types for Supporting the Fire Service**............................. 197 Margrethe Kobes and Ricardo Weewer	
13	**Cost-Benefit Analysis of Fire Safety Measures**................... 221 Henrik Jaldell	
14	**Sociodemographic Patterns in the Effectiveness and Prevalence of Preventive Measures**...................................... 243 Marcus Runefors	

Part III Implementing Evidence-Based Fire Safety Promotion

15	**Vision Zero for Fire Safety**................................... 259 Ragnar Andersson and Thomas Gell	
16	**Fire Safety Education Campaigns**............................ 271 Charles R. Jennings	
17	**Targeted Interventions Towards Risk Groups**................... 293 Johanna Gustavsson, Gunilla Carlsson, and Margaret S. McNamee	
18	**Residential Fires in Metropolitan Areas: Living Conditions and Fire Prevention**... 307 Nicklas Guldåker, Per-Olof Hallin, Mona Tykesson Klubien, and Jerry Nilsson	
19	**Early Responders as a Resource for Effective Response**........... 327 Björn Sund and Sofie Pilemalm	
20	**Swedish Strategies for Prevention of Residential Fires: The Case of the Swedish Fire Protection Association and the Swedish Civil Contingencies Agency**.................... 345 Mattias Delin, Maya Stål Söndergaard, and Björn Sund	

Part IV Conclusion

21	**The Road Ahead**.. 363 Marcus Runefors, Ragnar Andersson, Mattias Delin, and Thomas Gell	

Index.. 377

Part I
Determinants, Mechanisms and Risk Groups

Chapter 1
Fire-Related Mortality from a Global Perspective

Syed Moniruzzaman

Abstract Fire-related injury mortality is a major global public health concern. Although fire-related injuries are considered largely preventable, this category of injuries is still assumed responsible for more than 120,000 global deaths annually. This chapter presents the global fire-related injury mortality by demographic, geographic, economic, and temporal distributions. The problem with data limitations is also highlighted. The mortality rates are higher among the elderly population in most regions, with some exceptions in individual countries. Globally, women are overrepresented in fire-related mortality. When reviewing fire-related mortality by geographic regions and national income, the rates are generally higher in sub-Saharan African and Eastern European regions, as well as in low-income regions and countries with lower sociodemographic index. From 1990 to 2017, global fire-related mortality decreased by 46%, with large disparities across countries and regions. A standardized data reporting system and reliable national data collection procedures are needed to monitor global fire-related mortality adequately.

Keywords Fire · Burns · Mortality · Geography · Income · Global burden of disease

---

S. Moniruzzaman (✉)
Risk and Environmental Studies, Centre for Societal Risk Research, Karlstad University, Karlstad, Sweden
e-mail: syed.moniruzzaman@kau.se

1 Introduction

The human relationship with fire dates back to ancient times. Just as controlling fire has been vital for human civilisation and development, fire has also brought devastation and damage to human life. Despite technological progresses and advancements in rescue and health services, fire-related events are still causing many human deaths every year and remain threatening human health, safety, and well-being.

An accurate picture of the global fire-related mortality does not yet exist due to incomplete and inconsistent reporting systems in many countries, especially in poorer countries [1, 2]. Two major sources are generally available for international comparisons, data reported to the International Association of Fire and Rescue Services (CTIF) from national fire and rescue services agencies and data reported through the national cause of death records to the World Health Organization (WHO). Of these, the latter source is by far more complete and consistent since the reporting is coordinated and reviewed by the WHO and based on a uniform and internationally adopted classification system, the International Classification of Diseases (ICD).

The ICD classification separates fire-related deaths into three major categories: deaths due to unintentional fires, deaths due to fires deliberately ignited for the purpose of suicide, and finally, deaths due to fires deliberately ignited for the purpose of homicide. The medical cause of death from fire is usually burn or intoxication, but sometimes also mechanical in case of jumps/falls, collapsing structures, and the like. Mechanical causes are not always identified as associated with fires, and deaths from intentional fires are sometimes confused with unintentional cases due to inaccurate national autopsy procedures and forensic quality control [3]. These sources of error must all be taken into consideration when assessing the global fire-related mortality.

Based on WHO data, the Global Burden of Disease (GBD) study provides regular updates on the leading causes of death and disability worldwide [4, 5]. According to GBD, more than 120,000 people died from "Fire, heat and hot substances", in 2017. This number includes burn-related deaths from other causes than fire such as scalding and electrical injuries and excludes deaths from intentional fires (suicide and homicide). While these uncertainties exist, the assessment of around 120,000 global death toll annually from fire is, unfortunately, the best available estimate from the published literature at the current stage. National evidence from a handful of countries, including Finland, Sweden, Kuwait, the UK, and the USA, suggest that the mortality from burns other than fire-related is comparatively low [6–10], just like mortality from intentional fires (Fig. 1.1).

While this might be true at the global level, considerable deviations may exist in single countries. For example, in India, representing 17% of the global population, Bhalla and Sanghavi [11] disclosed a considerable underestimation of the true number of fire-related homicides in women.

Given that deaths covered under the category "Fire, heat and hot substances" can be accepted as a reasonable indicator of the true number of fire-related deaths, this chapter intends to present the global fire-related mortality by demographic, geographic, economic, and temporal distributions.

1 Fire-Related Mortality from a Global Perspective

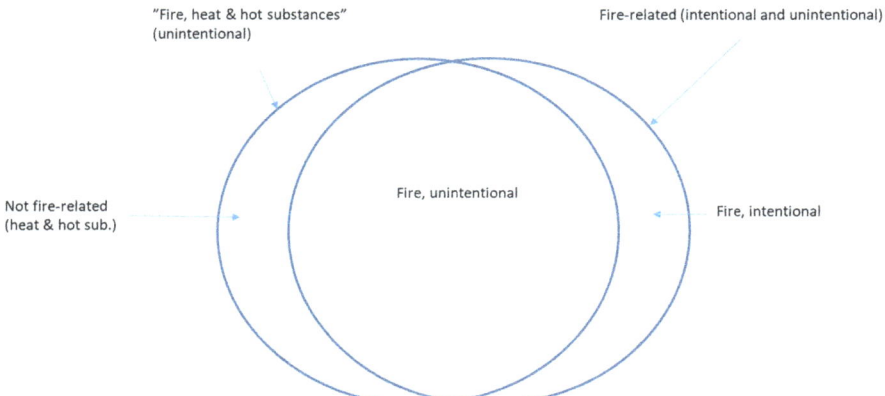

Fig. 1.1 Venn-diagram illustrating different types of fire/burn deaths

2 Fire-Related Mortality by Demography

The demography of fire-related mortality is a crucial aspect of fire safety since setting a successful fire prevention program presupposes the identification of vulnerable groups. Available reports show that global mortality rates of this category vary strongly between ages. In 2000, the mortality rates due to unintentional fire-related injury (here defined as flame burns and respiratory insult due to smoke inhalation) per 100,000 ranged from 2.5 in 5–14 years old to 12.5 in 80 years old and above [12]. Elevated rates were seen in the youngest children's group of 0–4 years old (6.6 per 100,000) and the elderly over 70 years of age (6.9 per 100,000) [12]. In 2013, the mortality rate due to fire, heat, and hot substances for children aged 1–14 years was 2.5 per 100,000 across 103 countries [13].

Elevated death rates in young children and the elderly are also seen in single regions. For example, in the European region, older adults are at excessive risk of dying from fatal fires [14, 15]. At the same time, fire-related mortality rates in the elderly over 75 years broadly vary between EU countries for the period 2005–2014 [16], with the highest in Latvia for both sexes (for males 19.9 and females 12.8 per 100,000) and lowest in Iceland for males and Malta for females, with no deaths recorded. This general age-specific pattern may differ significantly in other single countries [17, 18]. For example, in Cameroon, children under 10 years of age and the adult age group 21–40 years old shared the highest percentage of deaths due to fire, heat, and hot substances in a hospital burn study during 2008–2015 [18]. In an Indian study, an estimated 89% of people who die due to intentional and accidental fire and flames and electrocution were between 10 and 49 years old. The highest number is between 30 and 39 years – the lowest share of deaths among the elderly [17].

Generally, global mortality due to unintentional injury (all causes) is highly male-dominant (almost 2:1) [5]. However, this male-female disparity is less evident in fire-related injury mortality. In 2016, according to the WHO estimate, females had a higher number of deaths due to fire, heat, and hot substances than males on the world average, with a comparatively higher proportion in the South Asian region [5]. In 2004, globally, girls under 20 years of age had higher mortality due to fire, heat, and hot substances (4.9 per 100,000) than boys (3.0 per 100,000) [19], with the most significant disparities found in infants and adolescents 15–19 and in the South-Asian region.

In India, females share 65% of fire-related deaths, most of them aged 15–34 years [20]. In another study in India, this male-female ratio of deaths was 1:7, with 23.7% of victims being of child-bearing age [17]. Women's household activities combined with traditional cooking methods over open fire, unsafe cooking stoves, and often loose-fitting clothing might explain this higher share of young women's fire-related deaths in South Asian countries [17, 21]. Females in some countries in the Middle Eastern region, e.g., Iraq, Iran, and The United Estate of Arab Emirates (UAE), also experience higher fire-related mortality than males [5]. In the UAE, women mortality rates due to fire-related injuries are three times higher than men. On the other hand, males generally have higher fire-related mortality rates in Africa, the Americas, Europe, and the Western Pacific regions.

3 Fire-Related Mortality by Geographic Distribution

The number of people who die from fire, heat, and hot substances also varies by global regions and countries [4]. In 2017, mortality rates due to fire, heat, and hot substances were higher (around 4 per 100,000) in Sub-Saharan Africa and Eastern Europe compared to other global regions (Fig. 1.2). The rates were close to 3 per 100,000 population in Central Asia and generally lower in other regions. For example, in Latin American and Caribbean countries – all with age-standardized death rate (ASDR) close to 1 per 100,000 population and Western Europe and Southeast Asia, East Asia and Oceania less than 1 per 100,000 population. In Asia and the Pacific region, the highest rates were seen in the Philippines (0.9 per 100,000) and the lowest in Singapore (0.1 per 100,000). In North American countries – all with close to 1 per 100 000 population in the region. The rates were 0.9 and 1.2 per 100,000 population in Canada and the USA, respectively.

In Europe, the former Soviet region generally has the highest fire mortality rates. In 2017, five out of the top 10 ranked countries with mortality rates due to fire, heat, and hot substances represent former Soviet countries (Belarus: 4.6; Latvia: 4.1; Russian Federation: 3.6; Ukraine: 3.3, and Estonia: 2.9 per 100,000 population) [4]. In the same year, the mortality rates mainly were low in Western European countries (0.6 per 100,000), followed by Central Europe (1 per 100,000). Most of the fatal fire cases in European countries happen in the home environment. Similarly, according to CTIF, most fires and fire-related injuries (fatal and nonfatal) occur in the home environment as well [22].

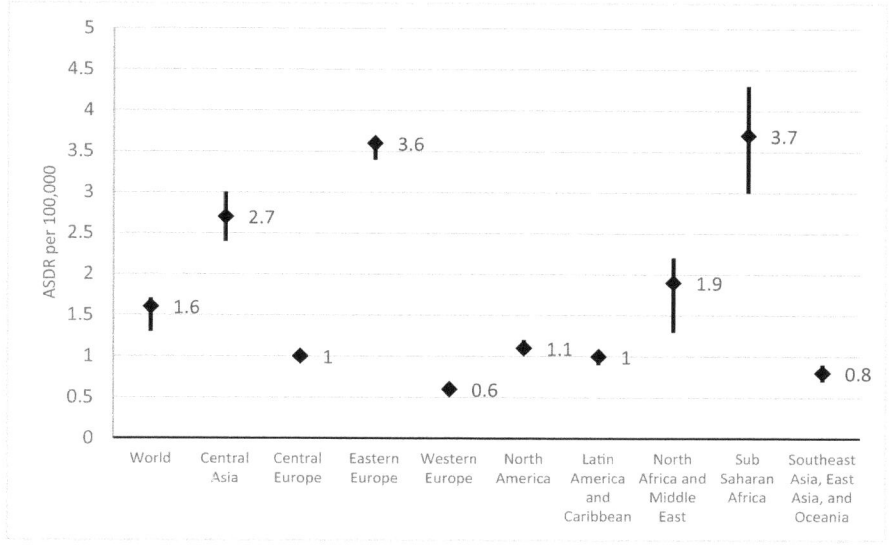

Fig. 1.2 Age-standardized death rates (ASDR) per 100,000 due to fire, heat, and hot substances and uncertainty interval by major WHO regions and subregions. (Data source: James, S.L., et al. [4])

In the global country list, in 2017, ASDR (per 100,000) due to fire, heat, and hot substances were lowest in Singapore: 0.2; Slovenia and Switzerland: 0.3; Colombia, Australia and New Zealand: 0.4, and highest in Lesotho: 7.2; Zimbabwe: 6.6; South Sudan: 6.5; Central African Republic: 5.3; and Burundi: 5.2 [4].

4 Fire-Related Mortality by Income Distribution

Economic development, often measured by income per capita, is regarded as "the best single indicator of living standards in a country" [23]. Like most unintentional injury causes, fire-related mortality rates are higher in lower-income countries and lower in higher-income countries. Globally, the association between income per capita measured by the gross domestic product (GDP) and fire-related mortality rates was found to be negatively correlated (r = −0.26) [24]. When this relationship was examined in detail for middle-income countries (MICs) and high-income countries (HICs) separately, the associations were found inverse for MICs, which means that there is a tendency towards increasing trends in this segment by increasing income [25].

ASDR data due to fire, heat, and hot substances are also available by Sociodemographic Index (SDI)[1] by combining income per capita, educational attainment and fertility rates [4]. Fire-related deaths generally decrease with higher SDI (Fig. 1.3). However, an individual country's rate can deviate remarkably from the average for a specific economic country grouping.

5 Changing Historical Trends

The mortality rates due to fire, heat, and hot substances have fallen gradually over the last decades in most countries. From 1990 to 2017, global mortality has decreased by 46.6% in age-standardized rates [4], and this declining tendency is highest in higher sociodemographic country groupings. In Fig. 1.4, ASDRs are shown for the countries that have experienced the lowest relative mortality changes (bars in light blue) and highest relative mortality changes (bars in dark blue), plus the few countries that had increasing changes (bars in red). The rest of the countries appeared between these two extremes. According to a report on the Swedish fire and flame mortality in an international comparison [25], mortality rates in high-income countries declined between 1985 and 2012 – except for the Baltic countries Estonia, Latvia and Lithuania, where peaking trends up to 14 per 100,000 were seen between 1991 and 1997 followed by declining trends. Among Nordic countries, Denmark, Finland, Norway and Sweden, the rates at the beginning of the period were below 2 per 100,000 and fell further below 1 per 100,000 at the end of the period. The rates per 100,000 fell below 1 in 1991 in the UK and in 2003 in Ireland. The rates were under 1 per 100,000 for France and Germany during the period. A recent study by Winberg [26] using the World Fire Statistics reports of the International Association of Fire and Rescue Services confirms steady declining trends of deaths due to fire and flames in Estonia, Germany, Great Britain, Latvia, Russia, and the USA, since 2002.

Especially, fire and burns mortality among children and adults have shown significant improvement in most HICs over the last decades [28–31]. This improvement in younger ages explains the key part of total mortality improvement and results in increasing skewness toward the elderly population, such as in Sweden [30]. In a US study, Pereira et al. showed a consistent improvement in mortality rates, except for older women 65–92 years between the two periods of 1989–1999 and 2000–2004 [32]. Similarly, substantial improvements were observed in survival rates of burn patients under 75 years during a study period of 20 years (1977–1996), but not in patients of 75 years and above [33]. It is predicted that the population older than 65 may increase by close to 1.5 times within the next three decades in HICs [34]. This demographic shift may accelerate the problem with fire-related deaths in the elderly further.

---

[1] SDI – a composite scale of the rankings and averaging the income per capita, educational attainment and fertility rates, expressed 0 to 1. This measure is developed and used by the Global Burden of Disease (GBD) researchers.

1 Fire-Related Mortality from a Global Perspective

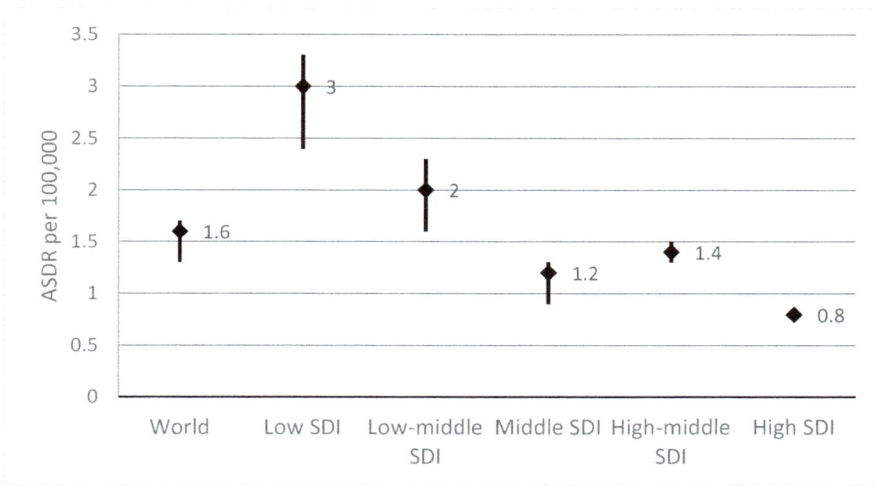

Fig. 1.3 Age-standardized death rates (ASDR) per 100,000 due to fire, heat, and hot substances and uncertainty interval by sociodemographic index (SDI). (Data source: James, S.L., et al. [4])

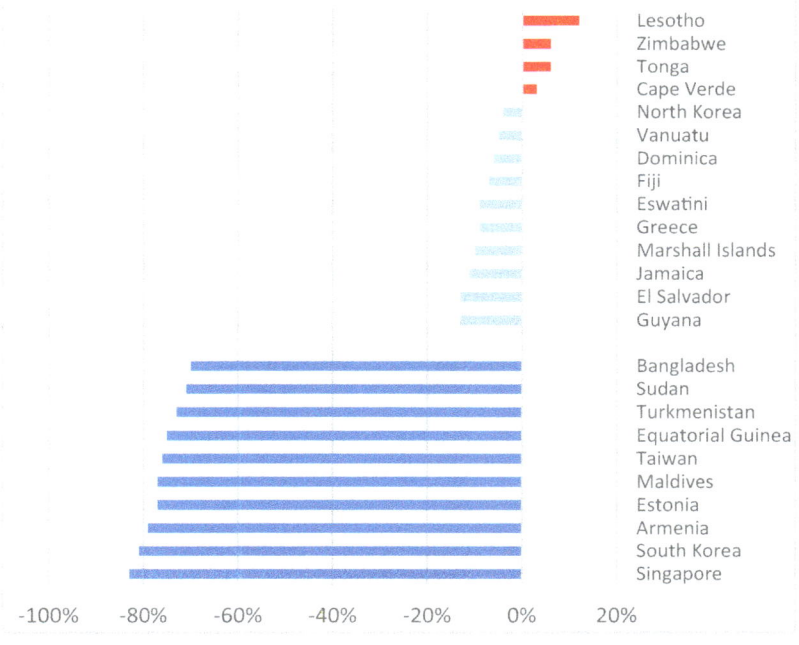

Fig. 1.4 Relative change of age-standardized death rates (ASDR) of fire, heat, and hot substances between 1990 and 2017. (Data source: Our World in Data [27])

6 Discussion and Conclusions

As stated initially, the international literature on fire-related mortality suffers from several limitations, such as confusion with other causes of burns, lacking coverage of mortality from both unintentional and intentional fires, and data validity problems due to weak data collection and reporting systems in many countries. Considering those limitations, this overview attempts to depict broader patterns and trends characterizing the global mortality from fires. These include:

- Declining trends have been reported all over the world with very few exceptions. The decline seems to follow generally improved living conditions as measured by GDP per capita and SDI. Peaking rates in some countries in Central and Eastern Europe coincided with socioeconomic strain in the 1990s and are since then declining.
- Small children and the elderly are at elevated risk, with an ongoing transition over time towards the elderly as the risk in early childhood seems to decline faster in children than in other age groups. In richer countries, the elderly now stands out as the most significant risk group, which demands adequate attention to prevent excess fire-related deaths in the future.
- Women are more at risk than men globally, due to significant overrepresentation in some countries in South Asia and the Middle East.
- Most fires and fire-related deaths and injuries occur in the home environment.

The generally weak and premature state of the international research in fire safety with regard to mortality and morbidity raises a number of challenges for future fire safety research. First of all, improved data collection and reporting systems are needed, based on internationally agreed classifications and procedures under the auspices of relevant organizations such as the WHO and CTIF. All patterns and trends identified above need to be confirmed in new studies based on more accurate and valid data. Secondly, new research questions need deeper analysis, such as why women are at excessive risk of dying from fire in certain countries and regions, and to what degree lifestyle factors like smoking and alcohol consumption contribute to the international patterns and trends identified.

References

1. Meacham BJ (2020) Developing a global standard for fire reporting. Published by the Royal Institution of Chartered Surveyors (RICS), London
2. Smolle C et al (2017) Recent trends in burn epidemiology worldwide: a systematic review. Burns 43(2):249–257
3. Buch AK et al (2018) Factors associated with autopsy rates in a 6-year sample of Danish suicides in the Capital area of Copenhagen. J Forensic Legal Med 60:50–55
4. James SL et al (2020) Epidemiology of injuries from fire, heat and hot substances: global, regional and national morbidity and mortality estimates from the Global Burden of Disease 2017 study. Injury Prev 26(Supp 1):i36–i45

5. WHO (2018) Global health estimates 2016: deaths by cause, age, sex, by country and by region, 2000–2016. World Health Organization, Geneva [November 25 2020]. Available from https://www.who.int/healthinfo/global_burden_disease/estimates/en/
6. Bang R, Saif JK (1989) Mortality from burns in Kuwait. Burns 15(5):315–321
7. Papp A (2009) The first 1000 patients treated in Kuopio University Hospital Burn Unit in Finland. Burns 35(4):565–571
8. Pruitt BA, Wolf SE, Mason AD (2012) Epidemiological, demographic, and outcome characteristics of burn injury. Total Burn Care 4:15–45
9. Afifi TO et al (2010) The relationship of gambling to intimate partner violence and child maltreatment in a nationally representative sample. J Psychiatr Res 44(5):331–337
10. Krishnan P et al (2013) Cause of death and correlation with autopsy findings in burns patients. Burns 39(4):583–588
11. Bhalla K, Sanghavi P (2020) Fire-related deaths among women in India are underestimated. Lancet 395(10226):779–780
12. Peden M, McGee K, Sharma G (2002) The injury chart book: a graphical overview of the global burden of injuries. World Health Organization, Geneva, p 5
13. Sengoelge M, El-Khatib Z, Laflamme L (2017) The global burden of child burn injuries in light of country level economic development and income inequality. Prev Med Rep 6:115–120
14. Brusselaers N et al (2010) Severe burn injury in Europe: a systematic review of the incidence, etiology, morbidity, and mortality. Crit Care 14(5):1–12
15. European Fire Safety Alliance (n.d.)EU-wide data on residential fires [12 August 2021]. Available from https://www.europeanfiresafetyalliance.org/our-focus/statistics/
16. Nilson F, Lundgren L, Bonander C (2020) Living arrangements and fire-related mortality amongst older people in Europe. Int J Inj Control Saf Promot 27(3):378–384
17. Kumar S et al (2013) Epidemiology and mortality of burns in the Lucknow Region, India – a 5 year study. Burns 39(8):1599–1605
18. Forbinake NA et al (2020) Mortality analysis of burns in a developing country: a CAMEROONIAN experience. BMC Public Health 20(1):1–6
19. Peden M et al (2009) World report on child injury prevention, vol 2008. World Health Organization, Geneva
20. Sanghavi P, Bhalla K, Das V (2009) Fire-related deaths in India in 2001: a retrospective analysis of data. Lancet 373(9671):1282–1288
21. Sawhney C (1989) Flame burns involving kerosene pressure stoves in India. Burns 15(6):362–364
22. Brushlinsky N et al (2021) World fire statistics. Center of fire statistics report of 2021. In: International Association of Fire and Rescue Services (CTIF)
23. Preston SH (2007) The changing relation between mortality and level of economic development. Int J Epidemiol 36(3):484–490
24. Peck M, Pressman MA (2013) The correlation between burn mortality rates from fire and flame and economic status of countries. Burns 39(6):1054–1059
25. Moniruzzaman S, Andersson R (2018) In: Andersson R, Nilsen P (red.) Towards an evidence based Vision Zero on residential fires – final report Swedish Contingencies Agency (in Swedish)
26. Winberg D (2016) International fire death rate trends
27. OurWorldInData (n.d.) Causes of death [24 November 2020]. Available from https://ourworldindata.org/causes-of-death#fire
28. Hoskin AF (2000) Trends in unintentional-injury deaths during the 20th century. Stat Bull (Metropolitan Life Insur Company:1984) 81(2):18–26
29. Göpfert A et al (2015) Growing inequalities in child injury deaths in Europe. Eur J Public Health 25(4):660–662
30. Jonsson A et al (2016) Fire-related mortality in Sweden: temporal trends 1952 to 2013. Fire Technol 52(6):1697–1707

31. Hu G, Baker SP (2009) Trends in unintentional injury deaths, US, 1999–2005: age, gender, and racial/ethnic differences. Am J Prev Med 37(3):188–194
32. Pereira CT et al (2006) Age-dependent differences in survival after severe burns: a unicentric review of 1,674 patients and 179 autopsies over 15 years. J Am Coll Surg 202(3):536–548
33. Wibbenmeyer LA et al (2001) Predicting survival in an elderly burn patient population. Burns 27(6):583–590
34. UN, United Nations, Department of Economic and Social Affairs, Population Division (2019) World population ageing 2019: highlights (ST/ESA/SER.A/430)

Dr. Syed Moniruzzaman is a senior lecturer at the Department of Risk and Environmental Studies and Centre for Societal Risk Research (CSR), Karlstad University, Sweden. He obtained his master's degree from Umeå University and PhD from Karlstad University in Public Health. Previously, as part of his research training, Dr. Moniruzzaman was affiliated with different universities and institutions, including Karolinska Institute, Stockholm; World Health Organization, Geneva; and Southampton University, UK. His research focus has mainly been on global injury death and development. Currently, he is coordinating a research collaboration between research institutions in Bangladesh and Karlstad University.

Chapter 2
Fire Fatalities and Fatal Fires – Risk Factors and Risk Groups

Anders Jonsson, Colin McIntyre, and Marcus Runefors

Abstract Knowledge of the relevant risk factors is a prerequisite for effective strategies to prevent fatal residential fires. The aim of this chapter is to present the most important known risk factors for residential fire fatalities.

This review of the literature concentrates on various characteristics of the individuals and households experiencing fatal residential fires. We have chosen not to include various types of fire safety measures in this review, such as smoke alarms, fire extinguishers, or mobile sprinklers, as these are the subject of another chapter.

The literature studied provides a reasonably consistent picture of several basic risk factors for death in a residential fire. With respect to age, the oldest have the highest risk. Among children, it is the youngest who have the highest risk. In all age groups, men are at greater risk than women. Smoking and alcohol have a large effect on risk. Certain socio-demographic factors are clearly associated with higher risk, such as living alone, having a low income, or being unemployed. In addition, individuals with functional limitations are at greater risk than others. These risk factors have been observed to hold true over an extended period of time in several countries, despite a gradual decrease in the mortality rate from residential fires in the last decades.

We note that much of the research on risk factors is relatively old, and many studies are of a descriptive nature. It is clear that many of the risk factors identified in the research are correlated. It is desirable that future studies take more account of covariation between the various risk factors and control for confounding factors. In addition, large-scale population-based case-control or cohort studies have the potential to provide a deeper understanding of risk factors for residential fire fatalities.

A. Jonsson (✉)
Risk and Environmental Studies, Centre for Societal Risk Research, Karlstad University, Karlstad, Sweden

Swedish Civil Contingencies Agency (MSB), Karlstad, Sweden
e-mail: Anders.Jonsson@msb.se

C. McIntyre
Swedish Civil Contingencies Agency (MSB), Karlstad, Sweden

M. Runefors
Division of Fire Safety Engineering, Lund University, Lund, Sweden

Keywords Unintentional fires · Fire mortality · Alcohol · Smoking · Socioeconomic factors · Sociodemographic factors

1 Introduction

Knowledge about risk factors plays a central role when formulating a fire safety strategy or designing a specific intervention to improve fire safety. The objective of such interventions may be to avoid fires by reducing the likelihood of a fire occurring in the first place, or to reduce the likelihood of an initial fire leading to serious outcomes such as a fatality. An understanding of risk factors will make it more likely that an intervention will be effective in fulfilling either of these objectives.

The aim of this chapter is to present current knowledge on risk factors for dying in a residential fire. Results from various research studies are presented, together with analysis in the form of reports from the fire authorities.

It would have been desirable to conduct a systematic review of all available literature, but there are some drawbacks to such an approach. Systematic reviews often have a high bar for academic rigour, with only a small selection of work being included. Important factors can be missed by this approach. However, research into risk factors has been ongoing for fifty years, so if the selection criteria are relaxed, then it is easy to end up with too much material to analyse.

This chapter is based on a more pragmatic approach. We make no claim to provide a comprehensive list of all the risk factors for death in a residential fire, but our intention is to include the most important factors identified over the last fifty years. We focus on the United States, Canada, Australia, New Zealand, the United Kingdom, and Scandinavia, as most of the published research comes from these countries.

A majority of research on risk factors with regard to residential fires has focused on fire death, in part perhaps because this is a well-defined fire outcome with a manageable number of cases to study. In addition, data are more readily available, since the police and medical authorities pay particular attention to these events, ascertaining the circumstances that lead to the fire and the cause of death.

Both early research [1] and research in recent years [2] have shown that there are significant differences between characteristics of the fires and the victims when different levels of residential fire outcomes are studied: death, non-fatal injury, and property damage. This would seem to indicate that there are different risk factors at play for the different fire outcomes. There are sufficient differences to warrant caution in assuming that fatal fires form part of the same spectrum as other fire outcomes.

This chapter focuses on risk factors for fatal residential fires, and it is important for the reader to note that a risk factor for one particular fire outcome will not necessarily hold true for other outcomes. There is more to read about these differences in

Chap. 3. Non-fatal Fires – The Injury pyramid, Socio-demographic Gradients and Protective factors.

2 Terminology

Most people have an intuitive understanding of what is meant by "risk factor". However, before proceeding with the main content of the chapter, it is worth defining some of the most important terms used in relation to risk factors.

A risk factor is any factor that precedes and is associated with a higher likelihood of a negative outcome (in our case, death due to a residential fire). Conversely, a protective factor is a characteristic associated with a lower likelihood of a negative outcome or an impact reduction of a risk factor. In many cases, a risk factor is the opposite of the protective factor. For example, while having a functional smoke alarm can be a protective factor, not having one can be a risk factor.

Some risk factors are fixed, which means that they cannot be manipulated and will not change over time. This type of risk factor is termed a *fixed marker* or *risk indicator*. Sex and race are examples of fixed markers.

Other risk factors are considered variable and can change over time. There are two types of variable risk factors. Those that when manipulated, change the probability of the outcome (*causal risk factor*) and those that do not change the probability of the outcome (*variable marker*). To reduce the incidence of the outcome of interest, interventions must focus on causal risk factors. Further, the focus should generally be on the causal risk factors having the greatest impact on their target population. The correlation between a causal risk factor and an outcome must not only be statistically significant but also be expected to produce a meaningful reduction in the outcome of interest. This does not mean that risk factors other than causal risk factors are of no interest. On the contrary, they are very useful, for example when identifying high-risk populations for prevention. However, changing them will not reduce the incidence of the negative outcome.

In order to ascertain whether a certain variable is a risk factor or not, the outcome must be related to something. If we, for example, want to study the factor sex, fatalities among men must be related to the number of men in the population under study, and this rate must be compared to fatalities among women in relation to the number of women in the population. These rates are compared for men and women to see if sex would appear to affect an individual's risk.

It is most common to search for risk factors related to individuals, but risk factors can also concern other subjects such as households, fires, or geographical areas. It is important to point out that risk factors are specific to their subject. For example, a relationship observed for a geographical area does not necessarily hold true for a particular individual living in that area. This common pitfall is called *the ecological fallacy*: an incorrect assumption about an individual based on aggregate data for a group.

Studies on risk factors often use the term *risk group*. Risk groups are used to describe individuals sharing traits that increase their probability of dying in a residential fire (or households with traits that increase their probability of being the scene of a fatal fire). One or more risk factors are used to divide the subjects into high-risk and low-risk groups.

Many studies of fire outcomes consider various circumstances without analysing them in relation to a relevant comparator. For example, there are many studies where it is observed that a large proportion of fatalities have a high level of alcohol in the blood. It is difficult to translate these observations into risk factors since we often lack a control group in the form of similar data for individuals not dying in fires. Circumstances which are observed often hold true but, without a clear indication of overrepresentation, are sometimes called *main characteristics*.

3 Delimitation

Many studies have shown that having a working smoke alarm in the home is associated with a lower fatality rate [3]. It has also been shown that smoke alarms are not evenly distributed across all households, and that households where fatal fires take place are less likely to have functional smoke alarms than households with reported fires or average households [4–6]. These observations indicate how important it is to continue the work of ensuring that more homes are protected by smoke alarms and also to understand in which situations a functional smoke alarm will not in itself be enough to avoid serious injury or death. However, we have chosen not to include various types of fire safety measures in this review (such as functional smoke alarm, fire extinguisher, or mobile sprinkler), even though not having them can be regarded as a risk factor. We refer the reader to the second part of this anthology, which goes into some detail about protective measures in the home.

4 Early Research

Residential fire research gained momentum in the 1970s in the wake of the report "America burning" from 1973 [7]. The report called for more emphasis on fire prevention and research to inform fire safety strategies. The background to the report was the Fire Research and Safety Act of 1968, which came in response to the marked increase in fire losses observed in the United States at the time.

Regarding fire deaths, early studies in the United States [8, 9] showed that the majority of fatalities occurred in residential fires. Toxic gases were identified as the primary cause of death, with carbon monoxide as an asphyxiant. Cigarettes were identified as a principal ignition source and alcohol was a significant contributory factor (particularly among men from 40 to 60 years of age). When comparing fatal fires with fires causing non-fatal injuries, it was noted that smoking was more prevalent as the cause for fatal fires, and that the highest proportion of deaths to total fire victims occurred in the younger and older age groups [1].

At about the same time, fire deaths were studied in Glasgow, Scotland [10–12] and the study was subsequently extended to cover the whole of the United Kingdom [13]. Most of the deaths occurred in residential fires in which the fires were restricted to the room or area of origin. The fatal fires occurred more often during the winter and at weekends. Old people were particularly vulnerable in these fires. Alcohol was identified as a factor across the United Kingdom in general, and this was particularly apparent in Glasgow.

At around this time, there was also an increased interest in the fire problem across the Nordic countries. In Sweden, a governmental investigation and a research paper [14, 15] called for improved statistical data and more research. Two studies in Denmark [16, 17] showed that fire deaths caused by smoking were a serious problem, particularly in nursing homes or settings where social problems, psychiatric disorders, or alcohol abuse were present.

These early studies were mostly exploratory and descriptive in nature. They were most often carried out by medical doctors and few went beyond the collection of vital statistics. However, one important observation from this early research was that fire deaths were clearly not randomly distributed in the population.

5   Age and Sex

Age and sex are the most commonly investigated risk factors for death in residential fires [18, 19]. Datasets for fire fatalities almost always include age and sex. Most countries produce high quality vital statistics for comparison, making, for example, cross-sectional studies easy to perform. Early research identified young children and elderly people as those most at risk, and also noted the over-representation of males in all age groups [8]. The disproportionate percentage of fire victims in the youngest and oldest age groups has been shown repeatedly over the years and in many different countries [20–23].

The long-term trend in fire fatality rates (deaths per million people) and in absolute numbers has been declining in most countries for many decades [24, 25] with the greatest reduction being observed among children [26]. In the United States, the youngest group (0–4 years) has gone from having a higher frequency of fire deaths than expected to now lying below the average for the general population [20].

It is clear that few small children die in residential fires in the countries studied. However, children up to four years of age have an elevated risk of fire death when compared to older children (aged 5–14). Several factors make small children more exposed to fatal fires. Playing with fire is a common cause for fires involving children [27–29]. They also lack an understanding of the dangers associated with fire and often lack the capability to escape from a fire. Small children are often reliant on parents or other older individuals for their safety if a fire starts in a home.

Several socio-demographic factors have been shown to be related to child mortality in residential fires. One study showed that substandard housing and overcrowding are associated with an increased fire mortality rate among children [30]. Another study showed that lower educational attainment of the mother, younger age of the child, and more children in the household all increased the risk of fire death for children [31]. In Philadelphia, USA, census tracts with low income levels, high proportions of households with single parents, and a higher proportion of housing built before 1939 were linked to higher levels of child mortality in fires [32]. In Ontario, Canada, children from families receiving help from the Children's Aid Society had a substantially higher risk of dying in a fire [28].

One study showed that smoke alarm functionality in fires involving child fatalities was low [28]. It has also been shown that smoke alarms do not seem to provide effectively protection against death or injury in fires caused by children playing with fire [27].

It is probable that the relationship between socio-demographic factors and child fire mortality is largely due to environmental factors and the behaviour of adults. A Scottish study showed that deaths among children were largely the direct result of the actions of an adult, with smoking and alcohol playing an important role [33].

The risk of death is highest among the oldest individuals (85 and older). However, excess risk in relation to the general population occurs already at fifty (relative risk >1). Impaired movement, hearing, and smell together with slower reactions and memory problems are all presumed to increase the risk of the elderly. It has also been observed that they have a lower prevalence of smoke alarms. One review study [34] points out that there are both medical and biological factors which can influence their risk. Existing illness associated with old age can increase the risk of death among the elderly, for example heart disease dramatically increases vulnerability to carbon monoxide, and presumably also other suffocating gases.

One risk factor which is less pronounced among the elderly is the consumption of alcohol. When compared with younger fatalities, the elderly were significant less likely to have alcohol detected in their blood [35, 36].

Many studies have shown that males are at higher risk of death from residential fires than females. This is true for all age groups, but is particularly pronounced in the middle-age population. It is unclear exactly what lies behind this observation. However, some explanations seem more likely than others. High consumption of alcohol is probably one. This dominance of male fatalities also applies when looking at the absolute numbers, except for the oldest population due to there being so many more females than males in that age group.

Age and sex are risk markers rather than causal risk factors. However, an understanding of how, for example, fire causes and injury mechanisms differ by age and sex is important for identifying specific risk groups and the prevention strategies that are most appropriate for them [37].

6 Smoking and Alcohol

Smoking and alcohol consumption are two lifestyle behaviours often observed to be associated with fire deaths [18, 19]. In several studies "smoking materials" is the leading known source of ignition in fatal residential fires [38]. Fires ignited by smoking more often result in a fatality than fires ignited by other means [39]. One study has shown that when comparing fires caused by smoking with fires ignited by other means, the victim was more often asleep, in the room of fire origin, intoxicated by alcohol or psychotropic drugs or sedated, suffering from mental illness and was aged between 18 and 65. Considering the room of origin, smoking-related fatal fires more often started in a bedroom or living room [40]. Another study showed that smoking-related fatalities can be grouped into two very different types of fire scenario. The first mainly involves older women where the clothing is ignited (these often start in the kitchen), while the second involves mainly middle-aged men, often intoxicated, where the bed or couch is most likely ignited by the cigarette (these often occur in a bedroom or living room) [21].

As mentioned above, child's play is a common cause in fires where young children die. The heat source is often a cigarette lighter or matches and, since the availability of those can be expected to be higher in homes with smoking, smoking could be considered an indirect cause of many of those fire deaths [27].

Non-smokers may be at increased risk due to fire from the presence of smokers in their environment [41]. An American study observed that one out of four fatalities in smoking-material fires was not the smoker who started the fire [42]. This is in contrast to a recent Swedish study [43] which did not observe a similar phenomenon among fire victims, indicating that the threat posed by smokers to non-smokers in their surroundings is unclear at present, due to the limited number of studies.

At the ecological level, an American study has shown that death rates in residential fires are high in states with a high proportion of smokers, and this relationship holds true even when taking account of socio-economic factors such as education and median household income [44].

The association between alcohol intoxication and death in residential fire is also well-documented [45, 46]. Understanding the role played by alcohol seems essential when trying to determine why fire deaths occur. The consumption of alcohol is an obvious contributory factor that can influence the risk of death in many ways. Alcohol can play a direct role, for example if it causes someone to become unconscious while smoking or fall asleep while cooking. Intoxication can also affect responsiveness to fire cues, preventing a victim from hearing or correctly interpreting a fire alarm. The consumption of alcohol can also affect the effectiveness of escape measures. Being under the influence of alcohol might affect judgement, making a person less likely to avoid inherently dangerous situations that could give rise to burns. Alcohol can further affect a person's balance, causing them to fall. There is some evidence that alcohol in the blood accelerates behavioural incapacitation from toxic gases, such as carbon monoxide [45]. In addition, several studies suggest that the probability of surviving serious burns is reduced for people with a history of alcohol abuse [45].

After a fire death, it is common for the blood alcohol content to be analysed in an autopsy. Several studies have observed a high proportion of adult victims testing positive for alcohol at the time of death. It is important to note the high level of intoxication in many of those testing positive for alcohol, one study estimating a mean value of 193.9 mg/dl [47].

It should be acknowledged that alcohol plays a role in more fires than those in which a victim tests positive for alcohol in the blood. It has been found that children and the very old account for 15% of the fatalities in alcohol-related fatal fires, without themselves drinking alcohol [48].

It is also interesting to note the differences between various age groups in the proportion of fatal fire victims testing positive for alcohol. The elderly are significantly less likely to have alcohol detected in their blood [46, 47, 49, 50]. The proportion of males testing positive for alcohol is higher than that for females [46, 49].

The consumption of alcohol has been shown to be more common in fatal fires caused by smoking or cooking than in fatal fires with other causes. The association between smoking and alcohol consumption in fatal fires has been pointed out in several studies [46, 51–53].

7 Living Alone or Being Home Alone at the Time of the Fire

When comparing fatal fires with non-fatal fires, early studies showed that being home alone at the time of the fire increases the risk of death [52, 54]. A similar association was later found at the individual level for the circumstance of living alone, by comparing individuals dying in residential fires with randomly selected individuals matched on sex and age [55] or with survivors in residential fires [56]. There are also many descriptive studies that have observed high percentages of victims in fatal fires with the characteristic of living alone or being home alone at the time of the fire, for example in London [57].

It is logical that being alone at home increases the risk of dying in a fire. If more than one person is present then it will be more likely that the fire is discovered and put out, or that a successful evacuation can take place. This is even more important if the person is especially vulnerable in a residential fire, for example due to old age in combination with impaired vision, hearing, or mobility. A recent ecological country-level study on older people (75 years and above) in Europe showed that when the share of older people living alone increased by one percentage point, the fire-related mortality increased by 4% [58]. It should, however, be noted that a part of the correlation between living alone and the risk of fatal fires is likely to be due to correlations with other important risk factors such as age and high alcohol consumption.

8 Socio-economic Factors

Low socio-economic status has been shown to be associated with an elevated risk of dying in a residential fire. Having low income [51, 55, 56], low educational attainment [51, 55], and being unemployed [55, 56] would all appear to be associated with greater risk of death. In addition, residents of rented housing [54–56, 59] may be at increased risk.

Consistent results have been observed, regardless of whether it is fires, individuals, or households that are being studied, and what they are being compared to. For example, low socio-economic status is associated with increased risk when:

- Comparing fatal with non-fatal fires [54]
- Comparing individuals dying in residential fires with survivors [56]
- Randomly selected individuals are matched on sex and age [55]
- Comparing households [51, 59]

Similar relationships have been observed at the ecological level. Studies from the United States have shown that the fire fatality rates were highest in areas where property rental values were low [60] and that housing age, the prevalence of mobile homes, and the proportion of the population in rented accommodation all have significant independent effects on fire death rates [61]. In New Zealand, the highest risk of death is observed in the most socio-economically deprived areas [62]. In England, fatal fire injury rates have been shown to increase with increasing levels of deprivation [63].

9 Race and Ethnicity

Studies in the United States report non-white populations to be at higher risk of both fatal and non-fatal injury, for both sexes and across all age groups [14]. In North Carolina, death rates for whites were one third of those for other races [64] and other US studies have shown that black individuals have a risk of fire death almost twice that of an individual of another race [39, 65].

However, the picture is far less clear when going beyond an analysis of crude death rates. For example, no association between race/ethnicity and fire fatalities was found when comparing victims with survivors from the same fire [47]. When comparing residential fire fatalities in Sweden with randomly selected controls matched on age and sex and taking socio-demographic factors into account, individuals born outside of Europe were found to have a lower risk [55].

Race and ethnicity are clearly associated with other factors that may have a greater impact on risk, for example socio-economic factors [66]. When large metropolitan counties in United States were studied at the ecological level, a significant interaction between the proportion of the population that was African American and median family income was observed. Counties with a high proportion of African

Americans in combination with low median family income showed extremely high fire death rates, suggesting the relationship to be multiplicative rather than additive [61].

10 Urban Versus Rural Residence

Studies have shown that living in rural areas is associated with a higher risk of residential fire death [55, 67]. A relationship that persists despite taking account of age, sex, and various socio-demographic factors [55]. When looking for plausible explanations, the longer response times of the emergency services in rural areas [68] and the lower presence of smoke detectors in fatal fires in rural locations [69] should be considered.

11 Functional Limitations

Physical and mental disabilities increase the risk of dying in a residential fire, making these groups particularly vulnerable. In the United States, it has been estimated that physical disability was a factor in 15% of home fire deaths [70]. Other international studies have also found that disability is a significant risk factor in unintentional residential fires. At least 21% of the victims in London suffered some form of disability [57]. In Denmark, one-fifth of the victims received disablement pension and two thirds of those over 67 years of age were disabled [71]. A recent Norwegian study observed that those over 67 years of age had reduced mobility, impaired cognition, and mental disorders as risk factors [23]. Fires where people with physical or mental disabilities were present were more likely to end up as a fatal fire [54]. At the individual level, when comparing people who died with survivors of the same residential fire, people with physical or cognitive disability have been shown to be at greater risk [48]. Another study compared survivors from residential fires where no one died with people who died in residential fires. This study showed that individuals who suffered some physical or mental illness or had some other pre-existing disability had a greater risk of dying in unintentional residential fires than those who did not [56]. Comparing residential fire fatalities with the general population matched on age and sex, no association could be observed between disability allowance and the risk of dying, once socio-demographic factors were taken into account [55].

In a study from Victoria, Australia, the mentally ill were overrepresented among fire fatalities. The association with known risk factors was assessed and it was highlighted that the mentally ill were much more likely to have combined alcohol and drugs prior to their death and to have a history of careless smoking [72]. See Chap. 5. The evacuation of people with functional limitations in residential fires for an overview on the role of functional limitations on self-evacuation possibilities in the event of fire in a residential building.

12   Discussion

The aim of this chapter is to give an overview of risk factors for death in a residential fire. An understanding of risk factors is essential for effective measures to reduce fire deaths. In this review, we have focussed on factors concerning various characteristics of the individuals and households experiencing fatal residential fires, in relation to relevant comparators, for example, those of the general population, households in general, or survivors of residential fires.

Many characteristics found to be associated with increased risk, such as age, sex, or ethnicity, are fixed and are not in themselves causal risk factors. However, knowledge about these fixed markers is still very important, as it will assist fire prevention program developers in targeting interventions for those with the highest risk.

Being old, male, or living with some kind of physical or cognitive functional limitations are all factors that increase the risk of dying in a residential fire. Sociodemographic factors such as having a low income, low educational attainment, being unemployed, or living alone are also associated with a greater risk of death. Smoking and the consumption of alcohol are clearly two very important behavioural risk factors. The earliest research into risk factors showed that a large proportion of fatal fires were smoking-related and that many of those who died were under the influence of alcohol at the time of their death.

Several risk factors appear to be resistant to change, having been observed in early research and confirmed in more recent work. However, it should be remembered that technological and social advances can mean that early research no longer holds true. Over the years, considerable improvements have been made in fire safety due to improved regulation and an increase in smoke alarm ownership. In several countries, there has also been a reduction in smoking among the general population.

It must also be remembered that a risk factor in one place and time cannot be automatically assumed to hold true in other settings. Most of the studies in this review have come from the United States, Canada, Australia, New Zealand, the United Kingdom, and Scandinavia. There are many differences between these countries, and it is not clear whether risk factors observed here will hold true in other countries.

Many of the risk factors identified in this review are correlated. For example, low socio-economic status has been shown to be associated with other risk factors, such as smoking and the consumption of alcohol. The correlations among risk factors make it difficult to isolate the effect that every individual factor has on the risk of death in a residential fire. Ideally, those responsible for risk-based targeting of fire safety interventions would have an understanding of individual factors and how they interact. However, at present the complexities are far from completely understood.

13 Conclusions

The literature studied in the course of this review provides a reasonably consistent picture of several basic risk factors for death in a residential fire. For many fire safety practitioners, knowledge of these risk factors will be of help in designing effective fire safety interventions. However, at present the evidence is somewhat limited and a deeper understanding of risk factors would be beneficial. As pointed out in the introduction, many of the studies only go so far as to point out main characteristics, where a more rigourous analysis of overrepresentation is needed to identify risk factors. It is also desirable that future studies take more account of covariation between the various risk factors and control for confounding factors. In addition, large-scale population-based case-control or cohort studies have the potential to provide a deeper understanding of risk factors for residential fire fatalities.

References

1. Levine MS, Radford EP (1977) Fire victims: medical outcomes and demographic characteristics. Am J Public Health 67(11):1077–1080
2. Gilbert SW, Butry DT (2018) Identifying vulnerable populations to death and injuries from residential fires. Inj Prev 24(5):358–364
3. Rohde D, Corcoran J, Sydes M, Higginson A (2016) The association between smoke alarm presence and injury and death rates: a systematic review and meta-analysis. Fire Saf J 81:58–63
4. Ahrens M (2015) Smoke alarms in US home fires. National Fire Protection Association. Fire Analysis and Research Division
5. Gilbert SW (2021) Estimating smoke alarm effectiveness in homes. Fire Technol 57(3):1497–1516
6. Runefors M, Nilson F (2021) The influence of sociodemographic factors on the theoretical effectiveness of fire prevention interventions on fatal residential fires. Fire Technol:1–18
7. National Commission on Fire Prevention and Control (1973) America burning. US Government Printing Office, Washington, DC. Available online from http://www.usfa.fema.gov/downloads/pdf/publications/fa-264.pdf
8. Berl WG, Halpin BM (1978) Human fatalities from unwanted fires. US Department of Commerce, National Institute of Standards and Technology, Gaithersburg
9. Birky MM, Halpin BM, Caplan YH, Fisher RS, McAllister JM, Dixon AM (1979) Fire fatality study. Fire Mater 3(4):211–217
10. Anderson RA, Watson AA, Harland WA (1981) Fire deaths in the Glasgow area: I General considerations and pathology. Med Sci Law 21(3):175–183
11. Anderson RA, Watson AA, Harland WA (1981) Fire deaths in the Glasgow area: II The role of carbon monoxide. Med Sci Law 21(4):288–294
12. Anderson RA, Harland WA (1982) Fire deaths in the Glasgow area: III The role of hydrogen cyanide. Med Sci Law 22(1):35–40
13. Anderson RA, Willetts P, Harland WA (1983) Fire deaths in the United Kingdom 1976-82. Fire Mater 7(2):67–72
14. SOU 1978:30 Brand inomhus
15. Magnusson SE (1978) Reducing life hazards due to fire-a governmental investigation
16. Trier H (1983) Fire fatalities and deaths from burns in Denmark in 1980. Med Sci Law 23(2):116–120

17. Gormsen H, Jeppesen N, Lund A (1984) The causes of death in fire victims. Forensic Sci Int 24(2):107–111
18. Warda L, Tenenbein M, Moffatt ME (1999) House fire injury prevention update. Part I. A review of risk factors for fatal and non-fatal house fire injury. Inj Prev 5(2):145–150
19. Turner SL, Johnson RD, Weightman AL, Rodgers SE, Arthur G, Bailey R, Lyons RA (2017) Risk factors associated with unintentional house fire incidents, injuries and deaths in high-income countries: a systematic review. Injury Prev
20. Ahrens M (2013) Home structure fires. National Fire Protection Association, Fire Analysis and Research Division, Quincy
21. Jonsson A, Bonander C, Nilson F, Huss F (2017) The state of the residential fire fatality problem in Sweden: epidemiology, risk factors, and event typologies. J Saf Res 62:89–100
22. Gummesen PB, Dederichs AS (2017) Residential fires in Denmark. In: Book of abstracts, p 62
23. Sesseng C, Storesund K, Steen-Hansen A (2018) Analysis of fatal fires in Norway over a decade – a retrospective observational study. Age 56(43.9):387
24. US Fire Administration (2011) Fire death rate trends: an international perspective. Top Fire Rep Ser 12(8):1–8
25. Winberg D (2016) International fire death rate trends
26. Jonsson A, Runefors M, Särdqvist S, Nilson F (2016) Fire-related mortality in Sweden: temporal trends 1952 to 2013. Fire Technol 52(6):1697–1707
27. Istre GR, McCoy M, Carlin DK, McClain J (2002) Residential fire related deaths and injuries among children: fireplay, smoke alarms, and prevention. Inj Prev 8(2):128–132
28. Chen YA, Bridgman-Acker K, Edwards J, Lauwers AE (2011) Pediatric fire deaths in Ontario: retrospective study of behavioural, social, and environmental risk factors. Can Fam Physician 57(5):e169–e177
29. Harpur AP, Boyce KE, McConnell NC (2013) An investigation into the circumstances surrounding fatal dwelling fires involving very young children. Fire Saf J 61:72–82
30. Parker DJ, Sklar DP, Tandberg D, Hauswald M, Zumwalt RE (1993) Fire fatalities among New Mexico children. Ann Emerg Med 22(3):517–522
31. Scholer SJ, Hickson GB, Mitchel EF, Ray WA (1998) Predictors of mortality from fires in young children. Pediatrics 101(5):e12–e12
32. Shai D, Lupinacci P (2003) Fire fatalities among children: an analysis across Philadelphia's census tracts. Public Health Rep 118(2):115
33. Squires T, Busuttil A (1995) Child fatalities in Scottish house fires 1980–1990: a case of child neglect? Child Abuse Negl 19(7):865–873
34. Eggert E, Huss F (2017) Medical and biological factors affecting mortality in elderly residential fire victims: a narrative review of the literature. Scars Burns Heal 3:2059513117707686
35. Elder AT, Squires T, Busuttil A (1996) Fire fatalities in elderly people. Age Ageing 25(3):214–216
36. Harpur AMYP, Boyce K, McConnel N (2014) An investigation into the circumstances surrounding elderly dwelling fire fatalities and the barriers to implementing fire safety strategies among this group. Fire Saf Sci 11:1144–1159
37. Graesser H, Ball M, Bruck D (2009) Risk factors for residential fire fatality across the lifespan: comparing coronial data for children, adults and elders. In: 4th international symposium on human behaviour in fire, conference proceedings. Interscie
38. Barillo DJ, Goode R (1996) Fire fatality study: demographics of fire victims. Burns 22(2):85–88
39. Ballard JE, Koepsell TD, Rivara FP, Van Belle G (1992) Descriptive epidemiology of unintentional residential fire injuries in King County, WA, 1984 and 1985. Public Health Rep 107(4):402
40. Xiong L, Bruck D, Ball M (2017) Unintentional residential fires caused by smoking-related materials: who is at risk? Fire Saf J 90:148–155
41. Sacks JJ, Nelson DE (1994) Smoking and injuries: an overview. Prev Med 23(4):515–520
42. Hall JR (2010) The smoking-material fire problem. National Fire Protection Association, Quincy, pp 50–57

43. Runefors M (2020) Fatal residential fires: prevention and response. Doctoral dissertation, Lund University
44. Diekman ST, Ballesteros MF, Berger LR, Caraballo RS, Kegler SR (2008) Ecological level analysis of the relationship between smoking and residential-fire mortality. Inj Prev 14(4):228–231
45. Howland J, Hingson R (1987) Alcohol as a risk factor for injuries or death due to fires and burns: review of the literature. Public Health Rep 102(5):475
46. Bruck D, Ball M, Thomas IR (2011) Fire fatality and alcohol intake: analysis of key risk factors. J Stud Alcohol Drugs 72(5):731–736
47. Barillo DJ, Goode R (1996) Substance abuse in victims of fire. J Burn Care Rehabil
48. Marshall SW, Runyan CW, Bangdiwala SI, Linzer MA, Sacks JJ, Butts JD (1998) Fatal residential fires: who dies and who survives? JAMA 279(20):1633–1637
49. Squires T, Busuttil A (1997) Alcohol and house fire fatalities in Scotland, 1980–1990. Med Sci Law 37(4):321–325
50. Miller I, Beever P (2005) Victim behaviours, intentionality, and differential risks in residential fire deaths. WIT Trans Built Environ 82
51. Ballard JE, Koepsell TD, Rivara F (1992) Association of smoking and alcohol drinking with residential fire injuries. Am J Epidemiol 135(1):26–34
52. Leth P, Gregersen M, Sabroe S (1998) Fatal residential fire accidents in the municipality of Copenhagen, 1991–1996. Prev Med 27(3):444–451
53. Waterhouse KB (2010) A review of fire-related deaths in Alberta. J Can Soc Forensic Sci 43(4):171–180
54. Runyan CW, Bangdiwala SI, Linzer MA, Sacks JJ, Butts J (1992) Risk factors for fatal residential fires. N Engl J Med 327(12):859–863
55. Jonsson A, Jaldell H (2020) Identifying sociodemographic risk factors associated with residential fire fatalities: a matched case control study. Inj Prev 26(2):147–152
56. Xiong L, Bruck D, Ball M (2015) Comparative investigation of 'survival' and fatality factors in accidental residential fires. Fire Saf J 73:37–47
57. Holborn PG, Nolan PF, Golt J (2003) An analysis of fatal unintentional dwelling fires investigated by London Fire Brigade between 1996 and 2000. Fire Saf J 38(1):1–42
58. Nilson F, Lundgren L, Bonander C (2020) Living arrangements and fire-related mortality amongst older people in Europe. Int J Inj Control Saf Promot 27(3):378–384
59. Goodsman RW, Mason F, Blythe A (1987) Housing factors and fires in two metropolitan boroughs. Fire Saf J 12(1):37–50
60. Mierley MC, Baker SP (1983) Fatal house fires in an urban population. JAMA 249(11):1466–1468
61. Hannon L, Shai D (2003) The truly disadvantaged and the structural covariates of fire death rates. Soc Sci J 40(1):129–136
62. Duncanson M, Woodward A, Reid P (2002) Socioeconomic deprivation and fatal unintentional domestic fire incidents in New Zealand 1993–1998. Fire Saf J 37(2):165–179
63. Mulvaney C, Kendrick D, Towner E, Brussoni M, Hayes M, Powell J et al (2008) Fatal and non-fatal fire injuries in England 1995–2004: time trends and inequalities by age, sex and area deprivation. J Public Health 31(1):154
64. Patetta MJ, Cole TB (1990) A population-based descriptive study of house fire deaths in North Carolina. Am J Public Health 80(9):1116–1117
65. Flynn JD (2010) Characteristics of home fire victims. National Fire Protection Association, Quincy
66. Ahrens M, Evarts B (2017) US fire death rates by state. National Fire Protection Association. Research, Date and Analytics Division
67. Chernichko L, Saunders LD, Tough S (1993) Unintentional house fire deaths in Alberta 1985–1990: a population study. Can J Publ Health. Revue canadienne de sante publique 84(5):317–320

68. Jaldell H (2017) How important is the time factor? Saving lives using fire and rescue services. Fire Technol 53(2):695–708
69. McGwin G, Chapman V, Rousculp M, Robison J, Fine P (2000) The epidemiology of fire-related deaths in Alabama, 1992–1997. J Burn Care Rehabil 21(1):75–83
70. Ahrens M (2014) Physical disability as a factor in home fire deaths. National Fire Protection Association, Fire Analysis and Research Division
71. Leth PM, Gregersen M, Sabroe S (1998) Fatal accidents in house fires. The most significant causes, such as smoking and alcohol abuse, multiplied by four the incidence during the last 40 years. Ugeskr Laeger 160(23):3403–3408
72. Watts-Hampton T (2006) Examination of risk factors and mental health status in an adult accidental fire death population 1998–2005. Doctoral dissertation, Victoria University

Dr. Anders Jonsson is since 2001 working as a statistician within the area of accident and injury analysis at the Learning from Accidents Section within the Swedish Civil Contingencies Agency. He took his PhD in Risk Management at Karlstad University, Sweden, in 2018 on "Fire-related deaths in Sweden: An analysis of data quality, causes and risk patterns".

Mr. Colin McIntyre holds a BSc in Mathematics from Edinburgh University. In the 1990s, Colin coordinated an analysis of what kind of statistics were needed to improve decision-making in the Swedish fire and rescue service. He then led the development of the system for data collection from fire service incident reports. He now works at the Swedish Civil Contingencies Agency with analysis of a range of statistics on fires, accidents and the emergency responses of the fire and rescue service.

Dr. Marcus Runefors is a Lecturer at the Division of Fire Safety Engineering at Lund University in Sweden, where he also finished his PhD in the beginning of 2020. The topic of his PhD was fatal residential fires from both a prevention and response perspective, focusing on the effectiveness of different measures to prevent fatal fires for different groups in the population.

Chapter 3
The Residential Fire Injury Pyramid

Finn Nilson

Abstract The injury pyramid is a commonly used model in order to illustrate the relationship between non-injurious events and fatal events, as well as the various injury-levels in-between. From a residential fire perspective, there is also the added aspect of whether fires are attended to or not. In practice, this means that the understanding of the residential fire problem is often understood merely from the perspective of fatal fires that are attended to by rescue services. However, as will be seen in this chapter, merely focusing on these incidents and the risk factors associated with these fires or victims produces a distinctly skew view of the residential fire problem. As such, it is important to attempt to assess and understand the entire residential fire injury pyramid.

Keywords Injury pyramid · Morbidity · Mortality · Non-fatal fires · Fatal fires · At-risk groups

1 Introduction

In terms of injury prevention, the concept of the injury pyramid has become well-established. While often used to illustrate the distribution of injuries, it has also come to function as a foundation to injury prevention interventions. Presented in 1931, in the book *Industrial Accident Prevention: A Scientific Approach* by Herbert Heinrich [1], the injury pyramid was the result of studying more than 75,000 industrial accidents. Heinrich's conclusions from these investigations were threefold. First, he declared that in terms of severity, the relationship between accidents resulting in serious injuries, accidents resulting in minor injuries and accidents resulting in no injuries was a 1:29:300 ratio (see Fig. 3.1). Second, he declared that in terms of causes, 88% of incidents were caused by the unsafe acts of people, 10% were

F. Nilson (✉)
Centre for Societal Risk Research, Karlstad University, Karlstad, Sweden
e-mail: finn.nilson@kau.se

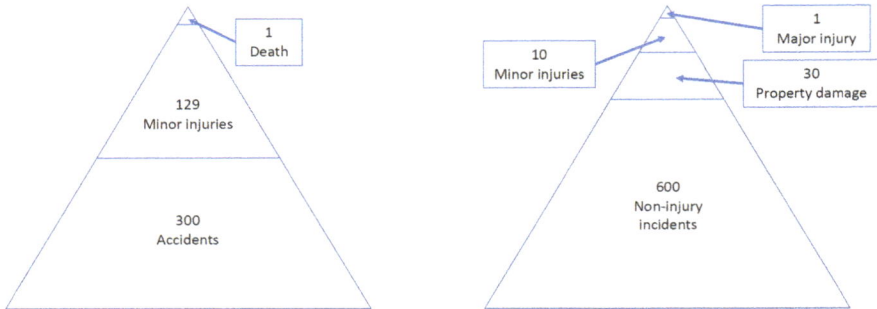

Fig. 3.1 Schematic injury pyramids according to Herbert Heinrich [1] and Frank Bird [3]

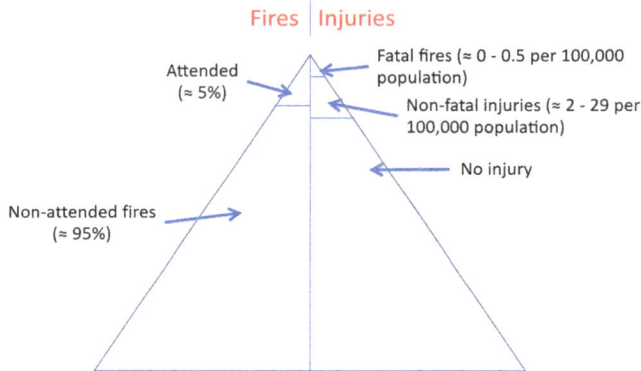

Fig. 3.2 A schematic injury pyramid of residential fires and the injury outcome

caused by unsafe conditions and 2% were not preventable. Third, Heinrich indicated that the causes of minor and major incidents are generally the same, stating that the repetition of non-injury incidents inevitably leads to major incidents [2].

Since the original claims, a number of authors (in particular within occupational and industrial safety) have continued to elaborate on Heinrich's conclusions. In particular, the 1966 book *Damage Control* by Frank Bird elaborated on the thoughts of Heinrich and presented a new ratio of 1 *major injury* to 10 *minor injuries* to 30 *property damage* to 600 *non-injury incidents* [3] (see Fig. 3.2). Also, in a later book *Practical Loss Control Leadership*, together with George Germain, the injury pyramid was further reiterated as was the concept that by reporting, investigating and preventing near hits or minor incidents, the pyramid can be flattened and the number of serious incidents can be reduced [4].

The presumption that minor incidents are simply potentially major incidents that have been luckily or skilfully avoided (based on the assumption that a large majority of incidents are caused by the unsafe acts of individuals) presides also today, not least within fire safety. It has been argued that *"unreported fires are important to note in the estimation of total fire hazards as they could have developed into potentially dangerous fires if they had not been detected or controlled early"* [5]. Despite the empirical evidence suggesting that hindering minor incidents will not hinder major incidents, both researchers and practitioners continue to (incorrectly) claim that a systematic approach of hindering near-misses will not only have an effect on the base of the pyramid (i.e. minor incidents), but also the top of the pyramid [6]. Similarly, the opposite is true. Reducing, for example, the incidence of fatal residential fires by focusing on the underlying causes of these incidents will not necessarily have an effect on the incidence rates of residential fires in general.

However, although there are considerable problems associated with the concept of the injury pyramid, there are practical uses in terms of residential fires. First and foremost, presenting injury data in an injury pyramid can be an illustrative exercise when comparing different countries or different injury types. Second, following an injury pyramid over time can give valuable insights into the successes of preventative measures as well as injury severity levels where more work is required.[1] Third (and ironically considering the original purpose of the injury pyramid), when combining the numbers in the injury pyramid with background data, the injury pyramid can effectively illustrate the differences between the severity levels in terms of who is at most risk, where these incidents can occur, which types of fires are overrepresented as well as differing contextual factors. As such, it is also possible to assess what potential effect different preventative measures will have on each level.

Despite the considerable problems with the original purpose and thinking behind the injury pyramid, this chapter aims to present a brief overview of the injury pyramid for residential fires. Focus will predominantly be on the qualitative differences in the severity levels, in accordance with the reasoning above. Importantly, given the differences in global fire mortality, in particular regarding determining factors for fire-related injuries [8, 9], this chapter will focus on the injury pyramid from a high-income country perspective.

2 Residential Fires Not Attended to by Rescue Services

The base of an injury pyramid is often composed of near-misses or incidents without injury. As such, the base of the pyramid regarding residential fires consists of residential fires that were extinguished without the need of help from rescue services.

Numerically, it is difficult to know exactly how regular such residential fires are given that no organisation has been present and therefore no registration has occurred. However, based on the results from a telephone interviews in the United

---

[1] N.b. in order for this to be possible it is important to have similar data collection procedures as well as taking into account changes in, for example, coding practices [7]

States in 2004 [10], it is clear that this level in the injury pyramid is by far the largest. According to the results, an estimated 7.2 million residential fires occur each year that are not attended to by rescue services and approximately 130,000 (usually minor) injuries are caused by these fires [11]. Importantly, compared to data from 1984, when an estimated 23.7 million residential fires occurred annually, the number of residential fires seems to have decreased dramatically [12].

Given the difficulty in collecting data regarding these types of fires, a limited number of studies have investigated this dimension of residential fires. However, despite this, the results are surprisingly similar regarding the socio-demographic groups that have a higher risk. An increased risk has been observed in households with members under 18 years [10, 13–17], those with a high educational level [10, 13–17], smokers [10, 13–16], those living in rented accommodation [10, 14], households with many family members [10, 16] and in immigrant households [17].

These results are in some senses surprising. Although individuals living in rented accommodation, smokers and ethnic minorities are known to have a high risk of fire-related mortality [18], high education as well as households with many family members and children have a distinctly lower risk for residential fire mortality [18–20]. One potential explanation as to why households with several individuals, high educational level and children are overrepresented in the risk of residential fires yet underrepresented in fatal fires is the preventative measures that are taken by different groups [21]. It is likely that in households with several individuals, high educational level and children, there is an increased chance of being alerted to a fire (either due to the presence of smoke alarms or simply due to the large number of individuals in the household) and the household having the equipment and training to handle the fire themselves.

While this may suggest that fatal fires are simply small fires that could have been stopped if the correct equipment had been in place, this would assume that the effectiveness of the intervention was the same in all groups and that the fires were of the same type. In regard to the higher risk of fire in households with children, it is well-known that children in the 6–12 year age group (that are the largest child risk group [17]) are more likely to experiment with matches and candles due to a lack of understanding of the potential consequences, thereby causing fires, compared to older age groups [22]. However, in terms of fatal fires, candles are only known to be a risk factor for elderly, often disabled, individuals [23]. Also, when analysing the potential of implementing different safety interventions on fatal fires, it is clear that interventions such as fire-safe cigarettes and flame-retardant clothes, bedding or furniture would be highly effective in reducing the fatal fire risk for the group that now dies in residential fires [24]. However, this type of equipment is almost completely absent from the households of those who to a larger degree have smaller fires that are handled independently [17]. Likewise, the equipment that is prevalent in low-risk homes (such as smoke alarms and fire extinguishers) have relatively low potential effect on reducing the risk of fatal fires in high-risk homes [24].

3 Non-fatal Fires Attended to by Rescue Services

The next stage in the injury pyramid is the level consisting of residential fires that the individual, or alternatively the individual's social network, was unable to extinguish. I.e., fires where the help of rescue services was required and where the victims survived.

On a yearly basis, again using the United States as an example, rescue services attend to approximately 360,000 residential fires [11], i.e., approximately 5% of all residential fires. Although the number of rescue service attended fires, at least in some respects, increased during the 1990s [25], in similarity to the risk of fatal fires [26, 27], the number of fires attended to by rescue services has decreased considerably during the last decades in Sweden, the United Kingdom and the United States [27–29]. Although this is obviously a positive development as it would suggest more fire-safe societies, there are also problems with such a development. For example, less residential fires means that rather than focusing on fires, a very large proportion of the rescue services' calls are either "false alarms" or related to other societal safety issues, such as traffic-related incidents [28, 29]. As such, at least in the UK, the maintaining of full-time stations is increasingly questioned [28] which is problematic in itself considering the importance of time in hindering fatalities [30].

In terms of comparisons, very few results exist regarding the differences between non-attended and attended residential fires or in relation to the general public. However, in general, smoke alarms seem to be more prevalent in homes that manage the fire themselves compared to those requiring help [31]. As such, this would indicate that an important difference between non-attended and attended residential fires is the size of the fire given that a smoke alarm will notify inhabitants of a smaller fire. As noted above, socio-demographic differences in safety equipment are considerable [21]. Therefore, it is unsurprising that rescue services are more often called out to areas with higher rates of unemployment, economic deprivation, low education and high rates of ethnic minorities [32, 33].

In terms of comparisons between fires attended by rescue services and fatal fires, it is clear that some characteristics increase the probability of being rescued. First, the presence of others seems to be an important element in increasing survival. Previous studies have shown that living with others is a strong protective factor against fire-related mortality [34] and this is also shown in a comparison between non-fatal and fatal fires [35, 36]. Similarly, living in an apartment is also protective [27, 35, 37], most likely due to the increased possibility of a fire being noticed early on in the process, as shown by the fact that neighbours are the most common individual to alert rescue services [35]. Combined with the fact that non-fatal fires are often attended to more quickly than fatal fires [35, 37], it is likely that the time from fire ignition to rescue is considerably shorter for non-fatal fires [37]. As such, urban dwellings are likely to increase the possibility of being rescued, a factor relatively unsurprising given the known increase in risk of fatal fires in rural locations [18, 30, 38].

The second factor visible in the published material is the physical and mental capabilities of the victim. Put simply, fires that occur in the homes of individuals who are under the influence of alcohol or drugs, have physical or mental disabilities or are of high age are considerably more likely to result in fatalities compared to those with the opposite characteristics [35, 37]. Interestingly, also circumstantial aspects that reduce the individual's awareness and capabilities also severely affect the outcome. Most notably, if the victim is awake when a fire starts, the chance of survival is considerably greater, irrespective of whether there were functioning smoke alarms [36].

A third factor is the type of fire. Smoking-related fires are a considerable cause of fatal fires [23], despite the fact that smoking-related fires account for a relatively small number of attended residential fires [11]. However, in terms of electrical and cooking-related fires, these are considerably more common among non-fatal rescue service attended fires than in fatal fires [35, 36]. It would seem, therefore, that focusing on minimising the number of electrical and cooking-related fires would most likely have a limited effect on the total number of fatal fires though would affect the number of rescue service-attended fires.

A final element that is interesting to note in regard to this level in the incident pyramid is that elderly individuals, as also shown in the lower risk of having a residential fire without needing the help of rescue services [17], are less likely to be involved in a non-fatal fire requiring the help of rescue services [33]. Given the increased risk of elderly being involved in a fatal fire compared to younger populations [18, 39], this would clearly indicate that the mortality risk is less related to the risk of experiencing a fire and more related to the consequences once a fire has started.

4 Non-fatal Injurious Residential Fires

Residential fires that lead to injury, though are not fatal, can be seen to be the next step in the injury pyramid. Obviously, these injuries are a part of either of the first two categories. However, in the previous two levels, individuals who have not sustained an injury are a clear majority meaning that if injured individuals have specific individual or fire characteristics, the previous levels may not be representable. Given that the primary goal for fire safety is the protection of human lives, it is therefore important to distinguish this perspective of fire safety despite them being included in several levels.

There are some aspects that are important to note before presenting this level. First, studies on fire-related injuries are often focused on burns, regardless of whether these were caused by an unintentional or intentional fire and regardless of whether the fire was residential or non-residential. Although some studies present the proportion of burns in relation to the type of fire, this is only in the descriptive statistics, not in the later analyses. This means that it can be difficult to ascertain exact socio-demographic factors for residential fire-related injuries. As such, much of the presented material in this section is related to burns in general. Also, the category of "non-fatal fire-related injuries" includes a broad array of injuries; from injuries merely requiring first-aid to long-term care in specialised burn units. While it would be beneficial to differentiate between these groups, this is difficult for a number of reasons. First, given that some type of data collection is required, a common cutoff for studies is whether an individual visited an emergency department (ED). However, the criteria for whether individuals receive care at an emergency department or other medical institutions can vary between countries, making international comparisons difficult. Second, there seems to have been a change in policies in many countries with more minor burns being admitted to specialised burn units than previously, not least as a consequence of a greater acceptance of the psychological impact burns can have on victims [40]. Although the relationship between different injury severity categories seems to be relatively similar with approximately 5–10% [9, 41–43] of burn victims presented at an ED needing specialised care, these aspects mean that differentiating severity is difficult, as is clearly seen by the fact that the rates of burns treated in hospitals vary between 2 and 29 per 100,000 inhabitants in Europe [44].

Regardless of these issues, a decrease has been observed in the rates of ED visits for burns between the 1990s and 2000s in the majority of high-income countries [9, 40]. Likewise, the injury severity (i.e. burn depth) and length of stay in hospitals seem to have decreased in many countries [40], at least in part due to improved medical treatment [45].

In terms of socio-demographic factors, studies from the United Kingdom, the United States and Australia have shown injury rates to be considerably higher in low-income neighbourhoods compared to more well-off areas [46–49]. As such, similar background factors are seen in attended residential fires. Families with low income seem to be particularly at risk in terms of burn injuries in general [50] and for children in low-income families the risk of attaining a burn injury is over eight times the risk for a child in a middle-to-high-income household [51]. However, in terms of education, although low-education is a risk factor for burns in some studies, this factor seems to have less of an impact on risk than income [50], i.e. an opposite result from non-attended residential fires.

Ethnic minorities have also been shown to be overrepresented regardless of whether only residential fires are studied or all types of burns are included [49, 50]. Although it is most likely that at least some of this increase in risk can be explained by socioeconomic confounders [9], results from Australia indicate that injury reductions have been less prominent among indigenous groups compared to the rest of the population [52]. Therefore, this group deserves increased attention, not least considering a lower prevalence of safety equipment [53, 54]. Similarly, although the overrepresentation of burn victims in single-parent households [50] is most likely due to socioeconomic confounders and difficulties with supervision of children, this group also has less fire safety equipment in the home [21, 55] meaning that preventative measures aimed at this group could also be beneficial.

In terms of sex, men are considerably overrepresented [40] in all age groups despite small children (0–4 years and in particular 6–24 months) having by far the greatest risk of receiving burn injuries that require hospitalisation [9, 56], followed by the age group of 15–44 years [57, 58]. In terms of elderly individuals, although the risk of attaining a burn injury is lower compared to younger groups, they are generally less well-equipped to cope with a fire. Case-fatality rates are considerably higher [59] (which may account for the relatively low hospitalisation rates in this age group, i.e., fires may more often be fatal than non-fatal), and when individuals survive, they have a high risk of needing to move to assisted living [9]. As such, this group may be more at risk than the statistics would suggest.

5 Fatal Residential Fires

Fatal residential fires are obviously the top of the residential fire injury pyramid. In terms of mortality rates in a total population, these vary from 0 to 0.5 per 100,000 in high-income countries [60]. In terms of general fire mortality, one of the most prominent risk factors, at least in high-income countries, is age [23, 61]. From a European perspective, the average fire-related mortality rate among older adults between 2005 and 2014 was 2.86 per 100,000. Notably, however, there was considerable variation between countries (a low of 0.55 in Iceland to a high of 14.65 in Latvia) [34].

The fact that old age is such a considerable risk factor for mortality despite not being a risk factor for the majority of the other levels in the injury pyramid is an important aspect. Old age has considerable effects on the physical and cognitive abilities of an individual [62], meaning that evacuation or more complex fire extinguishing can be difficult or impossible. Therefore, an early detection becomes the only reasonable preventative measure for older adults with reduced capabilities and could explain why this group generally focus on smoke alarms rather than other safety equipment [21]. It also helps to explain the inadequacies of applying an injury pyramid perspective to residential fires. As is clear from the typologies of fatal residential fires [23], certain types of fires are considerably more common among fatal fires than fires in general, for example regarding smoking-related fires. Often, these are relatively small fires that for a younger, well-functioning individual are easy to manage. For a disabled (either due to illness or substances) individual, however, such fires can be near impossible to manage.

Although the risk factor of age differs between fatal fires and other levels, there are also a number of socio-demographic risk factors that are similar with previous levels. These include being male [23, 63], living alone [34, 63–65], belonging to an ethnic minority [20, 46, 66], having low educational attainment [19, 20], as well as other deprivation-related factors such as having a low disposable income, receiving social allowance, being unemployed, receiving health-related early retirement pension, etc. [19, 36, 39, 46, 64, 65, 67, 68]. Interestingly, many of these socio-demographic differences have been observed since the 1970s [69, 70], though seem to have become even more pronounced since then [36, 64].

6 Discussion

As is hopefully clear from this chapter, in terms of the quantitative relationship between the different levels in the residential fire pyramid, there are a number of uncertainties, not least given that certain levels include the same fires. Also, certain levels are related to the number of fires, while others are related to the number of individuals. However, despite this, the quantitative relationship is valid to present as it clearly illustrates the large base of the pyramid. Due to the fact that whether fires are attended to or not is not necessarily related to the fire's outcome, the pyramid needs to be divided and separated from the perspective of the fire and the outcome.

As is seen in the figure above, based on an approximate ratio of data from Europe and the United States, a number of interesting aspects are seen. First and foremost, it is clear that a very large number of residential fires are managed within the household without the help of rescue services. Practically, this means that in most cases rescue services, or other government organisations that are responsible for preventative interventions, have no knowledge regarding approximately 95% of all residential fires (n.b. this number varies somewhat between countries). Although this in itself is not necessarily a problem, given that rescue services should focus on those households that have difficulty in extinguishing or evacuating, it is important for rescue services to be aware that their preconceptions regarding residential fires are largely constructed from the most severe cases or those households that need help.

Second, a very large number of residential fires do not lead to injuries or fatalities and traditional risk measurements can be highly misleading. Most rescue service statistics are based on only the three highest levels and therefore the risk of injury or death per residential fire can be understood as considerable. By including the base, however, it is clear that this is not the case. In fact, from a community perspective, the risk of injury or death is very low per residential fire. However, this is not the case when specific socio-demographic groups are compared.

	At-risk groups			
	Fatal fires	Non-fatal injurious residential fires	Non-fatal fires attended to by rescue services	Residential fires not attended to by rescue services
Age	Elderly	Children	Adults	Adults and children
Sex	Men	Men	–	–
Income level	Low	Low	Low	–
Education level	Low	Low	Low	High
Ethnicity	Minority groups	Minority groups	Minority groups	Minority groups
Physical or mental function	Low[a]	–	–	High
Household characteristics	Single occupancy	Single-parent households	Multi-person households	Multi-person households
Type of accommodation	Houses/ rural areas	–	Apartment/urban areas	–

[a]Either caused by physical or mental illness, or due to effects of alcohol and/or drugs

As is evident from the literature review in this chapter, which in turn is compiled in the table above, the socio-demographic groups most at risk differ considerably between the different levels. From a national or population perspective, it is clear that there is a socio-demographic scale in regard to residential fires. Healthy individuals who have been educated and who live with others are considerably more likely to handle a fire themselves. If their socio-demographic level is slightly lower, they are also highly likely to remain uninjured despite needing help from rescue services.

The importance of socio-demographic factors is further supported by studies showing a significantly lower use of preventative measures or practices among ethnic minority families [21, 53, 54, 71, 72], single-households and low-income families [21, 55], families in rented accommodation [21, 73], individuals with a lower educational level [21, 74, 75] as well as those living in socially deprived areas [76, 77]. Fire protection, therefore, seems to follow a "sociodemographic protection maturity U-curve" in which younger individuals living in single households with low income tend to exhibit low levels of fire protection. The level of protection then increases with socio-demographic development, to peak during middle-age, to then decrease again with old age [21, 78].

Whether this is true from an individual perspective, i.e., that the level of protection varies throughout an individual's life, is unknown. However, previous studies have shown that risk-taking generally decreases as one gets older [79] and adding a child to a household greatly increases the probability of the household having an existing fire escape plan [80, 81], thereby indicating that individual development may occur. Regardless, socio-demographic factors seem to be possible to overcome [82] given the effectiveness of interventions such as smoke alarm installations, education or multifaceted programs [63, 82–84]. It could therefore be hypothesised that by ensuring that all households had the same level of protection, many of the problems would be eliminated.

However, this is oversimplifying the issue. Although many interventions are effective on a general level, the potential effectiveness varies considerably between different socio-demographic groups [24, 85]. For example, simple interventions such as smoke alarms are relatively ineffective for frail, disabled smokers [24]. Similarly, hinders in the ability to evacuate, i.e. a crucial step in the fire process to minimise the risk of both death and injury [86], due to illness, intoxication, living alone, living in rural areas, etc., are all factors that are overrepresented among fatal fire victims [18]. Put simply, while a functioning smoke alarm will most likely be highly effective for the most at-risk group for *Residential Fires Not Attended to by Rescue Services*, its effectiveness for the most at-risk group for *Fatal Fires* is low.

In conclusion and in accordance with previous research [87–89], differences in fire risk and the consequences of fires are clearly the results of complex interactions of individual, societal and structural factors. A very small and insignificant fire can in one contextual setting result in a non-attended fire, while in another setting it can be a fatal fire. As such, there are no one-size-fits-all strategies. Rather, holistic, multifaceted programs are required that take the different levels of the residential fire injury pyramid into consideration.

By understanding the construction and internal relationship of the residential fire injury pyramid, the societal risk picture also becomes clearer. Specifically, the very large majority of residential fires never come to the attention of rescue services. Those that do are generally not representative of the total population. Instead, the households in which help from rescue services is required, or where injuries and deaths most often occur, have innate elements that decrease their ability to handle a fire independently. The more this ability is reduced, the greater the risk of a residential fire becoming a fatal residential fire. As such, although the risk of fatality per fire is very low for a large majority, for some individuals with particular characteristics, the risk of fatality per fire is high.

References

1. Heinrich HW (1931) Industrial accident prevention. McGraw-Hill, New York
2. Manuele FA (2002) Heinrich revisited: truisms or myths. National Safety Council, Itasca
3. Bird FE Jr (1966) Damage control: a new horizon in accident prevention and cost improvement. Am Manag Assoc
4. Bird FE, Germain GL (1996) Practical loss control leadership. Det Norske Veritas (USA)
5. Tannous WK, Agho K (2017) Socio-demographic predictors of residential fire and unwillingness to call the fire service in New South Wales. Prev Med Rep 7:50–57
6. Rebbitt D (2014) Pyramid power: a new view of the great safety pyramid. Prof Saf 59(09):30–34
7. Nilson F, Bonander C, Andersson R (2014) The effect of the transition from the ninth to the tenth revision of the International Classification of Diseases on external cause registration of injury morbidity in Sweden. Inj Prev 21(3):189–194
8. Peck M, Pressman MA (2013) The correlation between burn mortality rates from fire and flame and economic status of countries. Burns 39(6):1054–1059
9. Peck MD (2011) Epidemiology of burns throughout the world. Part I: Distribution and risk factors. Burns 37(7):1087–1100
10. Greene MA (2012) Comparison of the characteristics of fire and non-fire households in the 2004-2005 survey of fire department-attended and unattended fires. Inj Prev 18(3):170–175. https://doi.org/10.1136/injuryprev-2011-040009
11. Ahrens M (2015) Home structure fires. National Fire Protection Association. Fire Analysis and Research Division
12. Greene MA, Andres C (2009) 2004–2005 national sample survey of unreported residential fires. Citeseer
13. Housing SoE. Fires in the home: findings from the 2004/05 survey of English housing. Office of the Deputy Prime Minister2006 Contract No.: Report, London
14. Simmons J. Fires in the home: findings from the 2002/03 British crime survey. Office of the Deputy Prime Minister2004 Contract No.: Report, London
15. Simmons J. Fires in the home: findings from the 2001/02 British crime survey. Office of the Deputy Prime Minister2003 Contract No.: Report, London
16. Commission CPS (1984) National sample survey of unreported residential fires: final technical report prepared. U.S. Consumer Product Safety Commission1985 Contract No.: Report, Princeton

17. Nilson F, Bonander C, Jonsson A (2015) Differences in determinants amongst individuals reporting residential fires in Sweden: results from a cross-sectional study. Fire Technol 51(3):615–626
18. Jonsson A, Jaldell H (2019) Identifying sociodemographic risk factors associated with residential fire fatalities: a matched case control study. Inj Prev 26(2):147–152
19. Duncanson M, Woodward A, Reid P (2002) Socioeconomic deprivation and fatal unintentional domestic fire incidents in New Zealand 1993–1998. Fire Saf J 37(2):165–179
20. Jennings CR (1999) Socioeconomic characteristics and their relationship to fire incidence: a review of the literature. Fire Technol 35(1):7–34
21. Nilson F, Bonander C (2019) Household fire protection practices in relation to sociodemographic characteristics: evidence from a Swedish National Survey. Fire Technol:1–22
22. Klein JJ, Mondozzi MA, Andrews DA (2008) The need for a juvenile fire setting database. J Burn Care Res 29(6):955–958. https://doi.org/10.1097/BCR.0b013e31818ba101
23. Jonsson A, Bonander C, Nilson F, Huss F (2017) The state of the residential fire fatality problem in Sweden: epidemiology, risk factors, and event typologies. J Saf Res 62:89–100. https://doi.org/10.1016/j.jsr.2017.06.008
24. Runefors M, Nilson F (2021) The influence of sociodemographic factors on the theoretical effectiveness of fire prevention interventions on fatal residential fires. Fire Technol:1–18
25. Guldåker N, Hallin P-O (2014) Spatio-temporal patterns of intentional fires, social stress and socio-economic determinants: a case study of Malmö, Sweden. Fire Saf J 70:71–80
26. Jonsson A, Runefors M, Särdqvist S, Nilson F (2016) Fire-related mortality in Sweden: temporal trends 1952 to 2013. Fire Technol 52(6):1697–1707
27. Ahrens M (2017) Trends and patterns of US fire loss. National Fire Protection Association (NFPA) report. Google Scholar
28. Knight K (2013) Facing the future: findings from the review of efficiencies and operations in fire and rescue authorities in England. London Communities and Local Government Publications
29. Danielsson S, Sund B (2016) UB Lägesanalys, December 2016. Beredskap MfSo, Karlstad
30. Jaldell H (2015) How important is the time factor? Saving lives using fire and rescue services. Fire Technol:1–14
31. Chubb M (2003) Wake up and smell the smoke. Fire Eng
32. Taylor MJ, Higgins E, Lisboa PJ, Kwasnica V (2012) An exploration of causal factors in unintentional dwelling fires. Risk Manage 14(2):109–125
33. Hastie C, Searle R (2016) Socio-economic and demographic predictors of accidental dwelling fire rates. Fire Saf J 84:50–56
34. Nilson F, Lundgren L, Bonander C (2020) Living arrangements and fire-related mortality amongst older people in Europe. Int J Inj Control Saf Promot 27(3):378–384
35. Runefors M (2020) Measuring the capabilities of the Swedish fire service to save lives in residential fires. Fire Technol 56(2):583–603
36. Xiong L, Bruck D, Ball M (2015) Comparative investigation of 'survival' and fatality factors in accidental residential fires. Fire Saf J 73:37–47
37. Kobes M, Van Den Dikkenberg R (eds) (2016) An analysis of residential building fire rescues: the difference between fatal and nonfatal casualties. Interflam
38. Nilson F, Bonander C (2020) Societal protection and population vulnerability are equally important in explaining local variations in fire mortality among older adults in Sweden. Fire Technol
39. Mulvaney C, Kendrick D, Towner E, Brussoni M, Hayes M, Powell J et al (2009) Fatal and non-fatal fire injuries in England 1995–2004: time trends and inequalities by age, sex and area deprivation. J Public Health (Oxf) 31(1):154–161. https://doi.org/10.1093/pubmed/fdn103
40. Smolle C, Cambiaso-Daniel J, Forbes AA, Wurzer P, Hundeshagen G, Branski LK et al (2017) Recent trends in burn epidemiology worldwide: a systematic review. Burns 43(2):249–257
41. Yamamoto LG, Wiebe RA, Matthews WJ Jr (1991) A one-year prospective ED cohort of pediatric burns: a proposal for standardizing scald burns. Pediatr Emerg Care 7(2):80–84

42. Banco L, Lapidus G, Zavoski R, Braddock M (1994) Burn injuries among children in an urban emergency department. Pediatr Emerg Care 10(2):98–101
43. Rawlins JM, Khan AA, Shenton AF, Sharpe DT (2007) Epidemiology and outcome analysis of 208 children with burns attending an emergency department. Pediatr Emerg Care 23(5):289–293
44. Brusselaers N, Monstrey S, Vogelaers D, Hoste E, Blot S (2010) Severe burn injury in Europe: a systematic review of the incidence, etiology, morbidity, and mortality. Crit Care 14(5):R188
45. Stylianou N, Buchan I, Dunn KW (2015) A review of the international Burn Injury Database (iBID) for England and Wales: descriptive analysis of burn injuries 2003–2011. BMJ Open 5(2)
46. Istre GR, McCoy MA, Osborn L, Barnard JJ, Bolton A (2001) Deaths and injuries from house fires. N Engl J Med 344(25):1911–1916
47. DiGuiseppi C, Edwards P, Godward C, Roberts I, Wade A (2000) Urban residential fire and flame injuries: a population based study. Inj Prev 6(4):250–254
48. Goltsman D, Li Z, Bruce E, Connolly S, Harvey JG, Kennedy P et al (2016) Spatial analysis of pediatric burns shows geographical clustering of burns and 'hotspots' of risk factors in New South Wales, Australia. Burns 42(4):754–762
49. Alnababtah K, Khan S, Ashford R (2016) Socio-demographic factors and the prevalence of burns in children: an overview of the literature. Paediatr Int Child Health 36(1):45–51
50. Edelman LS (2007) Social and economic factors associated with the risk of burn injury. Burns 33(8):958–965
51. Istre GR, McCoy M, Carlin D, McClain J (2002) Residential fire related deaths and injuries among children: fireplay, smoke alarms, and prevention. Inj Prev 8(2):128–132
52. Duke J, Wood F, Semmens J, Spilsbury K, Edgar DW, Hendrie D et al (2011) A 26-year population-based study of burn injury hospital admissions in Western Australia. J Burn Care Res 32(3):379–386
53. Hapgood R, Kendrick D, Marsh P (2000) How well do socio-demographic characteristics explain variation in childhood safety practices? J Public Health 22(3):307–311
54. Mulvaney C, Kendrick D (2004) Engagement in safety practices to prevent home injuries in preschool children among white and non-white ethnic minority families. Inj Prev 10(6):375–378
55. Kendrick D (1994) Children's safety in the home: parents' possession and perceptions of the importance of safety equipment. Public Health 108(1):21–25
56. Pruitt BA, Wolf SE, Mason AD (2012) Epidemiological, demographic, and outcome characteristics of burn injury. Total Burn Care 4:15–45
57. Chien W-C, Pai C-C, Lin C-C, Chen H-C (2003) Epidemiology of hospitalized burns patients in Taiwan. Burns 29(6):582–588
58. Åkerlund E, Huss FR, Sjöberg F (2007) Burns in Sweden: an analysis of 24538 cases during the period 1987–2004. Burns 33(1):31–36
59. Macedo JLS, Santos JB (2007) Predictive factors of mortality in burn patients. Rev Inst Med Trop Sao Paulo 49(6):365–370
60. James SL, Lucchesi LR, Bisignano C, Castle CD, Dingels ZV, Fox JT et al (2020) Epidemiology of injuries from fire, heat and hot substances: global, regional and national morbidity and mortality estimates from the Global Burden of Disease 2017 study. Inj Prev 26(Supp 1):i36–i45
61. Hasofer AM, Thomas I (2006) Analysis of fatalities and injuries in building fire statistics. Fire Saf J 41(1):2–14
62. Lexell J, Taylor CC, Sjöström M (1988) What is the cause of the ageing atrophy?: Total number, size and proportion of different fiber types studied in whole vastus lateralis muscle from 15-to 83-year-old men. J Neurol Sci 84(2–3):275–294
63. Marshall SW, Runyan CW, Bangdiwala SI, Linzer MA, Sacks JJ, Butts JD (1998) Fatal residential fires: who dies and who survives? JAMA 279(20):1633–1637
64. Jonsson A, Jaldell H (2018) PA 07-4-2351 Identifying sociodemographic risk factors associated with residential fire fatalities: a matched case-control study. BMJ Publishing Group Ltd
65. Holborn PG, Nolan PF, Golt J (2003) An analysis of fatal unintentional dwelling fires investigated by London Fire Brigade between 1996 and 2000. Fire Saf J 38(1):1–42

66. Chandler SE, Chapman A, Hollington SJ (1984) Fire incidence, housing and social conditions – the urban situation in Britain. Fire Prev 172:15–20
67. Ballard JE, Koepsell TD, Rivara F (1992) Association of smoking and alcohol drinking with residential fire injuries. Am J Epidemiol 135(1):26–34
68. Chhetri P, Corcoran J, Stimson RJ, Inbakaran R (2010) Modelling potential socio-economic determinants of building fires in south east Queensland. Geogr Res 48(1):75–85
69. Berl WG, Halpin BM (1978) Human fatalities from unwanted fires. US Department of Commerce, National Institute of Standards and Technology
70. Jonsson A (2018) Dödsbränder i Sverige (Fire-Related Deaths in Sweden). Karlstad University, Karlstad
71. Tannous WK, Agho K (2019) Domestic fire emergency escape plans among the aged in NSW, Australia: the impact of a fire safety home visit program. BMC Public Health 19(1):872
72. Vaughan E, Anderson C, Agran P, Winn D (2004) Cultural differences in young children's vulnerability to injuries: a risk and protection perspective. Health Psychol 23(3):289
73. DiGuiseppi C, Roberts I, Speirs N (1999) Smoke alarm installation and function in inner London council housing. Arch Dis Child 81(5):400–403
74. Tannous WK, Whybro M, Lewis C, Ollerenshaw M, Watson G, Broomhall S et al (2016) Using a cluster randomized controlled trial to determine the effects of intervention of battery and hardwired smoke alarms in New South Wales, Australia: home fire safety checks pilot program. J Saf Res 56:23–27
75. Sidman EA, Grossman DC, Mueller BA (2011) Comprehensive smoke alarm coverage in lower economic status homes: alarm presence, functionality, and placement. J Community Health 36(4):525–533
76. Durand MA, Green J, Edwards P, Milton S, Lutchmun S (2012) Perceptions of tap water temperatures, scald risk and prevention among parents and older people in social housing: a qualitative study. Burns 38(4):585–590
77. Roberts H, Curtis K, Liabo K, Rowland D, DiGuiseppi C, Roberts I (2004) Putting public health evidence into practice: increasing the prevalence of working smoke alarms in disadvantaged inner city housing. J Epidemiol Community Health 58(4):280–285
78. Smith R, Wright M, Solanki A (2008) Analysis of fire and rescue service performance and outcomes with reference to population socio-demographics – fire research series 9/2008. London, Department for Communities and Local Government
79. Rolison JJ, Hanoch Y, Wood S, Liu P-J (2013) Risk-taking differences across the adult life span: a question of age and domain. J Gerontol B Psychol Sci Soc Sci 69(6):870–880
80. Yang J, Peek-Asa C, Allareddy V, Zwerling C, Lundell J (2006) Perceived risk of home fire and escape plans in rural households. Am J Prev Med 30(1):7–12
81. Tannous W, Agho K (2018) Factors associated with home fire escape plans in New South Wales: multinomial analysis of high-risk individuals and New South Wales population. Int J Environ Res Public Health 15(11):2353
82. Kendrick D, Young B, Mason-Jones AJ, Ilyas N, Achana FA, Cooper NJ et al (2013) Home safety education and provision of safety equipment for injury prevention. Evid Based Child Health Cochrane Rev J 8(3):761–939
83. Ta VM, Frattaroli S, Bergen G, Gielen AC (2006) Evaluated community fire safety interventions in the United States: a review of current literature. J Community Health 31(3):176
84. Warda L, Tenenbein M, Moffatt ME (1999) House fire injury prevention update. Part II. A review of the effectiveness of preventive interventions. Inj Prev 5(3):217–225
85. Runefors M, Johansson N, van Hees P (2017) The effectiveness of specific fire prevention measures for different population groups. Fire Saf J 91:1044–1050
86. Runefors M, Johansson N, Van Hees P (2016) How could the fire fatalities have been prevented? An analysis of 144 cases during 2011–2014 in Sweden: an analysis. J Fire Sci 34(6):515–527
87. Jennings CR (1997) Urban residential fires: an empirical analysis of building stock and socio-economic characteristics for Memphis, Tennessee

88. Corcoran J, Higgs G, Rohde D, Chhetri P (2011) Investigating the association between weather conditions, calendar events and socio-economic patterns with trends in fire incidence: an Australian case study. J Geogr Syst 13(2):193–226
89. Nilson F, Bonander C (2020) Societal protection and population vulnerability: key factors in explaining community-level variation in fatal fires involving older adults in Sweden. Fire Technol. https://doi.org/10.1007/s10694-020-00997-9

Prof. Finn Nilson is a full professor of Risk Management within injury prevention and societal safety and the Director for The Centre for Societal Risk Research at Karlstad University, Sweden. His research primarily concerns injury prevention epidemiology and evaluation of interventions with a special interest in underlying sociodemographic risk factors.

Chapter 4
Fire-Related Injury Mechanisms

Fredrik Huss

Abstract Understanding medical and biological factors affecting survivability in fires provide a solid ground for safety and preventive measures.

Most fire deaths are due to (smoke) inhalation injuries alone or in combination with burns. Smoke is a complex mixture of compounds that cause harm through Asphyxia, Acute irritation, Physical exposure, and Long-term effects. Not only the present incident and the acute setting are important, the following period also holds a substantial morbidity and mortality. Risk groups such as men, smokers, alcohol–/drug-impaired, physically disabled or cognitively impaired, and elderly have been identified. The global number of elderly people has increased significantly and is projected to continue increase rapidly.

While considering their own safety, emergency medical services need to quickly identify injured patients to promptly initiate life-saving interventions such as securing airways and providing O_2 counteracting the effects of inhaled toxic gases. Minor burns and smoke expositions can be treated ambulatory with routine wound care or a short period of O_2 inhalation. However, larger burns and inhalation injuries are often serious and need advanced treatment in hospital.

Different biological and/or medical factors that can explain, or identify, persons more vulnerable than others to fire, smoke, or heat incidences are reviewed in this chapter.

Given the short amount of time at hand to escape a fire situation, measures to extend this time must be taken; however, prevention is really the key. Environmental modifications, safety rules promotion, etc. need to be tailored to specific groups; children do not function as adults, psychiatric disabled differ from physically disabled, etc.

F. Huss (✉)
Department of Surgical Sciences, Plastic Surgery, Uppsala University, Uppsala, Sweden

Burn Center, Department of Plastic and Maxillofacial Surgery, Uppsala University Hospital, Uppsala, Sweden
e-mail: fredrik.huss@surgsci.uu.se

Keywords Burn injury · Inhalation injury · Mortality · Burn care · Injury/trauma mechanisms · Intensive care

1 Introduction

At 03:00 the fire alarm goes off. Mum hears the annoying noise distantly. It was only an hour ago she took the sleeping pill, the wine didn't do it for her this night. The divorce is really taking a toll on her, she can't sleep any longer. She smells smoke, her heart starts to pound. Her head is spinning, she can hear the children cry in their room. She's terrified. Her dad recently moved in to help her after the divorce. She's thankful for that even though she's afraid that he is showing signs of Alzheimer and just recently recuperated from his third heart attack. Dad! She cries, while swearing to herself that he, of course, removed his hearing aid for the night. She stumbles out of bed and heads for the nursery. In the hallway thick black smoke is lingering in the ceiling. The little one stands clinging to the crib wall, crying. She picks him up while screaming to the older child to run outside. With the little one in her arms she heads for her dad. The smoke is thicker now, she can barely see where she's going in the hallway. Her lungs ache, she coughs heavily and can feel how it's becoming heavier to breathe. Mum reaches for her asthma-spray just to realize she's in her pyjamas and the spray is still on the night stand...

Who in the family will make it out safely? This small, typical, family and situation show several intrinsic factors that have severe impacts on the chances for them to escape the dangerous situation.

Fire, heat, and hot substances have since the beginning of times been risks, to all species, and in all societies. Even the *homo erectus* (approximately 1.8 million years ago) was in danger, e.g., from lightning and wildfires. The risks increased even more when hominins learned the ability to control fire (suggested to happen approximately one million years ago [1]). In parallel with mankind's evolution, of course also measures to avoid and handle dangers have been developed and implemented.

As society, with time, has become increasingly more complex, so have also the risks.

Can be seen as obvious, but what exactly are the mechanisms behind people being injured or dying due to fire, heat, and hot substances? Which are the medical and/or biological explanations that make some people (more) vulnerable to fire, smoke, or heat (that also could explain the increased morbidity and mortality in certain groups)?

A multidisciplinary approach to reduce, and possibly avoid, injury and death due to fire, heat, and hot substances has previously mostly prevailed. However, it is evident that an interdisciplinary approach would be more fertile. Given the fact that most victims belong to one, or several, specific risk groups, it is necessary to take on the whole chain; pre-, per-, and post-incident. What can be done from the medical/health care sector to reduce the risks for, and effects of, a fire-related incidence for the more vulnerable persons?

2 Causes of Death in Residential Fires

Preventing situations that can put people in risk of fire and burns is of course a prerequisite in decreasing fire-related morbidity and mortality, e.g., how buildings are built regarding material, escape routes, etc. Once a fire incident is at hand, another prerequisite is that the person is made aware of the danger. It is not obvious that the person can embrace the situation and rationally seek to escape. Elderly, children, and physically, psychiatrically, or alcohol/drug-induced debilitated individuals often need longer time to react, if they react at all, to the threat. Even if/when the threat is acknowledged and the person, hopefully, reacts to escape, other, fire-related, factors come at play.

The majority of residential fire deaths (75–80%) are due to smoke inhalation alone or in combination with cutaneous burns. Since only 26% of deaths are attributable to burns, smoke inhalation is deemed as the main killer [2–5].

Asphyxiation, heat stroke (core hyperthermia), and distributive shock as a result of incidences with fire, heat, and hot substances are examples of immediate causes of death [6]. Occurring, but less common, are associated trauma or even already dead (homicide, suicide, or disease). The cause of death can seemingly be obvious, but there is often a road to the deadly point that is not routinely evaluated in autopsies or forensic examinations. In the scope of this book, these are factors that need to be considered. Why did the person end up in this situation, i.e., why did/could the individual not flee? Incapacitation plays a large role. Smoke, heat, physical condition, illnesses, etc. all add up to the situation preventing the individual from escaping the danger zone, thus exposing himself to further harm or, eventually, death.

2.1 Inhalation Injury

Inhalation injury is defined as inhalation and/or aspiration of hot gases, vapors, liquids, or toxic/chemical substances (residues after combustion). The risk is higher if the fire incident occurs in a closed room. Inhalation injuries can be seen in 2–20% of the cases with (flame) burns. The combination burns and inhalation injury increases morbidity and mortality significantly and increases the patient's need for fluid resuscitation in the early resuscitation phase. Since the heat exchange is very effective in the upper airways, the vast majority of thermal inhalation damage is limited to the upper airways (above the glottis) [7].

Although anamnesis or findings indicate that inhalation of hot or harmful substances has occurred, there are no clear clinical acute signs of an actual inhalation injury. This means that the acute diagnosis is only based on a number of probability factors (an adequately performed and assessed bronchoscopy may help but is not conclusive in the acute setting). These factors are partly based on circumstances at the time of the injury itself and partly on symptoms of that the upper airways have been damaged. However, the main clinical problems resulting from an inhalation injury are mainly caused by effects at the alveolar level and these cannot be assessed initially, but always appear somewhat later in the process (5–7 days).

Signs of Inhalation Injury

- Fire accident (or similar) in a closed room.
- Soot in sputum.
- Burns to face/neck.
- Changed level of consciousness.
- Strained breathing.
- Hoarseness of voice.

If an inhalation injury is likely, or in anticipated major and early airway problems, immediate intubation (placement of a flexible plastic tube into the trachea to maintain an open airway) should be considered. Especially when there is:

- Deep burns to the neck and face.
- Burns in the mouth.
- Stridor, hoarseness, or swelling in the pharynx.
- Unconsciousness.
- Hypoxia/hypercapnea.

Clinical Entities of Inhalation Injuries

Three clinical entities of inhalation injury exist (and may exist simultaneously):

- Upper airway injury (above glottis).
- Lower airway injury (below glottis).
- Inhalation of toxic gases:

Upper Airway Injury (Above Glottis)

The airways cranially of larynx/glottis, that is, the uvula, pharynx, and epiglottis, can be damaged and thus also swell considerably. This always entails the risk of acute total upper airway obstruction. The patient has stridor, hoarseness, and/or changed pitch. The time for any possible total occlusion of the airways varies and can be unpredictable. Generous indication of intubation exists. Inhalation of hot gases (but also hot liquids or chemicals) is usually the pathogenesis.

4 Fire-Related Injury Mechanisms

Lower Airway Injury (Below Glottis)

Epithelial damage, increased secretion, inflammation, atelectasis, and obstruction occur when toxic substances reach beyond the larynx and the lung parenchyma is damaged. Due to the heat exchange in the glottic area, thermal damage is very rarely seen below the glottis, but they do occur (especially after explosions/explosive combustion). The presence of hot steam also increases the risk of thermal damage in the lower respiratory tract. The patient exhibits dyspnea, cough, wheezing voice, and abundant secretions. Bronchoscopy can reveal an image of edema, bleeding, and soot. Lower airway damage significantly increases mortality.

Inhalation of Toxic Gases

Results in more systemic effects than upper/lower airway damage, vide infra.

2.2 Smoke

Smoke is a complex, heterogeneous, mixture of many different compounds (gases and particles). Depending on the fuel (what's burning), temperature, time since ignition, oxygen supply, and more, the composition varies greatly, also over time.

Four major separate harmful pathways for smoke can be identified [5, 8–10] (Table 4.1):

- Asphyxia.
- Acute irritation.
- Physical exposure (heat, vision).
- Long-term effects.

2.3 Asphyxia

Since all cells of the body demand O_2 for their metabolism, i.e., to live and function, an adequate O_2 delivery is essential and is maintained by the cardiorespiratory systems. The air contains normally 21% O_2 and when inhaled O_2 diffuses, in the alveoli of the lungs, to the capillary blood where it binds to hemoglobin (>98%) or dissolves directly in the plasma (<2%). The heart pumps the blood into the systemic circulation and further eventually to the microcirculation of cells and tissues. There, the O_2 is released from the hemoglobin and diffuses into the cells where it enters the electron transport chain in the mitochondria to enable production of aerobic energy. Normally, the O_2 delivery to the cells is a demand-driven process.

Table 4.1 Table of selected important fire gases

	Type of component	Examples of sources	Principal risks
Asphyxiants			
CO_2, CO	Inorganic gas	All fires	Acute: asphyxia
HCN	Inorganic gas	Nitrogen containing fuel, e.g., nylon	Acute: asphyxia
Irritants			
NO, NO_2, (NO_X)	Inorganic gas	Nitrogen containing fuel, e.g., nylon	Acute: irritation Long term: lung damage
NH_3	Inorganic gas	Nitrogen containing fuel, e.g., nylon	Acute: irritation Long term: lung damage
HCl	Inorganic gas	Chlorine containing fuel, e.g., PVC	Acute: irritation Long term: lung damage
HF	Inorganic gas	Fluorine containing fuel, e.g., PTFE, PVDF	Acute: irritation Long term: lung damage
HBr	Inorganic gas	Bromine containing fuel, e.g., Br-flame retarded material	Acute: irritation Long term: lung damage
SO_2	Inorganic gas	Sulphur containing fuel, e.g., wool	Acute: irritation Long term: lung damage
Isocyanates	Volatile organic gas	Nitrogen containing fuel, e.g., mineral wool	Acute: irritation. Long term: asthma, cancer
Phenol	Volatile organic gas	Generally in many fires	Acute: irritation
Styren	Volatile organic gas	Polystyrene fuel	Acute: irritation
Benzene	Volatile organic gas	All fires	Long term: cancer
PAH	Semi-volatile/ condensed phase organics	All fires, aromatic fuels	Long term: cancer
Dioxins/ furans	Semi-volatile/ condensed phase organics	Chlorine or bromine containing fuels	Long term: cancer, immunotoxicity, etc.
Obscuring			
Soot particles	Particles	All fires	Acute: visual obscuration Long term: depositions in the lungs

After Blomqvist [8]

If the cells' O_2 demands cannot be met due to inability to acquire, transport, or deliver sufficient amounts through breathing/circulation asphyxia is present, cells and tissues become hypoxic and start to die.

Gases developed in fires can cause asphyxia in many ways [11], to mention a few:

- Displacement of O_2 in the inhaled air (less O_2 inhaled).
- Affect the diffusion of O_2 from lung to blood or blood to cells through.

    – (Soot) particles/debris depositions in the alveoli

- Thermal injury to the mucosa.
- Shifting of the dissociation curve of hemoglobin.

- Impair hemoglobin O_2 carriage (e.g., CO has 210 times higher affinity than O_2 to hemoglobin and thus blocks the bindings sites for O_2 leading to less O_2 being transported).
- Elicit metabolic acidosis and/or systemic ischemia.

Interference with the mitochondria's electron transport chain.

2.4 Acute Irritation

Mucous membranes in, e.g., eyes, mouth, nose, and respiratory system, react to chemical irritants in different ways, e.g., by increased secretion, bronchospasm, and cell damage. Some effects are acute and can result in, e.g., visual impairment or difficulties breathing rendering the person unable to escape the danger zone, whereas other effects are more long-term (lung damage, pneumonia, pneumonitis, lung edema) that may result in death some time later. The irritative effect that occurs directly is more related to the concentration than the dose of the irritant. However, in larger doses more long-term effects can be seen. Still, the critical doses and concentrations for humans are not easy to establish [8].

2.5 Physical Exposure (Heat)

The heat exchange in the upper airways is very effective. Thus, thermal inhalation injury is mostly limited to the upper airways (above the glottis). There, burns and resulting edema may quickly impair the airways' patency.

In escaping a fire scenario, the heat can also be incapacitating in the sense that the person is prevented to reach escape routes because of oppressing temperatures. The person may find himself trapped in a room because of fear of, or actual, injurious heat and succumbs due to additive harmful factors such as harmful gases.

2.6 Physical Exposure (Vision)

A person's vision may be impaired in a fire scenario not only by irritant gases. The aerosol of solid and liquid particles and gases that make up the smoke simply makes it difficult to see where one is going due to obscuration and darkening (light extinction) of the surroundings [8].

2.7 Long-Term Effects

Even though the acute effects of different smoke constituents probably pose the more important aspects regarding the context of this book. One also needs to consider more long-term effects. Several of the constituent gases, particles, and debris involved in fires can cause direct systemic and airway and lung tissue damage as well as trigger development of, e.g., cancer, immunotoxicity, and asthma later on. Deposition of solid particles, particularly those in the nm-range, are of concern regarding health effects long time after the fire incident [8].

3 Medical and Biological Factors Affecting Mortality

The global number of elderly people (>65 years) has increased. This is a result of advances in living conditions, social care, and medicine and is projected to continue increase rapidly from 0.7 billion people today and reach 1.6 billion in 2050 [12].

In 2019, the global death rate per 100 k population, all ages, regarding burns was 1.44. For people ≥65 years, the rate was more than 3-fold higher, ≥75 years more than 5-fold, and for ≥85 years more than 9-fold.[13].

The risk of injury and death in residential fires (at least in HMIC) has previously been shown increased in risk groups such as men, smokers, alcohol−/drug impaired, physically disabled or cognitively impaired patients, and elderly [14–19]. Cultural and sociodemographic differences along with behavioral factors aid in explaining this increased risk [19–22].

Can possible biological and/or medical factors be found that explain or identify one person being more vulnerable than another to fire, smoke, or heat incidences?

3.1 Carbon Monoxide

The major toxic gas that causes most deaths in residential fires is CO [8]. An inorganic color- and odorless, non-irritable gas, slightly lighter than air, present in basically all fires. The major acute effect is, due to CO's higher affinity to the heme proteins of hemoglobin, that CO competes out the O_2, thus less O_2 can be transported to cells and tissues. Furthermore, CO has high affinity also for other hemeproteins and thus binds to, e.g., myoglobin in myocardium and skeletal muscle [23, 24]. In the myocardium, the effect is cardiac dysfunction. The resulting tissue hypoxia increases the vascular permeability leading to an accumulation of interstitial fluid (edema). Depending on affected organ, the edema gives symptoms such as neurological/unconsciousness (brain), respiratory failure (lungs), arrythmias/heart failure (heart), and renal failure (kidneys). However, also several more delayed effects as neurological and other sequlaes like cognitive deficiency, anxiety, stubborn headache, sleeping disorder, balance problem, dizziness, impaired vision, neuropathies, mood disorders, muscular weakness, hearing loss and/or tinnitus, stroke, and autoimmune connective tissue diseases can be noted [25–30].

Persons with cardiovascular diseases are postulated to be more vulnerable to CO with incapacitation and death at lower and sublethal concentrations [3, 25, 31–35]. In 541 fire deaths, investigated by Birky et al., 60% of the victims died of CO alone (50% CO-hemoglobin set as lethal concentration), 20% due to CO along with pre-existing cardiovascular disease, and 11% of burns alone [4]. Regional abnormalities of heart wall movement, diagnosed with echocardiography, suggesting preexisting asymptomatic atherosclerosis leading to local ischemia when exposed to CO were found in an older subgroup of patients treated with hyperbaric oxygen for severe CO poisoning [36]. Satran et al. also found preexisting hypertension and male sex-predicted CO-induced myocardial injury [36]. Other studies on people with exertional angina pectoris who were exposed to (low concentrations) CO have established a relation between CO-hemoglobin concentration and time to angina [37].

Healthy adult humans can tolerate 10–15% CO-hemoglobin without symptoms, whereas individuals with coronary artery diseases can develop angina rapidly during physical effort already at CO levels of 2%. A deadly fire in a care home for elderly where 14/19 residents died was investigated by Purser [38]. He could show that the residents with cardiovascular diseases trended towards increased susceptibility to CO poisoning, and for heart disease alone, there was a statistically significant increase.

The treatment is to counteract the O_2 displacement by increasing the amount of O_2 inhaled, thus the increased amount of O_2 can compete with CO at the binding sites on hemoglobin and reduce CO-hemoglobin's half-time from about 4–5 h (room air) to approximately 1 h. Hence, (100%) O_2 should promptly be provided, preferably via a tight-fitting mask. In certain situations, hyperbaric O_2 therapy (100% O_2 under increased atmospheric pressure – commonly 2–3 atmospheres) can be used and will decrease CO-hemoglobin half-time to about 20 min. However, the indications and (side) effects of HBO treatment are debated.

3.2 Carbon Dioxide

Carbon dioxide, CO_2, is a color- and odorless, inorganic, non-irritable gas, heavier than air (1.5 times), present in basically all fires. CO_2 is well-tolerated in low concentrations, but in higher (>5%) acts mostly as a simple asphyxiant, by displacing O_2, but also as a toxicant [39].

In higher concentrations, hypercapnia and respiratory acidosis develop which affect the parasympathetic nervous system, thus depressing the respiration and circulation. At even higher concentrations, neurological symptoms as convulsions, coma, and death appear. In >30% CO_2, almost instant unconsciousness followed by cardiac arrest within minutes occurs. Thus, in situations with very high CO_2 concentrations, the toxic effect may well be the lethal cause and not the asphyxiating [39].

However, in residential fires, it is unlikely that the concentrations of CO_2 will rise fast enough to be the lethal gas since other, more fast-acting, gases will reach lethal concentrations sooner.

Symptoms present in CO_2 intoxication thusly vary depending on the concentration and tachy–/bradypnoea, tachy–/bradycardia, arrhythmias, convulsions, and cardiac stress can be noted. This is probably the reason for that hypercapnia due to CO_2 intoxication is more dangerous for people with cardiovascular deceases [40].

Another important mechanism of CO_2 is its effect of increasing the respiratory rate, thus increasing uptake of other (toxic) combustion products [3]. Especially elderly and people with cardio–/respiratory conditions are more vulnerable in fire incidents [41].

3.3 Oxygen Depletion

The three necessary constituents in a fire (the fire triangle) are fuel, energy, and an oxidizer [8]. As the process of combustion proceeds, the constituents are consumed. For O_2, this means that the atmosphere becomes O_2-depleted which, of course, even worsens the effects of the asphyxiant gases.

Oxygen deprivation alone can incapacitate a person at around 10% O_2 concentration and be lethal at <7%. However, without extreme heat, such as in a flash fire (room temperature high enough to autoignite most flammable materials and the room is engulfed in flames), this situation is unlikely. Furthermore, the temperature involved in a flash fire would probably, in itself, be lethal before the O_2 deprivation affects the person [42].

3.4 Hydrogen Cyanide

Hydrogen cyanide, HCN, is an inorganic colorless gas (boiling point = 25.6 °C) released when nitrogen containing fuel burns with mostly asphyxiating effects. To most people, it has a marked bitter almond odor; however, approximately one-third of the population lack the ability to smell HCN, possibly genetically controlled. HCN is approximately 35 times more toxic than CO, and basically all organs of the body, especially those sensitive to low O_2 levels, brain, respiratory, and cardiovascular systems, can be affected. Inhalation of HCN can be rapidly fatal [8]. Even though its role in fire deaths is somewhat debated, it is regarded as being an important asphyxiating gas that needs prompt treatment. HCN shows a molecular similarity to O_2 in the sense that it binds (reversibly) to cytochrome a3 and interferes with the oxidative metabolism at the cellular level (intracellular hypoxia occurs within the mitochondria), thus turning the metabolism into anaerobic, producing lactate that leads to systemic acidosis. HCN needs to be promptly treated with, e.g., hydroxocobalamine, but since there are no specific tests or symptoms the treatment indication is the suspicion of exposure and/or acidosis. Levels of HCN can be measured in blood, but the interpretation of the results is difficult since HCN is both produced and degraded in blood and body tissues, even postmortally [43, 44].

Even though data are lacking regarding increased vulnerability to HCN in any risk group, it can be safe to establish that there is enough synergy among asphyxiant gases and people with cardiovascular diseases to view them more vulnerable. Synergy between HCN and CO has been shown in animal models [45, 46].

3.5 Asphyxiation Synergy

The common effect of all asphyxiants, or narcotic gases as they are sometimes called, is that they ultimately lower the O_2 concentration in tissues and organs, be it by simple ambient O_2 displacement (lowers inhaled O_2 concentration) or by systemic effects. Carbon monoxide is probably the most studied asphyxiant and preexisting cardiovascular diseases seem to increase the vulnerability through cardiac ischemia. Other asphyxiants probably produce similar effects and may also act in synergy.

The common, most basic, treatment is to provide a surplus of O_2 to be inhaled, be it through normo- or hyperbaric ways.

3.6 Irritants

Irritant gases are most often (volatile) inorganic gases with the common feature of acutely inducing irritation of, preferably, the airways, but also eyes, skin, and mucous membranes generally. The irritants have an important role regarding lethality in fire situations. The irritants may not be acutely lethal, but the rapid physiological and resulting behavioral effects reduce the possibility to escape and lead to incapacitation, allowing the accumulating irritating effects or the asphyxiants, or heat, to become lethal [8, 47, 48].

The principal effects of irritants are similar and HCl may be the most studied irritant in fire and smoke situations. However, most data are from animal models and the human interpretation needs to be careful [49].

Most irritants also elicit long-term effects such as lung damage, asthma, cancer, and immunotoxicity.

As with the asphyxiants, preexisting conditions like pulmonary diseases or asthma render people more vulnerable to the irritants since their physiological reserves are already limited.

Irritant gases can cause pain in eyes, skin, or respiratory tract, bronchospasm, hypersecretion, and impaired vision.

3.7 Nitrogen Dioxide

Nitrogen dioxide, NO_2, is an inorganic, reddish-brown gas with a pungent acid smell. It is released when nitrogen-containing fuel burns with acutely irritating and to some degree asphyxiating effect and can, in the long-term, cause lung damage.

NO_2 is directly toxic to the respiratory tract and is easily absorbed through the lungs. NO_2 diffuses into the respiratory epithelial lining fluid and dissolves and chemically reacts. This reaction and its metabolites determine the health effects which include (acute and long-term) cardiovascular effects (triggering heart attacks), diffuse inflammation, bronchoconstriction, inflammation, reduced immune response, edema leading to bronchitis, pneumonia, or fulminant lung edema, and interstitial fibrosis [50].

Besides the asphyxiating effect of fluid accumulation in the lungs, the formation of methemoglobin blocks the O_2 transport in much the same way as CO [51].

3.8 Heat Exposure

Classic heatstroke can be caused by high surrounding temperatures [6]. Preexisting medical conditions and/or an inactive lifestyle with low aerobic capacity increase the vulnerability to heat (in)tolerance or heatstroke. Age itself seems not to be a decisive risk factor [52, 53]. In a fire incident, the rise in temperature is most often not that quick and other mechanisms of incapacitation, injury, and death occur before a classic heatstroke develops.

The amount of tissue damage inflicted by heat can be viewed as a simple relationship between how long the tissue is exposed to a certain temperature.

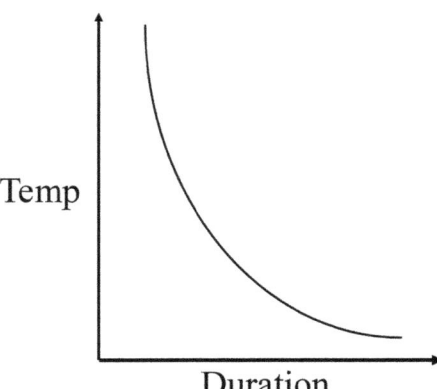

Considering that a prolonged exposition of the skin to 44 °C is enough to produce irreversible epithelial cell damage, it is easily understood that higher

4 Fire-Related Injury Mechanisms   57

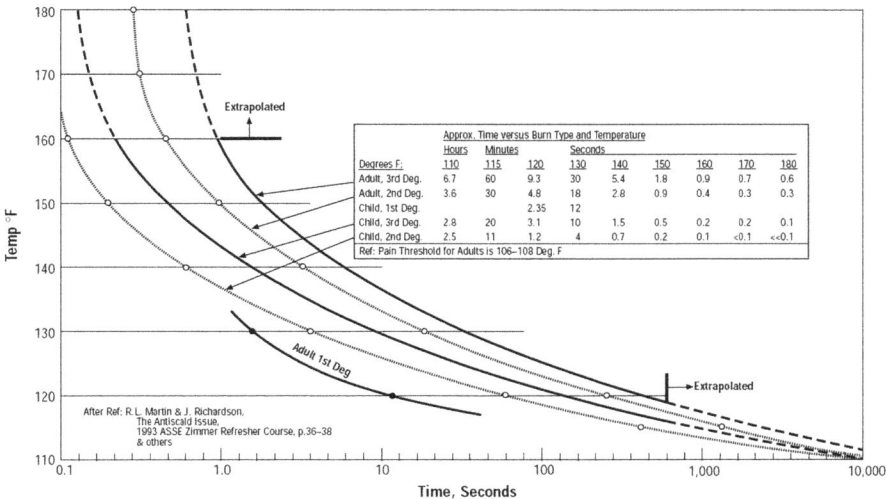

Fig. 4.1 Relationship temperature-time and suggested cut-offs for different burn depths in children and adults [55].

temperatures, such as those involved in a fire, can cause serious damage to the human body's deeper tissues rapidly [54] (Fig. 4.1).

Several, mostly mathematical, models have been used to estimate what temperature skin and tissue reach during a burn/heat incident [56–58]. There are a plethora of factors affecting the tissue response to heat; e.g., skin thickness varies depending on the body area and between persons due to age, gender, and more; blood perfusion of the tissue varies; skin is affected differently whether the heat source is radiation, flame, scald, or contact; type of clothing worn; moisture on the skin (sweat); air humidity; etc. To be exposed to a fire/heat incidence elicits several physiological responses and reactions that further complicate the prediction of tissue damage. For example, a decrease in heart function with decreased cardiac output and hypotension, e.g., due to effects of inhaled gases, lessens the blood perfusion to the skin, which is followed by both the heat exchange (by the flowing blood) being decreased, and thus more heat energy absorbed, giving deeper burns. A sustained hypotension with the sustained lessened blood flow in the skin creates a cellular environment lacking enough nutrients and O_2, leading to that cells that have been subjected to reversible damage from the heat insult may well succumb due to the cellular environment.

From these complicated conditions, it can be perceived as contradictory as to when and how tissue damage occurs. An ambient temperature of 90 °C can well be tolerated for 45 min or longer without resulting in cutaneous burns (compared to being in a sauna) [59]. Others indicate that tolerance to temperatures <120 °C is limited by hyperthermia, but at >120 °C pain is followed by cutaneous burns [10].

Increased ambient temperature (⩾31 °C) during exposure to CO was studied in healthy adults, indicating synergistic effects of the heat and gas probably leading to more rapid incapacitation of a person.

Considering mortality and morbidity by fire, heat, and hot substances, one frequently focuses on the incident itself and the acute setting. However, one must not forget the period that follows the insult.

3.9 (Cutaneous) Burns

Some of the main functions of the skin are:

- To be a barrier against the environment (both "physically" and against pathologic microorganisms).
- Temperature regulation.
- Fluid regulation.
- To be an interface to the surroundings (sensation, looks).

After having been exposed to fire, heat, and hot substances, it is common that the person has acquired cutaneous burns. The burnt skin then loses the above mentioned functions.

The burn trauma is a condition with many faces ranging from minor superficial blisters/wounds that heal uneventfully spontaneously to massive full-thickness burns covering large areas of the body necessitating advanced intensive care and surgery. Treatment of significant burns is often considered one of the costliest forms of hospital care.

The burn trauma itself induces a massive inflammatory reaction both locally and systemically and affects basically all organs and systems in the body. The open wounds, along with different (blood-, respiratory-, gastric-, urinary-, etc.) catheters needed for the (intensive) care, are gateways for pathological microbes easily leading to infections and sepsis with high morbidity and mortality.

The depth, surface extension of the burn wounds, age, and the presence of an inhalation injury are the major denominators determining the severity, treatment, and outcome of the burn trauma [60, 61].

The modern terms used are:

- Superficial burns (epidermal, previous 1st degree).

    - Only the epidermis is damaged.
    - Intense redness and pain.
    - Equivalent to a sunburn.
    - Intact sensation and capillary refill.
    - Heals in few days without scars.

- Superficial dermal burn (previous 2nd degree, a).
  - The entire epidermis and superficial parts of the dermis are damaged.
  - Often blisters, moist surface, redness, and painful wound surface.
  - Intact sensation and capillary refill.
  - Usually heals within 2 weeks with proper wound care and without scars, but with possible changes in pigmentation.
- Deep dermal burn (previous 2nd degree, b).
  - The entire epidermis and deep parts of the dermis (hair follicles, sweat glands, and other adnexae) are damaged.
  - Marbled, dark red-white, dry, or moist wound surface.
  - Usually no blistering.
  - Diminished sensation and capillary refill.
  - Surgery with skin transplantation is usually required.
- Full-thickness burn (previously 3rd degree).
  - The entire skin (epidermis and dermis) and sometimes also deeper tissues are damaged.
  - Pale-brown or black color, leathery texture.
  - Dry surface.
  - No sensation or capillary refill.
  - Surgery with skin transplantation is required for healing.

Burns affecting >20% of the total body surface area (%TBSA) are usually considered major, or significant. Full-thickness burns are more serious than superficial. However, also larger superficial burns cause systemic (inflammatory) reactions that can be detrimental.

To predict the mortality in burn patients, professor Serge Baux presented, in 1961, the Baux-score: mortality rate = age + %TBSA [62]. However, advances in burn care and the appreciation of an inhalation injury's deleterious effect have rendered the original Baux-score too pessimistic. Thus, in 2010, Osler et al. revised the Baux-score to mortality rate = age + %TBSA + plus 17 points if inhalation injury is present [63]. Today, the better burn centers regularly successfully treat burns with Baux-score > 130–140. This indicates that the question today is not to be whether the patient survives, especially not in younger age groups, but more to what kind of life the patient can be rehabilitated back to.

Looking at global in-hospital mortality due to fire, heat, and hot substances, one must carefully evaluate published data because of an obvious risk of selection bias since patients with a poor prognosis will probably not be referred to, and treated, in hospitals in resource-constrained areas.

4 On the Scene

Of all the destructive mechanisms involved in a fire, carbon monoxide and hydrogen cyanide may be the most sinister. Mortality is highly increased when these 2 gases are involved. Emergency medical services (ambulance etc.) need to quickly identify these patients and promptly initiate life-saving interventions such as securing airway and spinal control and provide O_2 and intravenous fluid resuscitation [9].

The patients may not present with classic signs of toxic exposure; thus, triage may be difficult. Textbook signs of cherry red skin (CO) or smell of bitter almond (CN) are mostly only found in the books. Due to the varying time of exposure and concentrations of toxic gases, a broad variety of signs and symptoms may be present: e.g., nausea, confusion, headache, loss of consciousness, cardiac arrest, etc. Thus, also potential risk factors and environmental findings that could indicate inhalation injuries, like fire incident in an enclosed space, should be sought after [9]. Routine examinations with, e.g., pulse oximetry are unreliable and more specific laboratory data are not available on the scene. EMS therefore should broadly initiate treatment. Equally important, though, is the safety of the EMS and others working on the scene. Irritant and toxic substances released in the fire may also affect them and proper protective equipment is necessary.

A cornerstone in the field work on site is to provide supportive and safe care while acknowledging, in order of priority, safety, patient extrication and decontamination, airway management, getting intravenous access, burn treatment, prevent hypothermia, and patient dispersion [9].

4.1 Treatment

Minor scalds, burns, and smoke expositions can preferably be treated in ERs or GP's offices. Routine wound care or a short period of O_2 inhalation is often sufficient. However, larger burns and inhalation injuries are most often serious and need advanced treatment in hospital.

4.2 Isolated Inhalation Injuries

The medical issues with an (isolated) inhalation injury can be summarized as toxic effects (local and systemical), increased secretion, and obstructivity. If the patient cannot maintain a patent airway or the oxygen exchange, intubation and connection to a ventilator is necessary. The patient is treated in the intensive care unit. Symptomatic treatment with O_2, bronchodilators, and bronchial toilet is often sufficient. Complications as pneumonia and sepsis are treated with systemic antibiotics and other necessary organ supportive treatment.

4.3 Burn Injuries With/Without Inhalation Injury

More extensive burns should be treated in specialized burn units/centers. A burn trauma patient is a special type of trauma patient and should, in the acute phase, be treated according to Emergency Management of Severe Burns (EMSB) or Advanced Burn Life Support (ABLS), and Advanced Trauma Life Support (ATLS) [64–68].

The burn trauma itself elicits a massive systemic inflammatory response, leading to basically all organ systems and cascade systems becoming affected. (vide supra) The treatment involves securing a patent airway and organ-supportive measures. The cornerstone of the acute treatment is, besides ordinary intensive care (organ support), the fluid resuscitation, where the fluids that escape the bloodstream into the soft tissue due to the inflammatory reaction are compensated. This is to ensure that critical organs (kidneys, brain, heart, etc.) have enough circulation ("permissive hypovolemia") to maintain their primary functions. According to the Parkland formula, the patient is to be given 2–4 ml × body weight (kg) × %TBSA intravenous fluid the first 24 h after trauma [69]. Thus, for a 100 kg patient with 50% burns, the calculated required amount of resuscitation fluid for the first 24 h is 10–20 l! Still, the Parkland formula only calculates a predictive fluid amount and the individual volume should be adjusted according to the patient's circulatory status and urine production aiming for "permissive hypovolemia" [7, 70]. A concomitant inhalation injury usually increases this amount with >50% (i.e., >30 l in the example). A massive general swelling/edema thus follows that can lead to serious complications such as compartment syndrome in extremities, abdomen, eyes, or brain. The burned skin/tissue is no longer viable and should be removed within the first days. Surgically, the burned tissue is removed and resulting wounds covered with, preferably, split-thickness skin grafts from the patient's unburned areas. However, already at 20–30% TBSA (and above), the amount of unburned skin may not be sufficient to cover all wounds. In these cases, different techniques such as re-harvesting skin when donor sites have healed or in vitro culture of autologous epithelial grafts can be used.

Commonly, one estimates approximately 1 hospital day per % TBSA burned. The early hospital phase, though, is only the start of a long marathon. Months, and even years, follow with physiotherapy and rehabilitation.

5 Discussion

Globally, incidences with fire, heat, and hot substances compose a serious general public health problem. More than 300,000 deaths occur annually from fire incidents alone [71]. Add to that even more deaths from scalds, electrical−/, chemical−/, and contact burns. Furthermore, millions of persons involved in incidences with fire, heat, and hot substances suffer from long-term issues as disabilities or disfigurements, let alone issues as destroyed homes and belongings and other secondary personal and economic effects.

The absolute majority (>95%) of the global fire-related deaths and injuries occur in LMICs where health care systems often are not as developed [71]. Many fire/burn prevention strategies have been introduced over the years and results are seen. However, in the global sense, strategies that have been proven successful in HICs may not be transferable to LMICs as the epidemiology and trauma panorama is substantially different.

Through different modellings based on inter alia experimental data from human and animal studies, time to human incapacitation in fire situations can be calculated. Commonly, approximately 3–4 min since start of fire are mentioned as time to incapacitation, and around 5–6 min to death [10, 72, 73].

Obviously, different physical properties of the fire (fuel, time, etc.) and where the fire occurs (same room as person, further away, etc.) as well as different biological (age, gender, etc.) and physical properties (diseases, disabilities, etc.) of the person allow this time to vary greatly.

Fire incidents have always happened and will also continue to happen in the future. Given the short amount of time at hand, once there is a fire incident, to escape the threatening situation, one comes to the conclusion that, of course, measures need to be taken to extend this time period, but that prevention is really the key. However, it has become increasingly evident that there is no "magic bullet" when it comes to prevention. Common preventive measures like modification of the environment, safety rules promotion, and suggested changes in behavior pre- and peri-incident can be effective, but need to be individually tailored to specific (risk) groups both in how measures are taken and how information is given; children do not function as adults, psychiatric disabled persons differ from physically disabled, etc. [74–79].

References

1. Berna F, Goldberg P, Horwitz LK et al (2012) Microstratigraphic evidence of in situ fire in the Acheulean strata of Wonderwerk Cave, Northern Cape province, South Africa. Proc Natl Acad Sci U S A 109:E1215–E1220. https://doi.org/10.1073/pnas.1117620109
2. Alarie Y (1985) The toxicity of smoke from polymeric materials during thermal decomposition. Annu Rev Pharmacol Toxicol 25:325–347. https://doi.org/10.1146/annurev.pa.25.040185.001545
3. Shusterman DJ (1993) Clinical smoke inhalation injury: systemic effects. Occup Med Phila Pa 8:469–503
4. Birky MM, Clarke FB (1981) Inhalation of toxic products from fires. Bull N Y Acad Med 57:997–1013
5. Eggert E, Huss F (2017) Medical and biological factors affecting mortality in elderly residential fire victims: a narrative review of the literature. Scars Burns Heal 3:205951311770768. https://doi.org/10.1177/2059513117707686
6. Kenttämies A, Karkola K (2008) Death in sauna. J Forensic Sci 53:724–729. https://doi.org/10.1111/j.1556-4029.2008.00703.x
7. Burn Center, Uppsala University Hospital (2019) Brännskadekompendium (Burn manual). https://pdf-flip.se/Akademiska_Sjukhuset/Brannskadekompendium/
8. Blomqvist P (2005) Emissions from fires consequences for human safety and the environment. Lund University, Lund

9. Gold A, Perera TB (2020) EMS, asphyxiation and other gas and fire hazards. In: StatPearls. StatPearls Publishing, Treasure Island
10. Purser DA, McAllister JL (2016) Assessment of hazards to occupants from smoke, toxic gases, and heat. In: Hurley MJ, Gottuk D, Hall JR et al (eds) SFPE handbook of fire protection engineering. Springer, New York, pp 2308–2428
11. Prien T, Traber DL (1988) Toxic smoke compounds and inhalation injury—a review. Burns 14:451–460. https://doi.org/10.1016/S0305-4179(88)80005-6
12. World Population Prospects – Population Division – United Nations. https://population.un.org/wpp/Graphs/Probabilistic/POP/65plus/900. Accessed 4 Jan 2021
13. Institute for Health Metrics and Evaluation In: Inst Health Metr Eval. http://www.healthdata.org/institute-health-metrics-and-evaluation. Accessed 4 Jan 2021
14. Elder AT, Squires T, Busuttil A (1996) Fire fatalities in elderly people. Age Ageing 25:214–216. https://doi.org/10.1093/ageing/25.3.214
15. Marshall SW, Runyan CW, Bangdiwala SI et al (1998) Fatal residential fires: who dies and who survives? JAMA 279:1633. https://doi.org/10.1001/jama.279.20.1633
16. Beaulieu E, Smith J, Zheng A, Pike I (2020) The geographic and demographic distribution of residential fires, related injuries, and deaths in four Canadian provinces. Can J Public Health 111:107–116. https://doi.org/10.17269/s41997-019-00256-7
17. Svee A, Jonsson A, Sjöberg F, Huss F (2016) Burns in Sweden: temporal trends from 1987 to 2010. Ann Burns Fire Disasters 29:85–89. https://www.ncbi.nlm.nih.gov/pmc/articles/PMC5241198/
18. Jonsson A, Bonander C, Nilson F, Huss F (2017) The state of the residential fire fatality problem in Sweden: epidemiology, risk factors, and event typologies. J Saf Res 62:89–100. https://doi.org/10.1016/j.jsr.2017.06.008
19. Istre GR, McCoy MA, Osborn L et al (2001) Deaths and injuries from house fires. N Engl J Med 344:1911–1916. https://doi.org/10.1056/NEJM200106213442506
20. Miller I (2005) Human behaviour contributing to unintentional residential fire deaths 1997–2003. New Zealand Fire Service, Wellington
21. Nilson F, Bonander C (2020) Societal protection and population vulnerability: key factors in explaining community-level variation in fatal fires involving older adults in Sweden. Fire Technol 57(1):247–260. https://doi.org/10.1007/s10694-020-00997-9
22. Purcell LN, Bartley C, Purcell ME et al (2020) The effect of neighborhood Area Deprivation Index on residential burn injury severity. Burns S0305417920304733. https://doi.org/10.1016/j.burns.2020.07.014
23. Lim M, Jackson T, Anfinrud P (1995) Binding of CO to myoglobin from a heme pocket docking site to form nearly linear Fe-C-O. Science 269:962–966. https://doi.org/10.1126/science.7638619
24. Kinoshita H, Türkan H, Vucinic S et al (2020) Carbon monoxide poisoning. Toxicol Rep 7:169–173. https://doi.org/10.1016/j.toxrep.2020.01.005
25. Weaver LK (2020) Carbon monoxide poisoning. Undersea Hyperb Med J Undersea Hyperb Med Soc Inc 47:151–169
26. Mazo J, Mukhtar E, Mazo Y et al (2020) Delayed brain injury post carbon monoxide poisoning. Radiol Case Rep 15:1845–1848. https://doi.org/10.1016/j.radcr.2020.07.048
27. Garcia JH, Khanna S (2020) Severe vision loss and intracranial hypertension presenting as delayed sequelae of "Mild" carbon monoxide poisoning. J Neuroophthalmol. Publish ahead of print. https://doi.org/10.1097/WNO.0000000000001104
28. Huang C-C, Ho C-H, Chen Y-C et al (2020) Autoimmune connective tissue disease following carbon monoxide poisoning: a nationwide population-based cohort study. Clin Epidemiol 12:1287–1298. https://doi.org/10.2147/CLEP.S266396
29. Kwak K, Kim M, Choi W-J et al (2021) Association between carbon monoxide intoxication and incidence of ischemic stroke: a retrospective nested case-control study in South Korea. J Stroke Cerebrovasc Dis 30:105496. https://doi.org/10.1016/j.jstrokecerebrovasdis.2020.105496

30. Liu J, Si Z, Liu J et al (2020) Clinical and imaging prognosis in patients with delayed encephalopathy after acute carbon monoxide poisoning. Behav Neurol 2020:1–5. https://doi.org/10.1155/2020/1719360
31. Ernst A, Zibrak JD (1998) Carbon monoxide poisoning. N Engl J Med 339:1603–1608. https://doi.org/10.1056/NEJM199811263392206
32. Stefanidou M, Athanaselis S, Spiliopoulou C (2008) Health impacts of fire smoke inhalation. Inhal Toxicol 20:761–766. https://doi.org/10.1080/08958370801975311
33. Balraj EK (1984) Atherosclerotic coronary artery disease and "low" levels of carboxyhemoglobin; report of fatalities and discussion of pathophysiologic mechanisms of death. J Forensic Sci 29:1150–1159
34. Wright J (2002) Chronic and occult carbon monoxide poisoning: we don't know what we're missing. Emerg Med J 19:386–390. https://doi.org/10.1136/emj.19.5.386
35. Balzan MV, Cacciottolo JM, Mifsud S (1994) Unstable angina and exposure to carbon monoxide. Postgrad Med J 70:699–702. https://doi.org/10.1136/pgmj.70.828.699
36. Satran D, Henry CR, Adkinson C et al (2005) Cardiovascular manifestations of moderate to severe carbon monoxide poisoning. J Am Coll Cardiol 45:1513–1516. https://doi.org/10.1016/j.jacc.2005.01.044
37. Allred EN, Bleecker ER, Chaitman BR et al (1991) Effects of carbon monoxide on myocardial ischemia. Environ Health Perspect 91:89–132. https://doi.org/10.1289/ehp.919189
38. Purser DA (2017) Effects of pre-fire age and health status on vulnerability to incapacitation and death from exposure to carbon monoxide and smoke irritants in Rosepark fire incident victims: effects of pre-fire age and health status on fire victims. Fire Mater 41:555–569. https://doi.org/10.1002/fam.2393
39. Permentier K, Vercammen S, Soetaert S, Schellemans C (2017) Carbon dioxide poisoning: a literature review of an often forgotten cause of intoxication in the emergency department. Int J Emerg Med 10:14. https://doi.org/10.1186/s12245-017-0142-y
40. Langford NJ (2005) Carbon dioxide poisoning. Toxicol Rev 24:229–235. https://doi.org/10.2165/00139709-200524040-00003
41. Sharma G, Goodwin J (2006) Effect of aging on respiratory system physiology and immunology. Clin Interv Aging 1:253–260. https://doi.org/10.2147/ciia.2006.1.3.253
42. Alarie Y (2002) Toxicity of fire smoke. Crit Rev Toxicol 32:259–289. https://doi.org/10.1080/20024091064246
43. Huzar TF, George T, Cross JM (2013) Carbon monoxide and cyanide toxicity: etiology, pathophysiology and treatment in inhalation injury. Expert Rev Respir Med 7:159–170. https://doi.org/10.1586/ers.13.9
44. Barillo DJ, Goode R, Esch V (1994) Cyanide poisoning in victims of fire: analysis of 364 cases and review of the literature. J Burn Care Rehabil 15:46–57. https://doi.org/10.1097/00004630-199401000-00010
45. Levin BC, Paabo M, Gurman JL, Harris SE (1987) Effects of exposure to single or multiple combinations of the predominant toxic gases and low oxygen atmospheres produced in fires. Fundam Appl Toxicol Off J Soc Toxicol 9:236–250. https://doi.org/10.1016/0272-0590(87)90046-7
46. Norris JC, Moore SJ, Hume AS (1986) Synergistic lethality induced by the combination of carbon monoxide and cyanide. Toxicology 40:121–129. https://doi.org/10.1016/0300-483x(86)90073-9
47. Purser DA (2010) Hazards from smoke and irritants. In: Stec A, Hull R (eds) Fire toxicity. WP, Woodhead Publishing, Oxford, pp 51–117
48. (2001) International study of the sublethal effects of fire smoke on survivability and health (SEFS) : phase I final report. National Institute of Standards (NIST)
49. Hull T, Stec A, Paul K (2008) Hydrogen chloride in fires. Fire Saf Sci 9:665–676. https://doi.org/10.3801/IAFSS.FSS.9-665
50. US EPA National Center for Environmental Assessment RTPN Integrated Science Assessment (ISA) for Oxides of Nitrogen – Health Criteria (Final Report, Jan 2016). https://cfpub.epa.gov/ncea/isa/recordisplay.cfm?deid=310879. Accessed 13 Jan 2021

51. Hoffman RS, Sauter D (1989) Methemoglobinemia resulting from smoke inhalation. Vet Hum Toxicol 31:168–170
52. Pandolf KB (1997) Aging and human heat tolerance. Exp Aging Res 23:69–105. https://doi.org/10.1080/03610739708254027
53. Kenney WL (1997) Thermoregulation at rest and during exercise in healthy older adults. Exerc Sport Sci Rev 25:41–76
54. Moritz AR, Henriques FC (1947) Studies of thermal injury: II. The relative importance of time and surface temperature in the causation of cutaneous burns. Am J Pathol 23:695–720
55. Bynum Jr D, Petri VJ et al (1998) Domestic hot water scald burn lawsuits – the who, what, when, why, where how. A Seminar and Technical Paper for the 25–28 Oct. 98 Annual ASPE Meeting at the Indianapolis Convention Center in Indianapolis, Indiana. Reprinted by Watts Regulator Company with permission of Dr. D. Bynum Jr. https://mail.inspectapedia.com/plumbing/DHW_Scald_Seminar_Reprint.pdf
56. Abraham JP, Plourde B, Vallez L et al (2015) Estimating the time and temperature relationship for causation of deep-partial thickness skin burns. Burns J Int Soc Burn Inj 41:1741–1747. https://doi.org/10.1016/j.burns.2015.06.002
57. Ng EYK, Tan HM, Ooi EH (2010) Prediction and parametric analysis of thermal profiles within heated human skin using the boundary element method. Philos Trans R Soc Math Phys Eng Sci 368:655–678. https://doi.org/10.1098/rsta.2009.0224
58. Majchrzak E, Jasiński M (2003) Numerical estimation of burn degree of skin tissue using the sensitivity analysis methods. Acta Bioeng Biomech 2003:93–108
59. Yeo TP (2004) Heat stroke: a comprehensive review. AACN Clin Issues 15:280–293. https://doi.org/10.1097/00044067-200404000-00013
60. Sheppard NN, Hemington-Gorse S, Shelley OP et al (2011) Prognostic scoring systems in burns: a review. Burns 37:1288–1295. https://doi.org/10.1016/j.burns.2011.07.017
61. Colohan SM (2010) Predicting prognosis in thermal burns with associated inhalational injury: a systematic review of prognostic factors in adult burn victims. J Burn Care Res 31:529–539. https://doi.org/10.1097/BCR.0b013e3181e4d680
62. Baux S (1961) Contribution a l'etude du traitement local des brulures thermiques etendues. Thesis
63. Osler T, Glance LG, Hosmer DW (2010) Simplified estimates of the probability of death after burn injuries: extending and updating the baux score. J Trauma 68:690–697. https://doi.org/10.1097/TA.0b013e3181c453b3
64. Stone CA, Pape SA (1999) Evolution of the Emergency Management of Severe Burns (EMSB) course in the UK. Burns 25:262–264. https://doi.org/10.1016/S0305-4179(98)00161-2
65. ABLS Program – American Burn Association. https://ameriburn.org/education/abls-program/. Accessed 9 Mar 2021
66. Kearns RD, Hubble MW, JamesH H et al (2015) Advanced burn life support for day-to-day burn injury management and disaster preparedness: stakeholder experiences and student perceptions following 56 advanced burn life support courses. J Burn Care Res 36:455–464. https://doi.org/10.1097/BCR.0000000000000155
67. Advanced Trauma Life Support In: Am Coll Surg. https://www.facs.org/quality-programs/trauma/atls. Accessed 9 Mar 2021
68. Sims JK (1979) Advanced trauma life support laboratory: pilot implementation and evaluation. J Am Coll Emerg Physicians 8:150–153. https://doi.org/10.1016/S0361-1124(79)80342-1
69. Baxter CR, Shires T (1968) Physiological response to crystalloid resuscitation of severe burns. Ann N Y Acad Sci 150:874–894. https://doi.org/10.1111/j.1749-6632.1968.tb14738.x
70. Saffle JR (2007) The phenomenon of "fluid creep" in acute burn resuscitation. J Burn Care Res 28:382–395. https://doi.org/10.1097/BCR.0B013E318053D3A1
71. Mock C, Peck M, Krug E, Haberal M (2009) Confronting the global burden of burns: a WHO plan and a challenge. Burns 35:615–617. https://doi.org/10.1016/j.burns.2008.08.016
72. Gann RG (2004) Estimating data for incapacitation of people by fire smoke. Fire Technol 40:201–207. https://doi.org/10.1023/B:FIRE.0000016843.38848.37

73. Purser D (1989) Modelling toxic and physical hazard in fire. Fire Saf Sci 2:391–400. https://doi.org/10.3801/IAFSS.FSS.2-391
74. Committee on Injury and Poison Prevention (2000) Reducing the number of deaths and injuries from residential fires. Pediatrics 105:1355–1357. https://doi.org/10.1542/peds.105.6.1355
75. Smith GA, Kistamgari S, Splaingard M (2020) Optimizing smoke alarm signals: testing the effectiveness of children's smoke alarms for sleeping adults. Inj Epidemiol 7:51. https://doi.org/10.1186/s40621-020-00279-6
76. Kegler SR, Dellinger AM, Ballesteros MF, Tsai J (2018) Decreasing residential fire death rates and the association with the prevalence of adult cigarette smoking — United States, 1999–2015. J Saf Res 67:197–201. https://doi.org/10.1016/j.jsr.2018.06.001
77. Shokouhi M, Nasiriani K, Cheraghi Z et al (2019) Preventive measures for fire-related injuries and their risk factors in residential buildings: a systematic review. J Inj Violence Res 11:1–14. https://doi.org/10.5249/jivr.v11i1.1057
78. Gielen AC, Frattaroli S, Pollack KM et al (2018) How the science of injury prevention contributes to advancing home fire safety in the USA: successes and opportunities. Inj Prev J Int Soc Child Adolesc Inj Prev 24:i7–i13. https://doi.org/10.1136/injuryprev-2017-042356
79. Istre GR, McCoy MA, Moore BJ et al (2014) Preventing deaths and injuries from house fires: an outcome evaluation of a community-based smoke alarm installation programme. Inj Prev J Int Soc Child Adolesc Inj Prev 20:97–102. https://doi.org/10.1136/injuryprev-2013-040823

Dr. Fredrik Huss is an Associate Professor in Plastic Surgery at Uppsala University and the Director of Uppsala Burn Center, Uppsala University Hospital, Sweden. He is a burn expert for the Swedish National Board of Health and Welfare's Stödstyrkan (Swedish Response Team) and for the Swedish National Air Medevac. He is the current Secretary of the European Burns Association. He received his PhD at Linköping University in 2005 with his thesis titled "In vitro and in vivo studies of tissue engineering in reconstructive plastic surgery."

Chapter 5
The Evacuation of People with Functional Limitations

Enrico Ronchi, Erik Smedberg, Gunilla Carlsson, and Björn Slaug

Abstract This chapter presents an overview on the role of functional limitations on self-evacuation possibilities in case of fires in residential buildings. This is performed highlighting the links between functional limitations, predominant activities, and fire evacuation. This study makes use of the International Classification of Functioning, Disability and Health (ICF) by the World Health Organization with application to the activities performed during a fire evacuation scenario and how those can be affected by functional limitations. Quantitative and qualitative data concerning the egress of people with functional limitations are also discussed. The findings are presented making use of the engineering egress timeline commonly adopted in fire safety engineering applications and attempting to translate consolidated concepts of the research in the field of accessibility to the fire evacuation field. This chapter highlights that most researches on the evacuation of people with functional limitations have so far focused on addressing mobility limitations, particularly on the movement phase. Current knowledge gaps concern the impact of cognitive limitations, the ability to smell smoke, and how speech impairments can affect communication during an evacuation scenario.

Keywords Egress · Disability · ICF · functional limitations · Evacuation · Ageing

1 Introduction

Current buildings are to a large extent designed to fit a population with average characteristics, and therefore it should come as no surprise that people with functional limitations will have issues in navigating such environments. It is argued that emphasis should be placed on both characterizing the capabilities of individuals and

E. Ronchi (✉) · E. Smedberg
Division of Fire Safety Engineering, Faculty of Engineering, Lund University, Lund, Sweden
e-mail: enrico.ronchi@brand.lth.se

G. Carlsson · B. Slaug
Department of Health Sciences, Faculty of Medicine, Lund University, Health Sciences Centre (HSC), Lund, Sweden

on the design of the environment, in order to increase egressibility for all. Extensive research has in fact shown that disability is a risk factor when it comes to fatal residential fires [1–3].

Regulatory and design guidance in emergency evacuation scenarios are often based on the general assumption of addressing the needs of "people with disabilities" [4]. Mirroring the initiative of disability rights movements, fire safety standards have started introducing recognition that people with functional limitations would not only need to access a building, but also be able to have equal rights when it comes to fire safety [5]. Nevertheless, limited knowledge is available in this area [6] and oversimplifications may be performed when assessing the characteristics of the population.

From an evacuation perspective, the building population has often been divided into two main groups: those able to self-evacuate and those needing assistance [7]. Examples of those strategies in residential settings include the use of the defend-in-place strategy and areas of refuge, both relying on occupants being rescued by first responders [8]. The use of suitable egress components has also started being adopted in fire evacuation design, e.g. occupant evacuation elevators [9]. The present chapter focuses on the case of self-evacuation. This is in line with the premise that residential buildings should be designed in a way so that people are able to live their lives independently, rather than rely on help from others. For this reason, the main focus is here on residential settings in which people with functional limitations may live alone or with their family, but without a dedicated mechanism for evacuation aid in case of emergencies. In other words, this study considers the case in which building management would not provide organizational aid in case of an evacuation scenario.

It should be noted that the term egress is generally used to refer to the movement out of the building, while the term evacuation is specifically used in the context of emergencies. In the present chapter, the two terms are used interchangeably since the only focus of interest is movement, perception, and decision-making in case of emergency. In addition, the term egressibility is also adopted as it allows referring to the accessibility of means of evacuation.

1.1 *Historical Background on Disability*

Disability, impairments, functional limitations, handicap – there have been many ways to describe functional capacity among individuals, and the terminology is changing over time in accordance with different aspects of the construct and the way society evolves. Previously, handicap (and later disability) was considered as a characteristic of the individual linked to a medical condition [10]. A person who was born with leg paresis had a mobility disability, and a person who suffered a stroke might have a disability affecting fine motor skills. However, the disability rights movement has contributed to change the perspective towards disability. This includes disability not being considered as a characteristic of the person, but rather the inability of society to accommodate the needs of all individuals, regardless of functional capacity [11]. It is therefore essential to understand the social, attitudinal, and environmental barriers in society linked to disability.

The way we see and define disability and the subsequent implications on fire evacuation can be related to different models of disability [12]. Traditionally, the *Medical model of disability* has had a large influence on collective efforts to address the needs of people with impairments [13]. The medical model assumes that disability can be explained through the underlying medical conditions of the individual. This means that, in order to mitigate the negative effects of disabilities, the individual needs to be cured. This could for example involve developing prosthetics for people with mobility impairments that otherwise could not independently walk out of a building in case of an emergency or conducting eye surgery on people with visual impairments who could not see emergency signage. However, not all disabling conditions can (or should) be cured. In the *Social model of disability*, the characteristics of the built and social environment are considered to cause disabilities. That is, it is the inability of society to accommodate the needs of people that creates a disability. This includes the environment (e.g. inaccessibility due to the type of egress components, technical installations/systems, communication, etc.), attitudes (e.g. prejudice, stereotyping, discrimination, etc.), and organization (e.g. inflexible evacuation procedures and practices). A person in a wheelchair is not disabled in an emergency if the escape routes do not include steps, etc., and people with cognitive impairments are not disabled as long as emergency way-finding is not too complicated to perform. However, Mike Oliver, one of the more prominent figures in the early days of the Social model of disability, has stated that the social model was never intended to be an all-encompassing model of disability [11]. Instead, the aim was to transform the picture of disability in society. The social model has had a large influence on society's view of disability and can be applied in all contexts, including residential settings.

Another model that has gained interest in recent years is the *Biopsychosocial model of disability* [14]. This model combines the medical and social model and recognizes that disability is both a social and medical phenomenon. The biopsychosocial model is used in the International Classification of Functioning, Disability and Health (ICF) developed by the World Health Organization (WHO) [15]. This classification aims to describe disability in terms of functioning, and not medical conditions. As such, the classification is diagnosis-agnostic and can be useful in many different fields, including fire evacuation. For this reason, this model and the associated term functional limitations [16] are used in this chapter. A schematic representation of the biopsychosocial model used in the ICF is presented in Fig. 5.1. This highlights the links between body function and structures (for example impairments linked to cognitive functions, sensory functions and pain, neuro-musculoskeletal, and movement-related functions), activity (for example activity restrictions linked to purposeful sensory experiences, communicating, walking, and moving), and participation (involvement in different life situations). Those are related to environmental and personal factors that can affect egress. Examples of environmental factors include natural and human-made environments that may be inaccessible due to egress components, technical installations/systems,

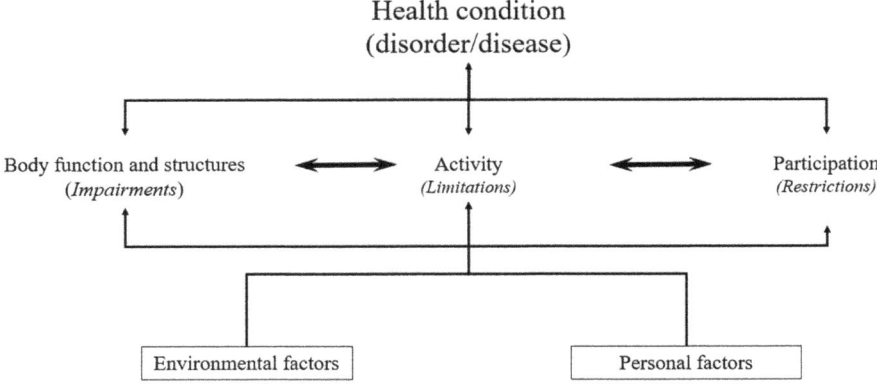

Fig. 5.1 A schematic representation of the International Classification of Functioning, Disability, and Health. (Redrawn from Ref. [15])

communication, etc.; attitudes such as prejudice, stereotyping, discrimination, etc.; and services, systems, and policies such as inflexible evacuation procedures and practices. Personal factors include, for instance, age, past experience, etc.

1.2 Chapter at a Glance

This chapter highlights the benefits of using the ICF in the egress context. Regulatory frameworks and ethical aspects related to people with functional limitations are also discussed in the context of residential fires. The issues linked to egress are presented within the framework of the engineering egress timeline [17], which is commonly adopted in the fire safety engineering world for the study of the required safe egress time (RSET) (intended here as the time needed by building occupants to reach a safe place) in performance-based design. This is generally used both to provide a simplified explanation of the egress process as well as calculate evacuation times (either with hand calculations [18, 19] or modelling tools [20]). The chapter then introduces how evacuation activities can be linked to ICF, presenting a list of key activities based on ICF, which can be connected to egress. This is deemed useful as it allows identifying how the accessibility and egressibility domains can be connected to each other and the benefits of getting familiarized with the ICF for fire safety stakeholders. The chapter then presents a set of quantitative and qualitative information related to the evacuation of people with functional limitations. Information is largely based upon two reviews [6, 21] and studies aimed at addressing the egress perspective of people with functional limitations [22, 23]. The review studies have their main focus on public environments, thus they have been complemented with studies concerning residential settings (e.g. [1, 2, 24]). It should also be noted that even data collected on public environments often contain information that are relevant for residential buildings.

2 From Accessibility to Egressibility in Residential Buildings

Residential settings present a set of specific characteristics from an evacuation standpoint both from a building design perspective as well as concerning the population involved. For example, building occupants may be asleep, thus creating further delay in the evacuation process. People are generally familiar with the environment, but this can also create an emotional tie to the building, personal belongings, and other residents, potentially leading to hazardous behaviour, such as re-entry or reluctance to leave the property during a fire emergency [7]. In addition, today, many people in need of assistance live at home rather than in care facilities and may not be able to perform self-evacuation.

The ability of people with functional limitations to evacuate has been the subject of several studies in the last decades. For instance, seminal studies [25–27] have been performed in the late 90s concerning a set of key egress activities and their link with prevalence, type, and abilities of people with functional limitations. A review of more recent studies can be found in [4, 21]. It is evident though that the majority of studies have investigated individual issues in isolation, while it is well-known that populations may have multiple functional limitations, especially in older ages [6, 28]. In fact, the increase in both number and severity of functional limitations that is associated with the ageing process is likely to affect evacuation performance and the ability to perform self-evacuation [29]. It is therefore important to identify not only how single functional limitations can affect the evacuation process, but also instances of combined functional limitations. This leads to the need for a systematic approach in assessing individual functional capacity in relation to the egress activities.

For a person with functional limitations, a personal emergency evacuation plan can also be a relevant approach [30]. The aim of those plans is to identify specific needs of individuals and link those with an individual escape plan. While personal emergency evacuation plans may be mandated or recommended in public buildings by regulatory guidance [31], this may not be the case in residential buildings. In many cases, the impact of functional limitations can be mitigated through the assistance of others. In addition, different aids that require the assistance of others are offered, such as movement assistance devices (e.g. stair-descent devices [32] or evacuation chairs [33]), buddy systems, etc. However, in a residential setting, these measures may be unaccompanied and self-evacuation is often the only possibility available to reach safety.

Progresses in the accessibility field have shown that different technical and non-technical solutions increase people's possibilities to live an independent life, regardless of functional capacity [34]. It is therefore crucial to investigate to which extent the fire safety among individuals with functional limitations is addressed, and what opportunities they have to evacuate independently. A key step to achieve this goal is reviewing the current data availability concerning the evacuation of people with functional limitations. This would allow identifying what we currently know and do not know concerning the impact of functional limitations on evacuation performance from a quantitative standpoint and aid future research accordingly.

Several efforts have been placed over the years to provide guidance on assessing and addressing the needs of people with functional limitations in residential settings. The accessibility field has seen a transition from the use of checklists and reports on home visits to more systematic assessment tools. A known example is the Housing Enabler [35, 36], an instrument used to perform a systematic assessment of accessibility in residential settings. To apply such tools to the evacuation field is already rendered complicated by the dynamic factors that are particular to an evacuation situation, such as potential changes in the environment (circulation paths getting crowded, visibility impaired by smoke, etc.) as well as the person (state of fear and stress affecting physical and cognitive functioning for instance). However, the applicability of those tools relies especially on the need to include one key variable, which is extremely relevant in case of evacuation: time. In fact, while accessibility does not explicitly take into consideration how long it will take for an individual to perform a certain activity, the time variable has a crucial impact on life safety during an emergency evacuation. It is therefore important to identify: (1) the key activities that take place during an evacuation, (2) how functional limitations can affect the ability to perform such activities including the temporal aspects of it.

3 Linking Egress Activities and Functional Limitations

A useful tool to characterize the temporal aspects linked to evacuation is the engineering egress timeline (see Fig. 5.2). This is often used in fire safety engineering [37] to approximate the different stages of an evacuation and identify the variables affecting them. The engineering egress timeline is a simplification of the

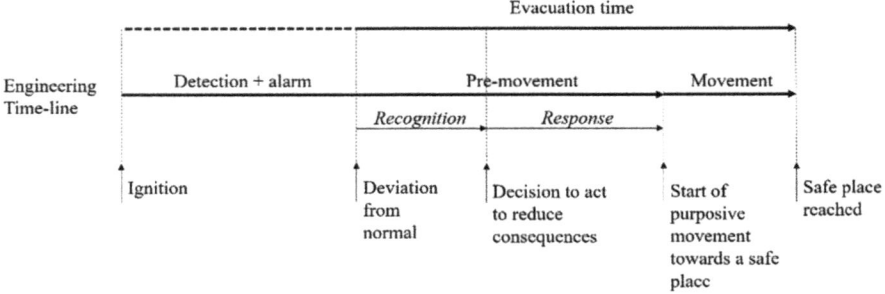

Fig. 5.2 The engineering egress timeline used in fire safety engineering. (Redrawn from Ref. [17, 37])

behavioural timeline, which represents the different protective actions that people may undertake during an evacuation scenario. Those actions can be interpreted according to different human behaviours in fire theories [38–40], generally aiming at explaining the decision-making process of evacuees and their interactions with others and the environment.

The timeline can be broadly divided into three phases (detection + alarm, pre-movement, and movement). After fire ignition, the timeline considers a first stage of detection/alarm (often indicated only as alarm) in which building residents are still not aware of the fire. Once a deviation from normal is identified, the so-called pre-movement phase (sometimes indicated as pre-evacuation or pre-travel phase to indicate that movement can take place during this phase) starts. This includes both the time to recognize what is happening (recognition phase) and the time to respond. The latter starts once a decision to act to reduce consequences is taken and lasts until the start of the purposive movement towards a safe place occur. The last phase concerns movement (this is also called travel phase) and it is concluded once safety is reached. Functional limitations may have an impact on the different phases of the timeline. It should be noted that the present timeline represents the case of people with self-evacuation possibilities (which is the core subject at study), while different timelines/sequence of events may take place in case of assisted evacuation. The latter is deemed less relevant in a residential context given the fact that building residents may not have assistance always available in case of an emergency.

A recent review by Bukvic et al. [6] has linked predominant activities in terms of ICF as well as functional limitations with evacuation activities. According to ICF, activity is the execution of a task or action by an individual [15], and by predominant activities, the aspects of functioning that are required to execute the tasks or actions are referred to. The predominant activities include ICF block such as purposeful sensory experiences (e.g. listening, watching), communicating, carrying, moving and handling objects, walking and moving, changing and maintaining body position, and applying knowledge. Those and the functional limitations (hearing, visual, mobility, upper extremity, cognitive and other functional limitations) were subsequently linked to evacuation activities (e.g. hearing alarm, seeing emergency cues, locating exit signs)in accordance with the engineering egress timeline, considering alarm [A], pre-movement [P], and movement [M] phases.

The suggested classification included visual, hearing, mobility, upper extremities, cognitive, and other functional limitations. A clear example is the distinction between mobility limitations (intended as limitations affecting the ability to move) in contrast with upper extremity limitations. The authors deemed relevant to split those aspects as the latter may affect the ability of an individual to operate doors or equipment, being those aspects particularly relevant in an evacuation scenario, thus being worthy of being analysed in isolation. In this section, a short overview of the key implications of functional limitations on evacuation activities in a home setting (based on ICF activities) is presented. This has been done by adapting the findings of the review by Bukvic et al. [6] for residential buildings.

Another important aspect to consider is that several life safety strategies may be adopted in residential settings (e.g. defend-in-place, total evacuation, phased evacuation, delayed evacuation) [7]. Given the scope of this chapter, this part discusses mainly predominant activities associated with strategies including evacuation.

Hearing limitations can have a significant impact on the ability to respond promptly to an evacuation alarm (evacuation activity *hearing alarm* in [A] and [P] phases) [24, 41]. For example, building residents with age-related hearing limitations (presbycusis) may have issues in hearing frequencies higher than 2000 Hz [42]. There may therefore be unwanted delays in response since alarms are often emitting sounds in the mid to high frequency range [24, 41–43]. In a residential setting, people may also be asleep, thus hearing limitations may challenge even further the effective response to an alarm [44, 45]. Another aspect that may delay response is that fact that people may be under the influence of prescription drugs which may affect their likelihood to wake up to an alarm [44]. This may be addressed with vibrating devices for alert such as bed/pillow shakers [45]. Visual limitations would affect the ability of residents to see visual cues of a fire [46] (activity *seeing emergency cues* in [A] and [P] phases). Similarly, a home fire can be sensed through smelling, but the impact of functional limitations on this issue was identified as a research gap by Bukvic et al. [6].

Visual, hearing, and cognitive limitations can affect the ability of *locating exit signs*; this activity belonging to both [P] and [M] phases. The degree of severity of the functional limitations of the building population has a strong impact on this activity and can affect the likelihood of successful implementation of an evacuation strategy. In fact, several research studies have investigated the design of exit signs for people with this type of functional limitations, such as addressing technological solutions to aid way-finding [27, 47–50], including the use of tactile surfaces [47]. While a residential setting is deemed to be a familiar environment, thus potentially decreasing the issues in locating exit signs and its impact on evacuation outcome, cognitive limitations can also be associated with difficulties in reading, understanding, and interpreting information, including those in signs [50]. In contrast, visual and hearing limitations would have a lower impact on locating signs in a familiar setting, such as a residential building.

Concerning *orientation, maintaining/changing direction,* and *finding architectural elements* (these activities are linked to all [A], [P], and [M] evacuation phases), a residential setting is deemed to present lower issues than a public building (given the lack of background noise that could interfere with audible way-finding systems and a higher degree of familiarity with the environment) for people with visual limitations [48]. Nevertheless, the presence of neurogenerative disorders linked to cognitive limitations (e.g. Alzheimer) would affect the ability of building residents to memorize the way-out of a building during a residential fire, and/or orientating themselves by recognising/understanding emergency cues. This in turn would make evacuation a challenging task even in a home environment which is deemed to be familiar [51, 52].

The evacuation activity *communication with others/rescue services* (linked to the [P] phase) is mostly relevant (although not exclusively) in case of a defend-in-place evacuation strategy rather than self-evacuation [53, 54], although hearing, cognitive, or other limitations (e.g. speech impairments) may affect the ability to communicate with other people present in the home environment during the fire evacuation emergency. This activity may also play an important role in case of evacuation strategies which include crowd management procedural solutions (e.g. phased or delayed evacuation strategies).

Visual, mobility, and upper extremity limitations can have a strong impact on the evacuation activity *using stairs* (related to the [P] phase). This is one of the most investigated issues in the literature on people with functional limitations [6]. People with visual limitations tend to move slower on staircases due to their interaction with the space during the navigation [7, 47, 53, 55, 56]. For instance, the identification of the stair treads and the end of the stairs is known issue [47], although it is likely to be less associated with issues in a familiar setting. The design of handrails has been indicated as one of the key factors for people with visual and mobility limitations [56]. The severity of the limitations will have a strong impact on the ability of people to perform self-evacuation and their eventual need for aid to use stairs [32, 57–62]. Permanent health conditions such as cardiovascular diseases, diabetes, cancer, arthritis, and osteoporosis can increase the prevalence of functional limitations, leading to decreased mobility affecting the use of stairs [4].

A set of activities are strictly linked to mobility limitations. This includes the *getting out of bed* activity (similar issues could be found to an activity such as getting out of a seat). This activity is linked to the [P] phase and is particularly relevant in evacuation scenarios in a residential setting as people may more often be in bed than in other settings. A known issue linked to this activity is the risk of falls [63] which may in turn delay or impede the evacuation. Other activities affected by mobility limitations include *moving to wheelchair*, *moving to escape mattress*, and *moving to stair-descent devices*. These activities will likely be less relevant to a single family dwelling (apart from *moving to wheelchair*), while they could be more relevant in apartment blocks. Those activities all refer to aids adopted to facilitate movement ([M] phase) and may or may not need assistance to be performed, with varying degree of preparation times for their use [64]. It should be noted that, if available, the familiarity with those devices is deemed to be higher in a home environment than in a public setting (e.g. an evacuation chair in a residential building or other similar stair-descend devices [58]). Additional activities affected by mobility limitations include *moving on horizontal*, *moving on incline*, and *traversing 90° bend* (all related to the [M] phase). Several evacuation studies have investigated different conditions (e.g. with or without movement aids), leading to varying evacuation performance during those activities [29, 56, 65].

In residential settings, it is less common to have elevators available for evacuation. This is in contrast with public building such as high-rise buildings or underground metro stations in which the use of occupant evacuation elevators is becoming more common, especially for people with mobility limitations [22]. It should be noted though that using elevators for evacuation can be challenging for people with cognitive limitations [52] and may also be problematic for people with upper extremity limitations. In any case, the *using evacuation elevators* activity is often not relevant for an evacuation in residential setting given their limited use in those settings.

Visual limitations, mobility limitations, and upper extremity limitations can all affect the evacuation activity *opening doors*. This activity is generally performed in every stage of evacuation, so it is assumed to belong to all three [A], [P], and [M] evacuation phases. The use of opening devices can be an issue for blind people [43] and people on a wheelchair or users of other aids [66], while operating door knobs and/or pushing pulling doors might be an issue for people with upper extremity limitations [55, 65, 66].

It should be noted that there may occur evacuation activities that cannot be directly derived from ICF, which are impacted by functional limitations. An example could be activities linked to attempting to fight the fire during an evacuation.

4 Data for Evacuation Design

One of the methods to perform evacuation design is to rely on engineering methods (including performance-based design) rather than following prescriptive design rules [67]. This method requires data for the study of the safety conditions of a building in case of fire. This includes the estimation of the different sets of values used to characterize the inputs for the engineering egress timeline and eventually calculate the Required Safe Egress Time (RSET). This data requirement is present for any type of building (including residential) and populations (including people with functional limitations). To address this issue, the handbook of the Society of Fire Protection Engineering (SFPE) has included a chapter [68] reporting the key datasets available in the literature for this purpose, covering the different phases of the timeline. Nevertheless, the majority of the data available in this document refers to people without functional limitations. The same can be said regarding general design values found in building codes (e.g. [69]). Following up this issue, a recent review was published [21] with the aim of reporting data available concerning people with functional limitations. This is deemed to feed the developments of the SFPE handbook and provide aid in the design of an inclusive fire evacuation strategy. Geoerg et al. [21] reviewed data concerning self-evacuation vs assisted evacuation possibilities. In addition, data were reported considering the two main egress phases, namely pre-movement and movement phase. It should be noted that it is a known issue in the evacuation literature that limited data on human behaviour are collected concerning the initial phase of an evacuation (e.g. pre-warning delays), thus this is generally considered implicitly within the pre-movement phase [70]. This phase may be particularly important in a residential setting when considering those with functional limitations as they may impact their ability to receive the alert (regardless of its type). Further information on the detection/alarm phase can be found in the chapter "Smoke Alarms" of this book.

4.1 Pre-movement Phase

Findings from Geoerg et al. [21] reported that a scarce body of literature is available on the impact of functional limitations on the pre-movement phase. In fact, while several studies have tried to characterize the pre-movement time of different populations under different conditions/scenarios [71], a very limited number of studies have specifically investigated populations involving people with functional limitations. Given behavioural uncertainty [72], existing data show a quite wide variation in terms of observed pre-movement times (ranging from seconds to approximately 30 min) [21]. It should be noted that these values are highly dependent on both the building under consideration as well as the population present in the building (as discussed when presenting the person-environment fit concept in the introduction). Pre-movement times are often represented making use of log-normal distributions to represent the set of occupants who may initiate their evacuation movement after a very long delay [73]. In residential buildings, people may be asleep at the beginning of an evacuation emergency [44], therefore pre-movement times may be affected by this issue. On the one hand, this issue is deemed to be further accentuated in presence of and for people with functional limitations, being a factor towards further delays. This issue can be associated with several actions such as extended time to get dressed, time to fix aids, transfer from chair/bed to aid, etc. In addition, attachments to belongings may result in behaviour that further delay response [74]. On the other hand, the familiarity with the residential environment is deemed to have a positive impact on pre-movement time, as people are generally familiar with the building and the technical installations concerning evacuation available in it [75]. In this context, it should also be noted that current research on people with functional limitations has mostly focused on the evacuation abilities with physical impairments in the lower body (e.g. mobility impairments), while the effect of cognitive impairments is rarely investigated [76].

4.2 Movement Phase

Several quantitative studies can be identified concerning the movement of people with functional limitations, focusing on different aspects, such as movement speeds in both vertical and horizontal egress components (e.g. [21, 60, 64, 77, 78]). In addition, a relatively large number of variables are considered in the literature such as the geometric layout of the egress path, type of movement (unidirectional vs counterflows), evacuation aids available, etc. Geoerg et al. [21] identified that the range of observed walking speeds that consider people with functional limitations varies between 0.23 and 1.95 m/s. This finding is deemed to be directly applicable to residential settings, given the fact that movement abilities would be comparable to those in public buildings (with the exception being linked to way-finding/route choice as it is deemed to be easier in a familiar residential setting and the more likely presence of obstacles and floor coverings). It should be noted though that a residential setting need also consider the case of people not being able to move at all on their own, thus completely relying on assistance for evacuation movement. This could cause additional delays due to the need to wait for assistance and is linked to several factors, such as number and skills of assistors, weight of the individual being assisted, assistive device, carry mode, etc. Given the scope of this chapter, the readers are referred to dedicated literature on this issue [79]. The difference in speed could be explained by several factors, such as the need for movement aid/devices or the general locomotion abilities of the building occupants with functional limitations [80]. Nevertheless, the current data available in the fire safety domain are rather limited when it comes to investigate the explanatory factors of movement speed rather than just reporting observed values [21]. In addition, experiments performed in laboratory settings are often based on several simplifications (especially concerning the heterogeneity of the population possibly involved in an evacuation [64]), thus leading to greater uncertainties when performing fire evacuation design for people with functional limitations.

5 Understanding the Impact of Functional Limitations

The previous sections have discussed how functional limitations represent a risk factor during fires in residential settings. However, less is known about why this is the case. It is reasonable to assume that it can partly be explained by a reduced ability to self-evacuate. Functional limitations come in many forms and shapes, such as limitations in vision, hearing, mobility, balance, cognition, etc.

5.1 Translating Knowledge on Public Buildings to Residential Buildings

Knowledge about the evacuation of people with functional limitations in residential buildings is limited, nevertheless research in the domain of public buildings could be useful. For example, Purser and Bensilum [76] investigated how people with various functional limitations consider their egress opportunities from historical buildings. The main findings of their study were that there are shortcomings in both the physical environment and the organization, and barriers for egress are dependent on the specific type of functional limitation. While organizational issues in a residential setting are generally associated with lower regulatory requirements on management, barriers are deemed to be a key issue in residential buildings as well. In addition, partnerships can be established between different stakeholders (e.g. fire services, social services, resident groups) to ensure that the guidance and support are available to those with functional limitations. This will translate in residents with functional limitations having necessary resources (equipment and human) to facilitate their receiving of the alert, communicating, and effecting their evacuation based on the emergency plans in place [81]. Research studies have also focused on specific aspects of evacuation, such as risk perception [82] and the impact of information campaigns [83], generally linking those with functional limitations rather than the building features, leading to non-inclusive design of the environment [84]. Evacuation from public buildings differs from evacuation in residential settings in many ways. Many older people may live alone in their homes, meaning that they have to rely solely on themselves in order to evacuate. Another aspect is that it is often the individual, or sometimes relatives or caregivers, that have the responsibility of any fire safety measures implemented, such as fire alarms. All of the above make it difficult to translate findings of public buildings (generally maintained by professionals) and residential settings. However, it is possible to identify commonalities in evacuation behaviour of people with functional limitations from public buildings that can be utilized in the context of residential settings. In qualitative research, generalizability is often facilitated by a "thick description of the participants and the research process" [85], which enables the reader to decide if the findings are transferable to another context than the one studied.

A study by Smedberg et al. [23] investigated in detail the perspectives of older people with functional limitations on egressibility. Although the focus was on public buildings, several findings could be directly applicable to residential settings. Semi-structured interviews were conducted with 28 older adults with different functional limitations to investigate their perspective on the possibilities to evacuate in case of emergency. The analysis was conducted using thematic analysis which is a well-known method to analyse qualitative data in the form of interview transcripts [86]. The method facilitated the construction of 'themes' which represent overarching patterns of meaning found in the data material. In their study, three themes were identified: Other people's difficulties in understanding, Strategies to cope with the limitation, and Uncertainty of evacuation.

The first theme, other people's difficulties in understanding, relates to how other people have issues understanding the limitation one might have, how they can help, and that certain types of limitations (those that are visible to others) would receive more consideration from others. In a residential setting, this could mean that caregivers and others might not know how the functional limitation of people affect them in an evacuation (e.g. their impact on evacuation response and movement), and subsequently would not know which aids are most adequate in such a situation. Nevertheless, in a residential setting, it is likely that this issue would be less prominent given the fact that family members would know exactly what functional limitations the individual has. This highlights that not only a caregiver or in general a person providing help would need knowledge of fire safety, but also of functional limitations, in order to suggest aids that would be helpful for a person with functional limitations during an evacuation.

The second theme, strategies to cope with the limitation, includes strategies, such as the person with a functional limitation adjusting their behaviour, avoiding inaccessible environments, using others, using the other senses, accepting the limitation, and pushing through. In residential settings, many of the above-mentioned strategies revolve around adjusting the personal component in the person-environment fit paradigm [87]. It is fair to assume that, in a residential setting, more effort would be aimed towards reducing environmental demands (such as removing thresholds, removing doors, etc.) since this is an environment encountered on a daily basis. The risk is however that fire safety is not included in the adaptation of the home environment because fire is not seen as a priority issue [88]. People with functional limitations encounter accessibility issues on a daily basis that need to be addressed, but fire and subsequent evacuation events can be seen as rare events. As someone is aging and functional ability declines [89], aspects not encountered on a daily basis are easily forgotten. The following excerpt from the above-mentioned study [23], extracted from an interview with an 78-year-old male with limitations in lower body movement, highlights this issue:

> Participant: "Yes, no I do not know... I am thinking about this and I guess I have thought about it myself as well, where I on the second floor have... the possibility to use a rope to climb down. And when I put it up 20 or 30 years ago, it wasn't weird, and I tried to climb it as well without issues. Today it would be significantly more difficult. I may come out... but how I get down I do not really know."

Even though this is purely anecdotal, it highlights some of the issues related to evacuation that may be found in the homes of older people. As people age, fire safety at home needs to be continually updated to fit the personal capacity of the individual. Such interventions could be facilitated through individualized fire safety interventions (see the chapter *Targeted Interventions towards Risk Groups*), recurring home visits by fire safety experts, occupational therapists, or other experts.

Uncertainty of evacuation, the third theme, reflects many of the uncertainties associated with the unusual situation of evacuation. In the study, many uncertainties relate more closely to public buildings, such as the uncertainty about the behaviour of others. However, participants reported uncertainty also in relation to the assessment of their own behaviour. This is likely linked to lack of understanding of the risks and lack of preparation [90]. The participants also stated that they generally did not worry about evacuation. The study argues that information campaigns addressing how evacuation from the home environment might develop would be helpful in aiding people, and in particular people with functional limitations, to better prepare for such situations. Another study, which coincidentally was conducted in the midst of a major disaster (the Kobe earthquake of 1995), found that the perceived ability to escape from the built environment decreased post-event [91]. So the fact that the participants in Smedberg et al.'s study [23] stated that they did not worry about evacuation should not be seen as an indicator that they in fact were well-prepared.

6 Discussion and Conclusion

To date, several steps are still missing towards the goal of an inclusive egress design, as limited attention is given to how elderly householders, especially those with limited mobility, would escape in the event of a fire [92]. First, it is necessary to move completely away from the medical model of disability in fire evacuation safety and transition towards more recent approaches that look more closely at enabling an equal egress without stigmatizing the needs of people with functional limitations. Second, to enable improvements towards an equal egress design of building, several research efforts are needed in the characterization of different populations and their interaction with the environment and technical/procedural evacuation solutions. Third, regulatory provisions should be reviewed in order to address in more detail the specific situations that different individuals with functional limitations may face. For example, potential areas in which regulatory changes could have a positive impact on the evacuation of people with functional limitations include provisions regarding inclusive alarm systems and the design of vertical evacuation means (e.g. stair design). While this process is ongoing and has done great progress in related fields (e.g. accessibility), fire evacuation safety seems to lag behind in a more comprehensive assessment of the individuals and the subsequent needed provisions to provide equal egress.

The studies discussed in this chapter can be used to identify the current state-of-the-art of egress of people with functional limitations in residential settings. This chapter highlights the need for a paradigm shift in the way egressibility is approached in fire safety at home. This includes moving away from generalizing this issue without considering the person-environment fit and addressing the interaction between a variety of functional limitations and egress activities. In addition, it appears evident that most research has so far focused largely on addressing mobility limitations, particularly on the movement phase, rather than providing a systematic investigation of all phases of the engineering egress timeline in relation to different functional limitations. In fact, investigations regarding the evacuation performance of people with functional limitations generally put an overemphasis on trying to characterize the population in terms of physical attributes such as movement speeds, especially in relation to quantitative research [84]. Limited research is conducted regarding the role of the environment and the presence of environmental barriers [84]. Recognizing that egressibility should be seen as a person-environment fit, there is little use in trying to measure the capabilities of people with functional limitations without considering to the full extent the environment in which the investigation takes place. Drawing parallels to other domains of human behaviour in fire research, there is a difference in trying to measure the walking speed of individuals in a smoke filled environment [93] and identifying design solutions aimed towards improving way-finding in such environments [94, 95]. It should be noted that the present chapter has fire engineers as primary (although not exclusive) target audience, thus the main emphasis has been placed here on identifying data availability rather than providing a full review of design and technological solutions for people with functional limitations. The readers are referred to dedicated studies (e.g. [45, 58, 79]) concerning this issue.

In a residential setting, people may be at home without assistance, thus self-evacuation possibilities are a key issue to be addressed. Considering people with functional limitations as a homogenous group that should be addressed in a single evacuation strategy or design solution is a commonly adopted approach, the work presented here highlights how this is likely not the best approach. This leads to the need for an interdisciplinary approach to address both improvements in design as well as partnerships with the different stakeholders which could contribute to a safer residential environment [81].

Regarding research gaps, to date, very limited information is available on the impact of functional limitations on the ability of people to sense smoke. This is surprising given the fact that smelling smoke is one of the key signatures to detect a fire and initiate protective actions, especially in a home environment [96, 97]. This is particularly relevant since deteriorating smell is also significantly associated with cognitive decline [98]. Another identified issue is that the process of ageing is often linked to a decrease of cognitive abilities, which in turn potentially affect several evacuation activities and increase risk behaviours [81]. In contrast, this type of limitations is the least investigated in the literature (often with a very limited number of participants in the studies conducted [51, 52]). This is probably associated with the ethical issues associated with conducting research with people with cognitive limitations (e.g. they may be unable to provide informed consent [99]). Another important aspect that needs further research is the study of the impact of cognitive limitations on the ability to communicate with others/rescue services during an emergency [100]. No dedicated research could be identified on the impact of speech impairment on the ability to communicate during an evacuation scenario.

In addition, there is a clear lack of qualitative research addressing functional limitations and egress in the residential setting. By collecting information from the source, i.e. people with functional limitations, important insights as to why they are vulnerable can be unveiled. Examples of such information could be linked to the identification of evacuation processes, actions, or procedures that may not be possible (or difficult) to perform by people with functional limitations. In addition, it is possible to obtain information concerning expected behaviour in their home situations [90]. Future research could focus on different types of functional limitations and how these affect the perceived ability to self-evacuate. Other aspects to investigate would be which aspects of the home environments are seen as barriers to egress, including the level of preparedness of those with functional limitations and other relevant factors. To address this issue, a qualitative approach with the user in focus might help to identify effective ways of improving egressibility at home.

In conclusion, this book chapter introduced the key concepts concerning the egress of people with functional limitations in residential settings. An overview of quantitative and qualitative literature has been performed along with a characterization of the possible impact of functional limitations on the engineering egress timeline. The framework of the International Classification of Functioning, Disability and Health has been connected to evacuation activities concerning residential settings to demonstrate the impact of functional limitations on the timeline. This chapter is deemed to provide a set of useful information for those interested in fire evacuation of people with functional limitations and shed lights on the specific aspects, which need to be taken into consideration to perform an inclusive design.

Acknowledgements Funding for the research in the area of egress of people with functional limitations was provided by Svenska Forskningsrådet Formas (Grant No. 2018-00575). This study was conducted within the context of the Centre for Ageing and Supportive Environments (CASE) at Lund University.

References

1. Brennan P (1999) Victims and survivors in fatal residential building fires. Fire Mater 23(6):305–310. https://doi.org/10.1002/(SICI)1099-1018(199911/12)23:6<305::AID-FAM703>3.0.CO;2-B
2. Marshall SW, Runyan CW, Bangdiwala SI, Linzer MA, Sacks JJ, Butts JD (1998) Fatal residential fires: who dies and who survives? JAMA 279(20):1633. https://doi.org/10.1001/jama.279.20.1633
3. Shokouhi M et al (2019) Preventive measures for fire-related injuries and their risk factors in residential buildings: a systematic review. J Inj Violence Res 11(1):1–14. https://doi.org/10.5249/jivr.v11i1.1057
4. Boyce K (2017) Safe evacuation for all – fact or fantasy? Past experiences, current understanding and future challenges. Fire Saf J 91:28–40. https://doi.org/10.1016/j.firesaf.2017.05.004
5. Shields T (1994) Fire and disabled people in buildings. J R Soc Health 114(6):304–308
6. Bukvic O, Carlsson G, Gefenaite G, Slaug B, Schmidt SM, Ronchi E (2020) A review on the role of functional limitations on evacuation performance using the international classification of functioning, disability and health. Fire Technol 57(2):507–528. https://doi.org/10.1007/s10694-020-01034-5
7. Ronchi E, Nilsson D (2013) Fire evacuation in high-rise buildings: a review of human behaviour and modelling research. Fire Sci Rev 2(1):7. https://doi.org/10.1186/2193-0414-2-7
8. Andrée K (2018) Utrymningshissar och utrymningsplatser utifrån de utrymmandes perspektiv [Evacuation elevators and refuge areas from the evacuees's perspective]. Lund University, Lund
9. Ronchi E, Nilsson D (2014) Assessment of total evacuation systems for tall buildings. Springer, New York
10. Imrie R (1997) Rethinking the relationships between disability, rehabilitation, and society. Disabil Rehabil 19(7):263–271. https://doi.org/10.3109/09638289709166537
11. Oliver M (2013) The social model of disability: thirty years on. Disabil Soc 28(7):1024–1026. https://doi.org/10.1080/09687599.2013.818773
12. Petasis A (2019) Discrepancies of the medical, social and biopsychosocial models of disability; a comprehensive theoretical framework. Int J Bus Manag Technol 3(4):42–54
13. Brisenden S (1986) Independent living and the medical model of disability. Disabil Handicap Soc 1(2):173–178
14. Wade DT, Halligan PW (2017) The biopsychosocial model of illness: a model whose time has come. Clin Rehabil 31(8):995–1004. https://doi.org/10.1177/0269215517709890
15. World Health Organization (2001) International classification of functioning, disability and health: ICF. World Health Organization, Geneva
16. Verbrugge LM, Jette AM (1994) The disablement process

17. Ronchi E (2020) Developing and validating evacuation models for fire safety engineering. Fire Saf J 120:103020. https://doi.org/10.1016/j.firesaf.2020.103020
18. Gwynne SMV, Rosenbaum ER (2016) Employing the hydraulic model in assessing emergency movement. In: Hurley MJ, Gottuk DT, Hall JR, Harada K, Kuligowski ED, Puchovsky M, Torero JL, Watts JM, Wieczorek CJ (eds) SFPE handbook of fire protection engineering. Springer, New York, pp 2115–2151. Accessed: Aug. 17, 2016. [Online]. Available: http://link.springer.com/10.1007/978-1-4939-2565-0_59
19. Predtechenskii VM, Milinskii AI (1978) Planning for foot traffic flow in buildings. Amerind Publishing, New Delhi
20. Lovreglio R, Ronchi E, Kinsey MJ (2019) An online survey of pedestrian evacuation model usage and users. Submitt Publ
21. Geoerg P, Berchtold F, Gwynne S, Boyce K, Holl S, Hofmann A (2019) Engineering egress data considering pedestrians with reduced mobility. Fire Mater 43(7):759–781. https://doi.org/10.1002/fam.2736
22. Butler KM, Furman SM, Kuligowski ED, Peacock RD (2016) Perspectives of occupants with mobility impairments on fire evacuation and elevators. National Institute of Standards and Technology, NIST TN 1923. Accessed 29 Aug 2016. [Online]. Available: http://nvlpubs.nist.gov/nistpubs/TechnicalNotes/NIST.TN.1923.pdf
23. Smedberg E, Carlsson G, Gefenaite G, Slaug B, Schmidt SM, Ronchi E (2021) A qualitative study on the perspectives on egressibility of older people with functional limitations. Submitt Publ
24. Moinuddin KAM, Bruck D, Shi L (2017) An experimental study on timely activation of smoke alarms and their effective notification in typical residential buildings. Fire Saf J 93:1–11. https://doi.org/10.1016/j.firesaf.2017.07.003
25. Boyce K, Shields T, Silcock G (1999) Toward the characterization of building occupancies for fire safety engineering: capabilities of disabled people moving horizontally and on an incline. Fire Technol 35(1):51–67
26. Boyce KE, Shields TJ, Silcock GW (1999) Toward the characterization of building occupancies for fire safety engineering: prevalence, type, and mobility of disabled people. Fire Technol 35(1):35–50
27. Boyce K, Shields T, Silcock G (1999) Toward the characterization of building occupancies for fire safety engineering: capability of people with disabilities to read and locate exit signs. Fire Technol 35(1):79–86
28. Tsuchiya-Ito R, Iwarsson S, Slaug B (2019) Environmental challenges in the home for ageing societies: a comparison of Sweden and Japan. J Cross-Cult Gerontol 34:265–289
29. Spearpoint M, MacLennan HA (2012) The effect of an ageing and less fit population on the ability of people to egress buildings. Saf Sci 50(8):1675–1684. https://doi.org/10.1016/j.ssci.2011.12.019
30. National Fire Protection Association (2016) Emergency evacuation planning guide for people with disabilities.
31. National Fire Protection Association (2018) NFPA 101, life safety code
32. Lavender SA, Mehta JP, Hedman GE, Park S, Reichelt PA, Conrad KM (2015) Evaluating the physical demands when using sled-type stair descent devices to evacuate mobility-limited occupants from high-rise buildings. Appl Ergon 50:87–97. https://doi.org/10.1016/j.apergo.2015.02.008
33. Sano T, Omiya Y, Hagiwara I (2004) Evacuation from high-rise buildings by using an evacuation chair. Fire Saf Sci 6:7b–1
34. Vaughan M, LaValley MP, AlHeresh R, Keysor JJ (2016) Which features of the environment impact community participation of older adults? A systematic review and meta-analysis. J Aging Health 28(6):957–978. https://doi.org/10.1177/0898264315614008
35. Carlsson G et al (2009) Toward a screening tool for housing accessibility problems: a reduced version of the Housing Enabler. J Appl Gerontol 28(1):59–80

36. Iwarsson S (1999) The Housing Enabler: an objective tool for assessing accessibility. Br J Occup Ther 62(11):491–497. https://doi.org/10.1177/030802269906201104
37. Proulx G (2002) Movement of people: the evacuation timing. In: SFPE handbook of fire protection engineering, 3rd edn. National Fire Protection Association, Quincy, pp 3-341–3-366 (Chapter 3–13)
38. Lindell MK, Perry RW (2012) The protective action decision model: theoretical modifications and additional evidence. Risk Anal 32(4):616–632
39. Canter DV (1990) Fires and human behaviour. Fulton, London
40. Tong D, Canter D (1985) The decision to evacuate: a study of the motivations which contribute to evacuation in the event of fire. Fire Saf J 9(3):257–265. https://doi.org/10.1016/0379-7112(85)90036-0
41. Huey RW, Buckley DS, Lerner ND (1996) Audible performance of smoke alarm sounds. Int J Ind Ergon 18(1):61–69
42. Proulx G (2002) Evacuation planning for occupants with disability. Fire Risk Management Program, Institute for Research in Construction
43. Kecklund L, Andrée K, Bengston S, Willander S, Siré E (2012) How do people with disabilities consider fire safety and evacuation possibilities in historical buildings?—a Swedish case study. Fire Technol 48(1):27–41. https://doi.org/10.1007/s10694-010-0199-0
44. Bruck D, Thomas I, Kritikos A (2006) Investigation of auditory arousal with different alarm signals in sleeping older adults. PhD thesis, Fire Protection Research Foundation
45. Smedberg E, Ronchi E (2021) Review of alarm technologies to wake sleeping people who are deaf or hard of hearing. Department of Fire Safety Engineering, Lund University, Lund
46. Kuligowski ED (2016) Human behavior in fire. In: SFPE handbook of fire protection engineering. Springer, New York, pp 2070–2114
47. Sørensen JG, Danmarks Tekniske Universitet, and DTU Byg (2015) Evacuation of people with visual impairments: PhD thesis. DTU Civil Engineering, Technical University of Denmark, Lyngby
48. Passini R, Proulx G (1988) Wayfinding without vision: an experiment with congenitally totally blind people. Environ Behav 20(2):227–252. https://doi.org/10.1177/0013916588202006
49. Proulx G, Kyle B, Creak J (2000) Effectiveness of a photoluminescent wayguidance system. Fire Technol 36(4):236–248. https://doi.org/10.1023/A:1015475013582
50. Slaug B, Schilling O, Iwarsson S, Carlsson G (2015) Typology of person-environment fit constellations: a platform addressing accessibility problems in the built environment for people with functional limitations. BMC Public Health 15(1):834. https://doi.org/10.1186/s12889-015-2185-4
51. Passini R, Pigot H, Rainville C, Tétreault M-H (2000) Wayfinding in a nursing home for advanced dementia of the Alzheimer's type. Environ Behav 32(5):684–710. https://doi.org/10.1177/00139160021972748
52. Passini R, Rainville C, Marchand N, Joanette Y (1995) Wayfinding in dementia of the Alzheimer type: planning abilities. J Clin Exp Neuropsychol 17(6):820–832. https://doi.org/10.1080/01688639508402431
53. Proulx G (1995) Evacuation time and movement in apartment buildings. Fire Saf J 24(3):229–246. https://doi.org/10.1016/0379-7112(95)00023-M
54. Roberts JL (2005) An area of refuge: due process analysis and emergency evacuation for people with disabilities. Va J Soc Policy Law 13:127–178
55. Boyce KE, Shields TJ, Silcock GWH (1999) Toward the characterization of building occupancies for fire safety: prevalence, type, and mobility of disabled people. Fire Technol 35(1):35–50
56. Boyce KE, Shields TJ, Silcock GWH, Sert F (1999) Toward the characterization of building occupancies for fire safety engineering: capabilities of disabled people moving horizontally and on an incline. Fire Technol 35:51–67. https://doi.org/10.1023/A:1015339216366

57. Butler K, Kuligowski E, Furman S, Peacock R (2017) Perspectives of occupants with mobility impairments on evacuation methods for use during fire emergencies. Fire Saf J 91:955–963. https://doi.org/10.1016/j.firesaf.2017.04.025
58. Hedman GE (2011) Travel along stairs by individuals with disabilities: a summary of devices used during routine travel and travel during emergencies. In: Peacock RD, Kuligowski ED, Averill JD (eds) Pedestrian and evacuation dynamics. Springer, Boston, pp 109–119. https://doi.org/10.1007/978-1-4419-9725-8_10
59. Hunt A, Galea ER, Lawrence PJ (2015) An analysis and numerical simulation of the performance of trained hospital staff using movement assist devices to evacuate people with reduced mobility: MOVEMENT ASSIST DEVICES TO EVACUATE PRM. Fire Mater 39(4):407–429. https://doi.org/10.1002/fam.2215
60. Kuligowski E, Peacock R, Wiess E, Hoskins B (2013) Stair evacuation of older adults and people with mobility impairments. Fire Saf J 62:230–237. https://doi.org/10.1016/j.firesaf.2013.09.027
61. Lavender SA, Hedman GE, Mehta JP, Reichelt PA, Conrad KM, Park S (2014) Evaluating the physical demands on firefighters using hand-carried stair descent devices to evacuate mobility-limited occupants from high-rise buildings. Appl Ergon 45(3):389–397. https://doi.org/10.1016/j.apergo.2013.05.005
62. Mehta JP, Lavender SA, Hedman GE, Reichelt PA, Park S, Conrad KM (2015) Evaluating the physical demands on firefighters using track-type stair descent devices to evacuate mobility-limited occupants from high-rise buildings. Appl Ergon 46:96–106. https://doi.org/10.1016/j.apergo.2014.07.009
63. Wickramasinghe A, Ranasinghe DC, Fumeaux C, Hill KD, Visvanathan R (2017) Sequence learning with passive RFID sensors for real-time bed-egress recognition in older people. IEEE J Biomed Health Inform 21(4):917–929. https://doi.org/10.1109/JBHI.2016.2576285
64. Geoerg P, Polzin RM, Schumann J, Holl S, Hofmann A (2018) Small-scale studies on evacuation characteristics of pedestrians with physical, mental or age-related disabilities. J Phys Conf Ser 1107:072006. https://doi.org/10.1088/1742-6596/1107/7/072006
65. Kesler RM et al (2017) Egress efficacy of persons with multiple sclerosis during simulated evacuations. Fire Technol 53(6):2007–2021. https://doi.org/10.1007/s10694-017-0668-9
66. Boyce KE, Shields TJ, Silcock GWH, Sert F (1999) Toward the characterization of building occupancies for fire safe engineering: capability of disabled people to negotiate doors, p 11
67. Meacham BJ, Custer RL (1995) Performance-based fire safety engineering: an introduction of basic concepts. Sage, Thousand Oaks
68. Gwynne SMV, Boyce KE (2016) Engineering data. In: Hurley MJ, Gottuk DT, Hall JR, Harada K, Kuligowski ED, Puchovsky M, Torero JL, Watts JM, Wieczorek CJ (eds) SFPE handbook of fire protection engineering. Springer, New York, pp 2429–2551. Accessed 18 Feb 2016. [Online]. Available: http://link.springer.com/10.1007/978-1-4939-2565-0_64
69. Boverket (2013) Boverkets ändring av verkets allmänna råd (2011,27) om analytisk dimensionering av byggnaders brandskydd (BFS 2011:27 med ändringar t.o.m. 2013:12). Boverket, Karlskrona
70. Gwynne S, Purser D, Boswell D (2011) Pre-Warning Staff Delay: A Forgotten Component in ASET/RSET Calculations. In: Peacock R, Kuligowski E, Averill J (eds) Pedestrian and Evacuation Dynamics. Springer, Boston, MA. https://doi.org/10.1007/978-1-4419-9725-8_22
71. Forssberg M, Kjellström J, Frantzich H, Mossberg A, Nilsson D (2019) The variation of pre-movement time in building evacuation. Fire Technol 55(6):2491–2513. https://doi.org/10.1007/s10694-019-00881-1
72. Ronchi E, Reneke PA, Peacock RD (2014) A method for the analysis of behavioural uncertainty in evacuation modelling. Fire Technol 50(6):1545–1571. https://doi.org/10.1007/s10694-013-0352-7
73. Purser DA, Bensilum M (2001) Quantification of behaviour for engineering design standards and escape time calculations. Saf Sci 38(2):157–182. https://doi.org/10.1016/S0925-7535(00)00066-7

74. D'Orazio M, Bernardini G (2014) An experimental study on the correlation between 'Attachment to belongings' 'Pre-movement' time. In: Weidmann U, Kirsch U, Schreckenberg M (eds) Pedestrian and evacuation dynamics 2012. Springer International Publishing, Cham, pp 167–178. https://doi.org/10.1007/978-3-319-02447-9_12
75. Kinateder M, Comunale B, Warren WH (2018) Exit choice in an emergency evacuation scenario is influenced by exit familiarity and neighbor behavior. Saf Sci 106:170–175. https://doi.org/10.1016/j.ssci.2018.03.015
76. Kecklund L, Andrée K, Bengtson S, Willander S, Siré E (2012) How do people with disabilities consider fire safety and evacuation possibilities in historical buildings?—a Swedish case study. Fire Technol 48(1):27–41. https://doi.org/10.1007/s10694-010-0199-0
77. Geoerg P, Schumann J, Holl S, Boltes M, Hofmann A (2019) The influence of individual impairments in crowd dynamics. Fire Mater 45(4):529–542
78. Kuligowski E, Peacock R, Wiess E, Hoskins B (2015) Stair evacuation of people with mobility impairments. Fire Mater 39(4):371–384. https://doi.org/10.1002/fam.2247
79. Hunt A, Galea ER, Lawrence PJ (2012) An analysis of the performance of trained staff using movement assist devices to evacuate the non-ambulant. In: 5th international symposium. Human behaviour in fire, pp 328–339
80. Hunt ALE (2016) Simulating hospital evacuation. PhD thesis, University of Greenwich
81. Cassidy P, McConnell N, Boyce K (2021) The older adult: associated fire risks and current challenges for the development of future fire safety intervention strategies. Fire Mater 45(4):553–563. https://doi.org/10.1002/fam.2823
82. Tancogne-Dejean M, Laclémence P (2016) Fire risk perception and building evacuation by vulnerable persons: points of view of laypersons, fire victims and experts. Fire Saf J 80:9–19. https://doi.org/10.1016/j.firesaf.2015.11.009
83. Diekman ST, Stewart TA, Teh SL, Ballesteros MF (2010) A qualitative evaluation of fire safety education programs for older adults. Health Promot Pract 11(2):216–225. https://doi.org/10.1177/1524839908318169
84. Christensen KM, Collins SD, Holt JM, Phillips CN (2006) The relationship between the design of the built environment and the ability to egress of individuals with disabilities. Rev Disabil Stud Int J 2(3):24–34
85. Korstjens I, Moser A (2018) Series: practical guidance to qualitative research. Part 4: trustworthiness and publishing. Eur J Gen Pract 24(1):120–124. https://doi.org/10.1080/13814788.2017.1375092
86. Braun V, Clarke V (2012) Thematic analysis. In: APA handbook of research methods in psychology, vol 2. American Psychological Association, Washington, DC
87. Lawton MP, Nahemow L (1973) Ecology and the aging process. In: Eisdorfer C, Lawton MP (eds) The psychology of adult development and aging. American Psychological Association, Washington, DC, pp 619–674. https://doi.org/10.1037/10044-020
88. de Wit R, Helsloot I (2021) Public perception in regard to fire services in the Netherlands. Fire Saf J 122:103343
89. Verbrugge LM, Jette AM (1994) The disablement process. Soc Sci Med 38(1):1–14
90. Karemaker M, ten Hoor GA, Hagen RR, van Schie CHM, Boersma K, Ruiter RAC (2021) Elderly about home fire safety: a qualitative study into home fire safety knowledge and behaviour. Fire Saf J 124:103391. https://doi.org/10.1016/j.firesaf.2021.103391
91. Yoshimura H (1998) Sounding out the disabled in the lower-extremities on their escape behavior in building fire for safer fire escape design. In: Human behavior in fire-proceedings of the first international symposium. Belfast, pp 353–359
92. Harpur A, Boyce K, McConnel N (2014) An investigation into the circumstances surrounding elderly dwelling fire fatalities and the barriers to implementing fire safety strategies among this group. Fire Saf Sci 11:1144–1159
93. Fridolf K, Ronchi E, Nilsson D, Frantzich H (2015) The relationship between obstructed and unobstructed walking speed: results from an evacuation experiment in a smoke filled tunnel. Downing College, Cambridge, pp 537–548

94. Fridolf K, Ronchi E, Nilsson D, Frantzich H (2013) Movement speed and exit choice in smoke-filled rail tunnels. Fire Saf J 59:8–21. https://doi.org/10.1016/j.firesaf.2013.03.007
95. Ronchi E, Fridolf K, Frantzich H, Nilsson D, Walter AL, Modig H (2018) A tunnel evacuation experiment on movement speed and exit choice in smoke. Fire Saf J 97:126–136. https://doi.org/10.1016/j.firesaf.2017.06.002
96. Burian B (2005) Do you smell smoke? Issues in the design and content of checklists for smoke, fire, and fumes. Forth Worth, Texas
97. Lloyd M, Roen K (2002) 'When you smell smoke…': 'risk factors' and fire safety in action. Health Risk Soc 4(2):139–153
98. Windon MJ, Kim SJ, Oh ES, Lin SY (2020) Predictive value of olfactory impairment for cognitive decline among cognitively normal adults. Laryngoscope 130(4):840–847. https://doi.org/10.1002/lary.28166
99. Boyce K, Nilsson D (2015) Investigating ethical attitudes in human behaviour in fire research. In: 6th International Symposium Human Behaviour in Fire. Interscience Communications Cambridge, pp 585–596
100. Arias S, Fahy R, Ronchi E, Nilsson D, Frantzich H, Wahlqvist J (2019) Forensic virtual reality: investigating individual behavior in the MGM grand fire. Fire Saf J 109:102861

Dr. Enrico Ronchi is an Associate Professor in Evacuation Modelling at Lund University, Sweden. He is recognized for his numerous research contributions in a wide range of areas concerning human behavior in fire and evacuation. He is currently Associate Editor for the journals Fire Technology and Safety Science, and he is a member of the editorial board of the Fire Safety Journal and SFPE Europe, the European magazine of the Society of Fire Protection Engineering (SFPE). He has also translated his work into practice through his involvement with multiple committees and publications with International organizations (e.g. International Standards Organization).

Mr. Erik Smedberg is a doctoral student at Lund University, Sweden. He has a BSc in Fire Safety Engineering and an MSc in Risk Management and Safety Engineering, both from Lund University. The topic of his PhD as well as his main research interests are human behavior in fire and evacuation of older people and people with functional limitations.

Dr. Gunilla Carlsson is an Associate Professor in Occupational Therapy at Lund University with a focus on how the environment hinders or supports activity and participation in an aging population. Based on clinical experience and many years of research, her specific focus is how to address accessibility problems in the built environment for people with physical and cognitive impairments. Her research is primarily about housing, but also mobility in the public environment.

Dr. Björn Slaug is an Associate Professor in Health Sciences at Lund University, Sweden. He has a background in public health research, and his current research focus concerns the development of methods supporting societal efforts to make the built environment accessible for all, regardless of functional capacity. His latest research output includes the development of a new assessment tool for analysis of the physical accessibility to entrances in the public environment. He has a large international network of collaborators from Japan, Germany, and several other European countries.

Chapter 6
Fire Safety Surveillance: Theoretical and Practical Challenges

Colin McIntyre and Anders Jonsson

Abstract There is a long history of the systematic collection and analysis of data to inform public health policy. The World Health Organization (WHO) defines public health surveillance as "*An ongoing, systematic collection, analysis and interpretation of health-related data essential to the planning, implementation, and evaluation of public health practice.*"

The aim of this chapter is to identify important aspects of a coordinated approach to fire safety surveillance. If the theoretical and practical challenges identified in the chapter can be overcome and the various components of such a system put in place, it could lead to better-informed decision making and hopefully over time help to improve residential fire safety.

The material on definitions presented in this chapter is based on what has been learned when studying fatal fires and fire deaths in Sweden. In the immediate aftermath of the fire at a Halloween party in Gothenburg in 1998 where 63 teenagers died, it was decided that the central fire authority should work systematically to access all data concerning fatal fires known to the fire service, police, forensic pathologists, road accident investigators, national burn centres, and the health authorities.

The authors also relate to experiences gained from cooperation on fire statistics among the Nordic countries and Estonia. The definitions used in these countries are compared with descriptions and definitions in national fire statistics from Great Britain and the USA.

Keywords Surveillance · Fire statistics · Residential definition · Fire definition · Fire death definition · Fire injury measurements

---

C. McIntyre (✉)
Swedish Civil Contingencies Agency (MSB), Karlstad, Sweden
e-mail: Colin.McIntyre@msb.se

A. Jonsson
Swedish Civil Contingencies Agency (MSB), Karlstad, Sweden

Karlstad University, Karlstad, Sweden

1 Potential Uses of Fire Safety Surveillance Data

There is a long history of the systematic collection and analysis of data to inform public health policy. The World Health Organization (WHO) defines public health surveillance as "An ongoing, systematic collection, analysis and interpretation of health-related data essential to the planning, implementation, and evaluation of public health practice" [1].The WHO description of public health surveillance can easily be translated to the context of fire safety, which would benefit from an ongoing, systematic collection, analysis, and interpretation of fire-related data needed for the planning, implementation, and evaluation of fire safety practice.

In a study of the effectiveness of an intervention where domestic smoke alarms were provided to residents in a specific part of Oklahoma City [2], it was noted that surveillance data had been used in several studies to identify populations at high risk of injury or death from fire. However, surveillance data had rarely been used for the implementation and evaluation of programs aimed at reducing fire-related injuries.

Various actors could use surveillance data to inform decision-making concerning many different aspects of fire safety.

It is desirable to have products and buildings with a good fire safety record. It is also desirable that people behave in a way that minimises fire risk and act in the best possible manner in the unlikely event that a fire breaks out. If they cannot put the fire out themselves, then it is important that the fire service can get there reasonably quickly and use best practice to save lives and extinguish the fire with a minimum of damage to property and long-term effects on the environment.

Ideally, surveillance data would enable us to identify products which have started fires and show when fire safety aspects of the building regulations do not perform as expected.

It is important that surveillance data help us to identify vulnerable groups and learn how their behaviour puts them at risk of starting a fire. It is also important to know how they behave when threatened by fire.

The fire service wants to optimise the fire cover they provide in their area of responsibility. To do that, they need to identify the best locations for their fire stations and the most appropriate manning levels. In order to do this, they need to analyse where and when fires occur, as well as the people and building types involved. Surveillance data should be able to provide the information necessary for such risk analysis, when combined with geographical data from other sources.

Ideally, surveillance data will also provide information about fire outcomes – who is killed or injured and how – as well as levels of property damage. This information will help firefighters learn the most effective ways to extinguish fires. Good data on fire outcomes and vulnerable groups will also help politicians decide on an appropriate level of fire safety to aim for, either nationally or in the local community.

In several countries, the fire service does outreach to meet vulnerable people in their homes and give advice about fire safety. Surveillance data should help the fire service to identify which kinds of people to make the top priority for visits, and what information they need to hear when they open the door.

To summarise, the goal of surveillance data is to inform the wide range of work to prevent fires from starting as well as all the work to minimise the negative effects of the fires which, despite our best efforts, still occur.

2 Desirable Features of a System for Fire Safety Surveillance

Ability to Separate Data on Residential Fires
Most fire-related deaths and injuries occur in a residential setting, so it is important that a surveillance system allows the analysis of data relating specifically to residential fires.

Data from the Most Reliable Sources
Many countries rely on data from the fire service to inform fire safety policy. Fire officers know how fires behave in general, and at a specific fire incident they know what actions they took and how they influenced the development of the fire.

However, fire officers cannot be considered a reliable source of data concerning fire outcomes in the form of injuries, property damage, and environmental degradation.

In addition, it must be remembered that the fire service is not called to all residential fires. Fire service data cannot provide a complete picture of fire incidence in a residential setting. In order to get a comprehensive understanding of fire incidence, it is necessary to obtain data from other sources such as insurance companies, as well as surveys, to estimate the incidence level of residential fires and the proportion of the various kinds of residential fires which are to be found in fire service and insurance statistics.

The ideal surveillance system would combine data from the most reliable sources to provide a comprehensive view of the residential fire problem.

Data from Existing Administrative Systems
It is very expensive to build up new dedicated systems for data collection. It is much more cost-effective to acquire data from existing administrative systems. For example, in many countries the fire service is required by law to record what happened and what actions were taken after each emergency response. These incident reports are stored in a local or national records management system. Medical procedures in hospitals are well-documented, including external causes of any injuries. Insurance companies have systems for the administration of claims after fires. In Sweden, there are also regulations on the documentation of health status and actions taken by the ambulance service.

Acquiring data from existing systems minimises the burden of recording data. No one wants to waste time recording similar data in two parallel systems.

One challenge when using data from existing sources is that data objects are primarily intended for administration and do not necessarily correspond to what is needed in a statistical analysis. There are also challenges in matching data from various datasets.

3 Data Sources for Fire Safety Surveillance

3.1 Fire Service Incident Reports

In the Nordic countries, incident reports from the fire service contain a lot of useful information on the fires which they attend. These data include where and when the fire occurred, together with an assessment of the fire cause. Several countries describe the size of the fire on arrival and its subsequent spread in a simple qualitative scale. The incident reports also contain an assessment of injuries caused by the fire and some also have descriptions of actions taken by the fire service to rescue people threatened by the fire as well as the methods used by the fire service to extinguish the fire.

3.2 Investigations After Fatal Fires

Fatal fires warrant a more thorough investigation than other, less serious fire events. Usually, the police will be involved to ascertain whether a crime has been committed, and if so, to gather evidence for a future court case. Whether or not crime is involved, people working with fire prevention, protection, or emergency response will benefit from a more detailed understanding of the cause of the fire, how it could develop to become life-threatening, and how rescue attempts could have been more effective.

Occasionally, a fire occurs after a road crash. Sometimes a crash victim would have survived any impact injuries, but the victim is trapped in a burning vehicle. Research shows that in Sweden, on average about five road crash victims per year die in post-crash fires [3]. This would indicate that the help of road accident investigators is needed if our aim is a comprehensive dataset on all fatal fires.

3.3 Data from Forensic Pathologists on Fire-Related Deaths

It is often far from easy to ascertain the cause of death when someone dies in connection with a fire. Some visible injuries may have occurred after the moment of death. It is unreasonable to expect fire officers, police investigators, or ambulance personnel to provide reliable information. However, in most countries, forensic pathologists investigate all non-natural deaths and they are often able to assess whether the death was caused by burns or toxic gases. They can often see if the victim has been exposed to smoke before death occurred. They can also provide data on blood alcohol levels and the presence of medicines or narcotics in the body.

All of this is invaluable knowledge if the aim is to reduce the number of fire deaths.

The Swedish National Board of Health and Welfare maintains a cause of death register. This contains data on all people who die in Sweden and, when available, data on Swedish residents who die in foreign countries. However, when comparing fire deaths in the three major data sources, it was apparent that the cause of death register does not provide useful data for fire safety over and above that which is available from the forensic pathologists [4].

3.4 Data from Ambulance Service

The ambulance service record data on patients who are taken to hospital from the scene of a fire. In particular, the ambulance personnel are much better qualified to assess the severity of a fire victim's injuries than fire officers.

In Sweden, ambulance personnel use the Rapid Emergency Triage and Treatment System (RETTS) for the triage of patients [5]. The system categorises patients into one of four colours based on the seriousness of the injury and risk of complications:

Red – Life-threatening condition, acute care
Orange – Serious condition/suspicion of serious condition
Yellow – No acute signs of life-threatening conditions, a need for investigation
Green – No acute signs of life-threatening conditions, no need for investigation

3.5 Data from National Patient Register on Fire-Related Injuries

Many countries maintain a national patient data repository with comprehensive data on diagnoses, external causes of injuries, and procedures for hospital in-patient care. WHO has a standard for the international classification of diseases (ICD). At present, most countries record data according to the tenth revision (ICD-10). The eleventh revision will come into effect in 2022, but it will take several years before it is implemented in most countries. ICD-10 has specific codes for fire-related injuries in Chap. 20, External causes of morbidity and mortality [6]:

Accidents, Exposure to smoke, fire, and flames (X00-X09):

    X00 Exposure to uncontrolled fire in building or structure
    X01 Exposure to uncontrolled fire, not in building or structure
    X02 Exposure to controlled fire in building or structure
    X03 Exposure to controlled fire, not in building or structure
    X04 Exposure to ignition of highly flammable material
    X05 Exposure to ignition or melting of nightwear
    X06 Exposure to ignition or melting of other clothing and apparel
    X08 Exposure to other specified smoke, fire, and flames
    X09 Exposure to unspecified smoke, fire, and flames

Intentional self-harm

    X76 Intentional self-harm by smoke, fire, and flames

Assault

    X97 Assault by smoke, fire, and flames

Event of undetermined intent

    Y26 Exposure to smoke, fire and flames, undetermined intent

Code positions four and five are intended to cover various general activities and locations. Unfortunately, when studying Swedish data, we have observed that quality in positions four and five is not always satisfactory, which among other things makes it difficult to identify injuries due to residential fires.

It is important to note that accidental exposure to smoke, fire, and flames includes separate codes for controlled fire.

3.6   Data on Fire Insurance Claims from Insurance Companies

It is important to consider economic losses due to fire when making decisions about investments to improve fire safety.

In several countries, fire service incident reports for building fires include a question on fire spread – the fire may be contained in the item of origin, room of origin, fire cell of origin, building of origin, or spread to other buildings. This provides a very rough indication of economic losses due to the fire.

Some countries, such as Finland, go further and get fire officers to estimate the economic losses due to a fire. However, it would appear unreasonable to expect a fire officer with little or no specific training to do something that can take months for specialists employed by insurance companies.

In the British Incident Recording System (IRS) [7], fire officers estimate the horizontal area of the building that was damaged by flame and/or heat. It is presumably hoped that this indirect measure provides a more reliable indication of the level of economic losses than a direct estimate by a fire officer.

The most comprehensive and reliable source for loss data would be the insurance companies.

Insurance data focus on claims, not fire events. Insurance data are recorded per claim and cannot easily be aggregated per fire. One fire can give rise to several claims, and these may be spread over various insurance companies.

The fire-related data from insurance companies are based on claims according to the fire clause in an insurance policy. In Sweden, the fire clause generally includes damage due to electrical faults in equipment which did not actually start a fire. Electrical faults without fire make up a significant proportion of the smaller claims, and this is particularly marked in years when there are many thunderstorms.

When studying insurance payments, it must be remembered that a claimant may face costs which are not covered by the insurance policy, and that most policies include an excess (an amount which is deducted from any insurance pay-out).

Regarding residential fires, it must be remembered that not all homes are insured.

In the past, the central fire authority in Norway has matched insurance pay-outs with fire service incident reports. The insurance companies were obliged to provide data on all pay-outs over a certain threshold.

3.7 Investigations After Residential Fires

It is clear that human behaviour plays a major role in how fires start, as well as the chances of an individual escaping from the fire, rescuing others threatened by the fire, or even extinguishing the fire before the fire service arrives.

Detailed information on people who experience a fire, their behaviour, and the factors which influenced their decision making is not recorded in fire service incident reports. It would therefore be valuable to carry out investigations after residential fires to collect this vital information.

In recent years, projects have been undertaken in both the UK and Sweden to collect more data on human behaviour in residential fires (Sect. 5.3).

3.8 Surveys on Residential Fires

Surveys can be used to study fire incidence in the home. However, fires in the home are relatively rare events, so an extremely large sample is needed to give reliable estimates of fire rates. If the survey is carried out in the form of a questionnaire, then non-response can be a significant problem. Response rates to questionnaire surveys have dropped markedly in recent years.

Since 1996, the central fire authority in Sweden has commissioned questionnaire surveys addressed to those aged between 18 and 79 roughly every five years. The latest study from 2018 shows that the fire service was called to about 51% of all residential fires, and an insurance company was involved after 44% of all residential fires [8].

In the Swedish survey, the fire service extinguished 37% of all residential fires. It is interesting to compare the Swedish estimate with the latest interview-based English Housing Survey from 2016 to 2017 [9] where 25% of residential fires were put out by the fire service. It should be noted that "fire" is not defined in the Swedish survey, whereas in the English survey interviewees were advised that "fire" means all sorts of fires, including chip pan fires and very minor fires and also fires in sheds, garages, or greenhouses on your property."

These two surveys indicate a much higher involvement of the fire service in residential fires compared with the 2004–2005 telephone survey of unreported residential fires in the USA [10]. Here it was estimated that only about 3.4% of residential fires were attended by fire departments. Fire in this survey was defined as "any incident – large or small – that resulted in unwanted flames or smoke, and could have caused damage to life or property if left unchecked."

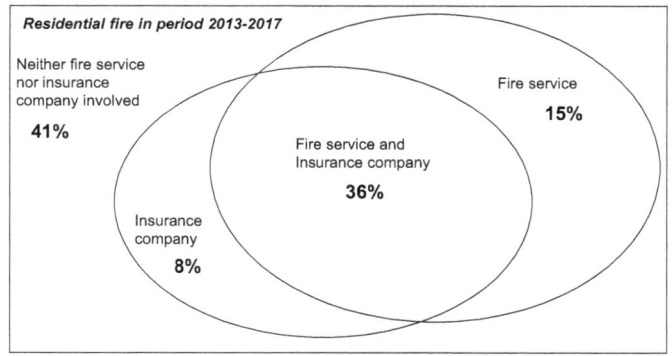

Fire service and insurance company involvement in residential fires, Sweden 2013-2017

Source: questionnaire survey for MSB by Statistics Sweden, 2018

3.9 Summary of Data Sources

Data Quality Summary Table

	Fire service Incident report	Fire service residential fire investigation	Fire service/police fatal fire investigation together with data from forensic pathologist	Cause of death register	Ambulance patient data register	Hospital patient data register	Fire insurance company claims data
Identity of victims	Low	High	High	High	High	High	Low[a]
Number of deaths	Medium[b]	–	High	High	–	–	–
Diagnoses of deaths	–	–	High	High	–	–	–
Number of serious injuries	Medium[b]	–	–	–	High	High	–
Diagnoses of serious injuries	–	–	–	–	–	High	–
Property damage	Low	Medium	–	–	–	–	High
Cause of fire	Medium	High	High[c]	–	–	–	Medium
Medicine/alcohol/drug use at time of fire	–	High	High	–	–	–	–
Human behaviour in actual fire	Low	High	High	–	–	–	–

[a]Identity of policyholder, who is not necessarily the victim
[b]Fire service not called to all fires causing injuries or deaths, and when called, the fire service will not always know the subsequent health outcomes
[c]Surprisingly high proportion of fatal fires with unknown causes. In Sweden the fire has often become fully developed, making the forensic investigation very difficult

4 Definitions

When comparing data from different sources within a country, or similar sources from different countries, it is important to know what definitions have been used in the various datasets. Similar terms can be used, but with different meanings. Even with similar terms, inclusion and exclusion criteria can differ significantly.

Clear definitions are important for comparing data from different sources, but are also vital for consistent reporting over time in any particular organisation. Without definitions to refer to, there is an obvious risk of interpretations of terms changing over time, in particular when new personnel are brought in to record or check the data.

For the surveillance of residential fire safety to be meaningful, there must be agreement on the central terms "residential" and "fire" as well as the negative outcomes that characterise a lack of fire safety, such as "death" and "serious injury."

Everyone has an intuitive understanding of what is meant by these terms. It is only when faced with borderline cases that two things become apparent. The first is that a logically sound theoretical framework is required for identifying which variables are most relevant for ongoing collection and analysis. The second is that when choosing appropriate variables, it is important to take into account the many practical challenges that arise when trying to capture your own data or access data from another organisation.

Data collected in the incident report forms used by the fire services in different countries vary according to what information is considered important to record and follow up. It could be expected that a small number of the most central variables would be common across all countries, but even with a common variable, the definition often varies or differences in the values that the variable can take make comparisons problematic.

This makes it very important to have clearly formulated definitions in any statistics. In particular, inclusion and exclusion criteria must be transparent for every definition.

Over the last 15 years, the central fire authorities in the Nordic countries have made efforts to improve comparability in their fire statistics and publish a common dataset [11]. In recent years, Estonia and Latvia have joined the work.

Despite cultural and climatic similarities between the Nordic and Baltic states, it is still a major challenge to identify a common core of data which allows reliable comparisons between the participating nations.

4.1 Definitions of "Residential"

What constitutes a home varies considerably between countries. It is therefore unsurprising that what is understood by the term "residential" also varies.

Winters in Sweden are generally colder than many other European countries. It is presumed that everyone has their permanent residence in a building. In the Swedish context, it is reasonable to consider residential fires as a subset of building fires.

This is in contrast to the UK or USA where a residence does not need to be a building. It is considered sufficient for the home to be in a "substantial structure" – for example a mobile home, caravan, or houseboat. However, a tent would not normally constitute a substantial structure.

Many people in the Nordic countries own or rent a summer cottage. While these are not normally considered their permanent residence, people can live in them for prolonged periods. In some cases, the owner improves the insulation, heating, and other facilities and the summer cottage becomes their permanent residence. It would be impractical for the fire service to differentiate between cottages for permanent residence and those only used on a temporary basis. Fires in all private summer cottages are therefore classed as residential fires. However, it should be noted that huts on a campsite would not be considered residential buildings.

The Swedish building regulations categorise buildings according to certain properties which influence fire safety. For example, it is expected that a person can find their way around a residential property. It is important to have a much stricter regulation of hotels, where it is much more difficult for guests to self-evacuate, as they would be trying to find their way out of an unfamiliar building. In Sweden, you would not expect people to have a hotel or guest house as a permanent residence and a fire in a hotel is not considered a residential fire.

This is in contrast to the USA, where some people live for prolonged periods in a hotel. Hotel fires are therefore classified as residential in the US Fire Administration's National Fire Incident Reporting System (NFIRS) [12].

The term "Dwelling" in English law refers both to the main house on the property and any outbuildings such as garages or sheds.

A significant proportion of all fires classified as "residential" in the Swedish statistics take place in outbuildings such as free-standing garages, saunas, or sheds. These fires are classified differently in the other Nordic countries and must be excluded for comparisons of residential fires in this region.

Many fires in blocks of flats take place in stairwells, cellars, or attics. Should these be considered residential fires?

One of the biggest challenges when comparing residential fire statistics is the variation in how institutional contexts are classified. For example, there is some confusion in the fire service when coding incidents in homes for the elderly. These can range from normal houses or apartments (with or without home help), to apartments in sheltered housing, to apartments in care- or nursing homes.

Clearly, incidents in normal houses or apartments should be considered "residential," as should sheltered housing, even if there are shared facilities such as dining rooms. In Sweden, residents in care- or nursing homes often rent their apartment, so it is not unreasonable to consider this a residential context. However, in the Nordic fire statistics cooperation, care- or nursing homes with staff on call 24/7 are classified in the "health care" category rather than "residential." A similar approach is used in NFIRS.

4.2 Definitions of "Fire"

The International Organization for Standardization in ISO 13943:2017(en) defines fire as a "process of combustion characterised by the emission of heat and fire effluent and usually accompanied by smoke, flame or glowing or a combination thereof." [13]

According to the National Fire Protection Association, the combustion reaction can be characterised by four components: the fuel, the oxidizing agent, the heat, and the uninhibited chemical chain reaction [14]. These four components are often referred to as the fire tetrahedron. Fuel can take many forms, but in most fires the oxidizing agent is oxygen in the surrounding air. Heat is needed to produce fuel vapours and cause ignition. The uninhibited chemical chain reaction ensures that sufficient excess heat from the exothermic reaction radiates back to the fuel to produce more vapours and cause ignition in the absence of the original source. The process will be self-sustained, allowing the fire to propagate, as long as the fuel or oxygen supply does not run out.

Fire can be described as a self-sustained combustion process. However, in a Swedish context, two additional conditions are implicit in the understanding of the term "fire": the lack or loss of control over a combustion process and negative consequences.

Unlike English, the French, German, and Scandinavian languages all have different words for controlled and uncontrolled fire.

This is dealt with in ISO 13943:2017(en) by going on to define controlled fire as "self-supporting combustion that has been deliberately arranged to provide useful effects and is limited in its extent in time and space" and uncontrolled fire as "self-supporting combustion that has not been deliberately arranged to provide useful effects and is not limited in its extent in time and space."

The challenge when defining "fire" is to get agreement on which combustion processes should be considered to constitute a fire. If "fire" includes the concept of a negative consequence, then there must also be agreement on the level of injury or damage that must be caused to say that a negative consequence has occurred.

When studying data from various national fire services, it is important to note that some countries require an open flame for the event to be considered a fire.

In Sweden, a flame is not a requirement for an event to be classified as a fire. A less rapid oxidation where the temperature does not rise above the ignition point may only give rise to charring, but a smouldering fire is still considered as a fire, as long as it results in damage of some kind.

A smouldering fire is a slow process. There are other combustion processes which occur very rapidly. For example, a dust explosion can take place when a solid substance is finely divided and mixed with air. In unfortunate circumstances, an ignition source such as a spark can ignite some dust particles which heat up the surrounding particles and start a very rapid chain reaction. This is a similar principle to a fire in other solid materials, but the speed of the process means that it is most often perceived as an explosion rather than a fire. Should dust explosions be considered a special case of a fire event?

In some fires, a flammable liquid is used as an accelerant to ensure the rapid development of a fire. However, sometimes the liquid evaporates quickly and the combustion of the vapour cloud occurs instantaneously in the form of an explosion and fails to ignite other surrounding material. Should an explosion of flammable vapours which does not start a more prolonged fire be considered a fire event?

Does the definition of a fire as a lack of control over a combustion process cause a problem when considering intentional fires? From the fire setter's perspective, the damage caused by the fire was a desired outcome. However, the arsonist has presumably little or no control over the fire's development once it has been started and so even intentional fires can be considered to constitute a fire event.

From a perspective of monitoring fire safety, it is important to be able to differentiate between accidental and intentional fires, as they demand completely different approaches to prevention.

Self-immolation is a specific kind of intentional fire which is important to follow up. It is not uncommon for such fires to take place without the fire service being called out. When all known fire-related deaths in Sweden were studied systematically, it became apparent that the fire and rescue service are unaware of about 20% of all deaths, and many of these were the result of self-immolation [4]. It would appear that self-immolation is more common than generally assumed, but often passes unremarked in Sweden and presumably many other European countries. It should be noted that the majority of these cases take place outdoors or in stationary cars, and only a small number can be considered residential fires.

If a fire is defined as a lack of control over a combustion process, does this include events where people are injured or die due to the toxic effects of combustion products? This could be caused by incomplete combustion in a faulty gas-powered heater or fridge, a flue which leaks combustion products into a room, or a charcoal grill which is placed in a room or tent.

There has clearly been some lack of control of a combustion process, but in the Nordic countries this would not be considered to constitute a fire.

Perhaps the greatest challenge when comparing fire service statistics from different countries is the various ways of classifying fire-related call-outs. There is a sliding scale of incidents:

- Events with no risk of combustion
- Events with the risk of a limited combustion process but without the potential to cause damage
- Events that give rise to a combustion process which could have damaged property or health, but where the chain of events was broken before any damage took place
- Fire events where a combustion process caused property damage or injury, but the fire was extinguished before the fire service arrived

– Fire events where the fire was still burning when the fire service arrived and the fire resulted in property damage or injury

These fire-related events are not classified in the same way by the fire services in the various Nordic countries. Classification problems are most apparent for chimney fires without fire spread and fire-related events in the kitchen – often with a hot-plate or microwave oven as heat source.

Another potential source of confusion is the term "fire incident." It can be taken to mean a fire event which the fire service was called to. It can also be understood in a different way: a fire event with the potential for negative consequences, where those consequences were avoided due to fortunate circumstances or a quick and effective response by people in the vicinity.

4.3 Definitions of "Fire Death"

There are large differences between what constitutes a fire death in the statistics published by the fire authorities in different countries.

It is not the term "death" which is problematic. The problems lie in how directly the fire caused the injuries that led to the death and how much time is allowed to pass between the fire and the death.

All countries agree on deaths due to a fire's toxic or thermal properties. Differences arise when considering deaths due to injuries sustained in other ways, for example when a building which is exposed to fire collapses, or when jumping from a window in an attempt to escape from a fire.

Sometimes people are injured when escaping from a fire in a crowded space. In Estonia, a death due to injuries sustained in a crush when trying to escape from a fire would be considered a fire death.

According to the definitions used in the British IRS, fire-related fatalities are those that would not have otherwise occurred had there not been a fire. On first inspection, this sounds reasonable, but is it really appropriate to classify a death in a road accident caused by a fire crew on their way to a fire as a fire-related death?

Different countries have different maximum allowed timeframes between exposure to the effects of a fire and the moment of death. A time limit of 30 days is quite common.

In principle, it would be best not to have any time limit. If the injuries sustained in a fire led to death, then it should be counted as a fire death however long the delay. Unfortunately, this is impractical. It is difficult to follow up specific patients over time, in particular if there are periods when they are allowed to go home in between getting treatment in hospital. In addition, the longer a patient survives, the greater the probability of dying in the meantime of something unrelated to the fire. In Sweden, the Civil Contingencies Agency (MSB) has decided to follow up individual patients for 90 days. Over the past six years, MSB are only aware of one patient who has died between day 31 and day 90.

4.4 Definitions of "Fire Injury"

Fire service statistics often have a grading of injury levels, for example "serious" and "minor," but it is unclear how a fire officer without medical training can make a reliable assessment of the injury level of a particular individual. In Sweden, all they know is whether an injured person left the fire scene in an ambulance or received treatment at the fire scene. Privacy regulations prevent ambulance personnel getting back to the fire service after a fire incident to let them know about a victim's injuries and whether the victim was admitted to hospital as an in-patient.

In the Swedish context, it would seem appropriate to define a minor injury as someone who received treatment from ambulance, fire service, or police personnel at the scene of the fire. The simplest definition of serious injury would be someone who left the fire scene in an ambulance. However, they might be treated as an out-patient in an emergency facility and then sent home, or just assessed and then sent home without treatment. A more satisfactory definition of serious injury would be someone who is treated in hospital as an in-patient for at least 24 h, using data from the National Patient Register [15].

5 Discussion

5.1 Matching Data from Different Sources

There would be clear benefits for analysis if it were possible to combine data from the various sources detailed above. For advanced research, it would be valuable to combine data from fire service incident reports with data on the fire victims in other national registers.

There are three fortunate circumstances in Sweden which, taken together, have the potential to provide a unique basis for fire safety research: the use of a national personal identification number [16], a common dispatch organisation for the ambulance and fire service, and the fire service's roll in salvage operations after a fire.

All Swedish residents have a national personal identity number and public authority databases on individuals in Sweden use the national personal identity number as key.

If a research project is approved by the relevant ethics board, and the researchers are somehow able to find out the personal identity numbers of the fire victims, then they can access a wide variety of data on the individuals concerned, such as diagnoses and treatment in hospital, country of birth, level of education, taxable income, and receipt of unemployment benefit or other social benefits.

It is difficult for the fire service to collect personal identity numbers of people involved in a fire. They are quite simply too busy rescuing people threatened by the fire, extinguishing the fire, and then initiating the salvage operation to minimise secondary damage to property.

The police will attempt to collect personal identity numbers of those involved, but they also face practical challenges with this.

However, there is a reliable source for personal identity numbers for all those who leave the scene of a fire in an ambulance. The number is almost always recorded by ambulance personnel together with health status data in the patient's medical documentation.

In Sweden, the ambulance service and fire service use the same dispatch system. A common case identity number is used for all organisations responding to a specific incident. It is therefore easy to match data from the fire service with patient data recorded by ambulance personnel.

The diagnosis, health status, and medical procedure data in the ambulance documentation are of interest in itself, but the patient's personal identification number also allows a researcher to follow what procedures the patient subsequently receives in hospital, as well as giving insight into any number of characteristics of the victim which are recorded in databases administered by other national authorities. It is therefore possible for the researcher to identify vulnerable groups with an elevated risk of fire-related injury. It is also possible to go further and study a patient's history of illness. A person in full health has a much better chance of surviving fire injuries than a person who is already suffering from some kind of ill health. It is possible to study the effects of comorbidity.

When studying economic losses due to fire, it is valuable to match fire service incident report data with data from insurance companies. This is particularly challenging as the focus for insurance companies is claims, not individual fires.

The fire service in Sweden commences initial salvage work as soon as possible during a fire incident. Their work plays an important role in minimising the secondary damage to property and saves the insurance companies a great deal of money. The insurance companies gladly pay for this work.

As mentioned above, it is a challenge to match fires and insurance claims – one fire can give rise to several claims with various companies. The Swedish Fire Protection Association has a salvage company which matches the data sets, acting as a clearing house between the municipal fire brigades and the insurance companies. The salvage company receives data from the fire service incident report and links it to the insurance claims involved in the specific fire.

This match made by the salvage company has the potential to allow the analysis of the economic outcome of fires related to any of the variables collected in the fire service incident report. For example, it would become possible for cost-benefit analysis to include the economic benefit of reduced response times or technological fire protection in the form of smoke evacuation or sprinkler systems.

5.2 Legal Basis for Access to Data

There would appear to be two major challenges to building up a comprehensive system for fire safety surveillance: cost aspects and access to data. It should be possible to obtain data from existing administrative systems without excessive costs for the organisation providing the data. As noted above, in Sweden there are common keys in the most important sources, which should enable efficient matching routines to be employed by the organisation hosting the combined data. However, it must be noted that data cannot be accessed from various sources without a clear legal basis which fulfils the requirements to respect privacy as specified in data protection and secrecy regulations.

MSB have relied on data from forensic pathologists to build a comprehensive dataset over fire fatalities for the period 1999–2015. Unfortunately, the National Board of Forensic Medicine has not provided data to MSB since then, due to secrecy and data protection considerations. It is necessary for the government to clarify the legal situation for MSB to be able to update the dataset.

It is even more controversial for an organisation such as MSB to have an ongoing procedure to obtain data from the National Patient Register. In this case, it may be more appropriate for MSB to store the key – the personal identity number – of those injured due to fire. MSB could provide a researcher with a list of the relevant individuals. It would then be relatively easy for the researcher to obtain the relevant data from the patient register or any other individual-based database of interest, on the condition that the research has been approved by an ethics board.

5.3 *The Importance of Investigation of Human Behaviour in Residential Fires*

It would appear to be a common assumption that fatal fires are the tip of an iceberg – that is to say, the people who die in fires are typical of those injured in fires as well as those who experience fires in their homes. This idea promotes the assumption that the same vulnerable groups are involved in all three types of fire with the corollary that if it is possible to reduce the total number of fires then the number of fire deaths will also be reduced. However, several studies conducted in different countries and time periods report that demographic characteristics, cause of fire, and primary diagnosis differ between non-fatal injuries and fatalities [17–19]. In a recent study, the main conclusion was that, holding ignition exposure constant, a proxy developed for vulnerability could explain the effects of age on the likelihood of death in fire for adults [20].

It is important to improve our knowledge of the various subsections of the population with an elevated risk of experiencing a residential fire, being injured in a residential fire, and dying in a residential fire. This knowledge is necessary to identify vulnerable groups to prioritise in fire safety work, but in order to improve their safety, we need to know how they behave in fires.

In recent years, a research project has been underway in the UK to learn about how people respond when a fire occurs in their home, with the goal of a better understanding of the range and causes of behavioural responses to dwelling fires and the outcomes of such incidents. The "Lessons in Fire & Evacuation Behaviour in Dwellings" (LIFEBID) project has evolved from a knowledge transfer partnership between Kent Fire & Rescue Service and the University of Greenwich to a collaborative effort involving many UK fire and rescue services, academics, and other relevant stakeholders [21]. Six insight themes were presented in 2015 to engage fire and rescue services in a discussion on the relevance of data on human behaviour in accidental dwelling fires for their work with fire safety [22]. The data collection phase was completed in 2018, resulting in a database with human behaviour in approximately 500 residential fires.

Research into this material and other projects to analyse human behaviour in residential fires has the potential to provide valuable insights into how fire safety can be improved.

The WHO definition of surveillance involves ongoing data collection. However, it is very labour-intensive and therefore costly to collect data on how people thought and behaved in actual fires. In this context, it would be more beneficial, as well as more cost-effective, to collect very detailed human behaviour data in projects at an interval of five or even ten years, rather than having an ongoing collection of superficial data.

5.4 More Advanced Measurements of Deaths

The Nordic countries all publish the number of fire-related deaths per year. However, there is a great deal of random variation in the numbers, which makes it very difficult to identify short-term trends. It is easy to fall into the trap of over-interpreting a rise or fall for a period of two or three years which subsequently can be assumed to be the result of random variation.

When comparing fire-related deaths between regions or countries, it is appropriate to relate the raw numbers to population statistics. It is relatively easy to use crude death rates based on mid-year population, but it is perhaps more relevant to work with age-standardised death rates.

Death rates are an important measure to compare between regions and countries, but do not give a complete understanding of the fire problem. Potential years of life lost is an alternative metric, which is well-established in other contexts. It is interesting to note that the Emergency Services Academy in Finland calculates the yearly sum and average of potential years of life lost due to fire.

5.5 More Advanced Measurements of Serious Injury

Being treated in hospital as an in-patient for at least 24 h is a reasonably clear definition which could be used in surveillance of serious injuries due to fire. However, it might be worthwhile to develop more advanced measurements of various levels of serious injury.

Concerning burns, it might be possible to study the percentage of the total body surface area (BSA) affected by a burn, together with first-degree, second-degree, or third-degree burns.

For injuries due to smoke inhalation, it might be appropriate to study whether the person is placed on a respirator.

In addition, there are two groups of measures of health outcomes used in Sweden in surveillance of road safety, which would be worth considering for the surveillance of fire injuries.

The first group of measures indicates the severity of injuries at the time of the event. They are based on an assessment of injuries to various parts of the body according to the Abbreviated Injury Scale, AIS, developed by The Association for the Advancement of Automotive Medicine [23]. AIS is an ordinal scale of 1 to 6, with 1 indicating a minor injury, 6 being maximal, and 3 being the threshold for a serious injury to a specific part of the body. A casualty that sustains an injury with any score of 3 or higher on the AIS is classified as clinically seriously injured according to the Maximum Abbreviated Injury Scale (MAIS3+). The AIS parameters can also be used to calculate an index providing an estimate of how near the combined injuries were to being fatal at the time of the accident (Injury Severity Score, ISS 9-).

The second group of measures provides an estimate of the permanent level of disability that the injuries are expected to lead to in the long term (Risk of permanent medical impairment, RPMI), calculated for two levels of medical invalidity: 1% and 10%.

Unfortunately, RPMI would need additional research to establish fire-specific values for some parameters.

Both measures would also require data over and above that which is available in the National Patient Register, so such surveillance would come at a high cost.

6 Conclusions

The level of fire safety in a particular context is the overall result of a multitude of actions taken by many different actors. These actions will reflect conscious or unconscious decisions made by those involved.

The collection of fire data and publication of fire statistics will not in itself lead to improved fire safety. For this to take place, the data must be used in some kind of analysis, and that analysis then be used by a decision maker who goes on to take some kind of action with a positive effect on fire safety.

An ongoing, systematic collection, analysis, and interpretation of fire-related data has the potential to improve the planning, implementation, and evaluation of fire safety practice. In this chapter, data sources relevant in the Swedish context have been identified, together with theoretical and practical challenges that will need to be overcome to realise all the potential benefits. Above all, the various actors in the field of fire safety need to agree on the relevant definitions, or if that is not possible, be very clear where there is divergence on definitions.

One major challenge will be access to data. If the central fire authority in a country is not able to use data from, for example insurance companies, pathologists, or the health authorities, then it may be necessary to rely on specific research projects. If this is the case, then hopefully the conclusions of any such project will remain a good basis for decision making for a number of years after the research is published.

In order to improve residential fire safety, we need a better understanding of human behaviour in fires. It is very labour intensive to collect data on how people thought and behaved in actual fires. It is unrealistic to expect an ongoing collection of such data, but detailed data could be collected in projects with 5-year or even 10-year intervals.

It is interesting to conclude by noting that the European Commission has observed that the nature and format of fire data collected across member states vary significantly, and that this poses an obstacle to data comparison, making it difficult to assess potential best practices and successful safety approaches. The commission has initiated an ambitious project to map the existing data and develop a proposal on how the lack of common data can be remedied to provide meaningful datasets to allow legislative decisions on fire safety at member state and EU levels. [24]

References

1. https://www.who.int/immunization/monitoring_surveillance/burden/vpd/en/. Accessed 1 Mar 2021
2. Mallonee S, Istre GR, Rosenberg M, Reddish-Douglas M, Jordan F, Silverstein P, Tunell W (1996) Surveillance and prevention of residential-fire injuries. New Engl J Med 335(1):27–31
3. Viklund Å, Björnstig J, Larsson M, Björnstig U (2013) Car crash fatalities associated with fire in Sweden. Traffic Inj Prev 14(8):823–827. https://doi.org/10.1080/15389588.2013.777956
4. Jonsson A, Bergqvist A, Andersson R (2015) Assessing the number of fire fatalities in a defined population. J Saf Res 55:99–103
5. Widgren BR, Jourak M (2011) Medical Emergency Triage and Treatment System (METTS): a new protocol in primary triage and secondary priority decision in emergency medicine. J Emerg Med 40(6):623–628
6. https://icd.who.int/browse10/2019/en#/XX. Accessed 1 Mar 2021
7. https://assets.publishing.service.gov.uk/government/uploads/system/uploads/attachment_data/file/922927/fire-statistics-definitions-011020.pdf. Accessed 1 Mar 2021
8. https://ida.msb.se/ida2#page=48651f02-1df3-4900-a4a6-0e337470033c. Accessed 1 Mar 2021
9. https://assets.publishing.service.gov.uk/government/uploads/system/uploads/attachment_data/file/724327/Fire_and_Fire_Safety.pdf. Accessed 23 May 2021
10. https://www.cpsc.gov/s3fs-public/UnreportedResidentialFires.pdf. Accessed 23 May 2021
11. http://nordicfirestatistics.org. Accessed 1 Mar 2021
12. https://www.usfa.fema.gov/downloads/pdf/nfirs/NFIRS_Complete_Reference_Guide_2015.pdf. Accessed 1 Mar 2021
13. https://www.iso.org/obp/ui/#iso:std:iso:13943:ed-3:v1:en. Accessed 1 Mar 2021
14. NFPA 921 Guide for Fire and Explosion Investigations (2008). National Fire Protection Association

15. https://www.socialstyrelsen.se/en/statistics-and-data/registers/register-information/the-national-patient-register/. Accessed 1 Mar 2021
16. Ludvigsson JF, Otterblad-Olausson P, Pettersson BU, Ekbom A (2009) The Swedish personal identity number: possibilities and pitfalls in healthcare and medical research. Eur J Epidemiol 24(11):659–667
17. Levine MS, Radford EP (1977) Fire victims: medical outcomes and demographic characteristics. Am J Public Health 67:1077–1080
18. Mulvaney C, Kendrick D, Towner E, Brussoni M, Hayes M, Powell J, Ward H (2008) Fatal and non-fatal fire injuries in England 1995–2004: time trends and inequalities by age, sex and area deprivation. J Public Health (Bangkok) 31:154–161
19. Jonsson A, Nilson F, Bonander C, Huss F (2018) Seriously injured due to residential fires in Sweden. Inj Prev:24
20. Gilbert SW, Butry DT (2018) Identifying vulnerable populations to death and injuries from residential fires. Inj Prev 24:358–364
21. https://fseg.gre.ac.uk/lifebid/about/index.html. Accessed 7 Feb 2021
22. Wales D, Thompson O, Hulse L, Galea E (2015) Human behaviour in fire. In: Proceedings 6th international symposium. Cambridge Interscience Communications Ltd, London, pp 465–476. ISBN:978-0-9933933-0-3
23. https://www.aaam.org/abbreviated-injury-scale-ais/. Accessed 20 May 2021
24. https://eufirestat-efectis.com/. Accessed 1 Mar 2021

Mr. Colin McIntyre holds a BSc in Mathematics from Edinburgh University. In the 1990s, Colin coordinated an analysis of what kind of statistics were needed to improve decision-making in the Swedish fire and rescue service. He then led the development of the system for data collection from fire service incident reports. He now works at the Swedish Civil Contingencies Agency with analysis of a range of statistics on fires, accidents and the emergency responses of the fire and rescue service.

Dr. Anders Jonsson is since 2001 working as a statistician within the area of accident and injury analysis at the Learning from Accidents Section within the Swedish Civil Contingencies Agency. He took his PhD in Risk Management at Karlstad University, Sweden, in 2018 on "Fire-related deaths in Sweden: An analysis of data quality, causes and risk patterns".

Chapter 7
Implications for Prevention

Ragnar Andersson and Marcus Runefors

Abstract This chapter summarizes Chaps. 1, 2, 3, 4 and 5 and introduces the principles of injury prevention. It is concluded that important aspects of human vulnerability appear largely overlooked in traditional fire safety practices and need to be addressed much more seriously if deaths and injuries are to be significantly reduced. When residential fires exceptionally lead to serious harm, it is often due to certain medical, functional, and/or social vulnerabilities of the victim. Since the same vulnerabilities tend to put residents at risk of many other health and safety hazards as well, the fire safety community should join efforts with health and social resources to develop broader programs for safer housing among vulnerable groups, including fire safety. As part of this, new and innovative fire-related solutions are urgently needed to better compensate for human shortcomings in the event of a fire at home.

Keywords Fire safety · Human vulnerability · Mortality · Morbidity · Collaboration · Home safety

1 Introduction – Empirical Summary

The preceding chapters all contribute to a richer understanding of the global fire safety problem. Chapter 1 identifies major data availability and validity problems in many countries, but from what is published on international fire mortality, patterns emerge which seem to reflect well-known global socioeconomic and gender

R. Andersson (✉)
Risk and Environmental Studies, Centre for Societal Risk Research, Karlstad University, Karlstad, Sweden
e-mail: ragnar.andersson@kau.se

M. Runefors
Division of Fire Safety Engineering, Lund University, Lund, Sweden

© The Author(s), under exclusive license to Springer Nature Switzerland AG 2023
M. Runefors et al. (eds.), *Residential Fire Safety*, The Society of Fire Protection Engineers Series, https://doi.org/10.1007/978-3-031-06325-1_7

inequalities as well as lifestyle and other cultural patterns such as smoking and alcohol habits, and clothing and cooking traditions. As countries develop, fewer people tend to die from fire, and a transition seems to occur from younger to older victims. Possibly, this also implies a shift over time from female to male victims, as females remain overrepresented mostly in low-income countries while men are at greater risk in high-income countries. Risk factors for residential fire death are explored more in-depth in Chap. 2, identifying both living alone and being under weaker socioeconomic conditions as significant determinants together with demographic and lifestyle factors such as alcohol consumption and smoking. Chapter 3 widens the scope to all residential fires, regardless of consequences, and concludes that most fires seem to be successfully handled by the residents themselves without injuries and without assistance from fire and rescue services. Only exceptionally, residential fires lead to serious harm, and when that happens, it is usually due to certain vulnerabilities related to the victim.

One critical aspect of vulnerability is evacuation ability, as described in Chap. 4. For residents with functional impairments, whether perceptual, cognitive, or motor, normal housing conditions may raise significant barriers for safe evacuation in due time. Chapter 5 identifies intoxication and burn as the leading injury mechanisms from domestic fire. In many cases, intoxication comes first and tends to gradually incapacitate the victim before the heat becomes critical. Both mechanisms covariate with the exposed individual's age, health, and functional status. Being under the influence of alcohol, medicines, or other substances (including CO from smoking) will accelerate the incapacitation process. The time frame for evacuation is short. Prompt and adequate care (prehospital and clinical) impacts survival and injury severity as well, which makes health care a complementary parameter in reducing death and severe injuries from fires. Finally, as pointed out in Chap. 6, proper surveillance of fire-related injuries and deaths is a fundamental prerequisite for the systematic prevention thereof.

2 General Accident and Injury Prevention Principles

This book concentrates on the prevention of deaths and injuries from fires. Experts in fire safety are usually well trained in fire engineering, but less trained in injury prevention. This gap is what we here wish to bridge with complementary perspectives and theoretical frameworks. When analysing accident and injury causation, a web of intertwined factors emerges behind both the events and their consequences. The consequences are always associated with more contributing factors since these also include vulnerability-related factors in addition to those leading up to the event. Deaths and injuries from fires are therefore not explained solely by the occurrence of the fire, but also by a number of additional factors determining the severity of its outcome.

Injury prevention is a discipline rooted in the medical sphere, taking human vulnerability to sudden external impacts as its point of departure. The nature of impacts varies by type of events; mechanical in case of traffic crashes or falls, thermal and toxic in case of fire, and so on. Humans, just as other species, entail intrinsic tolerances against external impacts to certain degrees, but if the thresholds are exceeded, injuries and death may follow. Moreover, tolerance varies from individual to individual depending on age, sex, health status, etc.

As we now recognize that most people manage fires without being injured and that those killed and severely injured increasingly appear among socially, functionally, and medically disadvantaged groups, the focus of interest will inevitably shift from an exclusive focus on the exposure (the fire) to the specific circumstances that exceptionally contribute to severe outcomes, that is toward the vulnerability side of the problem. The fire occurrence is clearly a necessary cause, but far from sufficient to explain why people die or sustain severe injuries from a fire. It is therefore the complementary causes determining the severe outcomes we need to identify, understand, and address to become able to seriously deal with the number of deaths and injuries from fires.

One of the most influential researchers on injury prevention, representing a human-centered and vulnerability-oriented approach, is undoubtedly Dr. William Haddon Jr. [1, 2]. He had a combined background in epidemiology, medicine, and engineering and published extensively on the principles of prevention, while, at the same time, serving as the first appointed director of the then newly established American federal traffic safety agency in the 1960s [3]. Haddon built his conceptualization of injury causation and prevention on existing frameworks in public health and epidemiology, especially the so-called epidemiologic triad; the host (the exposed individual), the agent (the hazard), and the environment [4]. Accordingly, illness, including injuries, is generally seen as emanating from an interaction between these three components. What distinguishes injuries from diseases is the agent factor, which in the case of injuries consists of a sudden release of energy (or the sudden absence thereof), in contrast to biological or other health hazards. Fractures result from mechanical energy, burns from thermal etc. if exposures occur at amounts and intensity exceeding thresholds for human tolerance. Understanding human tolerance (the vulnerability side) is, therefore, just as important as understanding the sudden hazard exposure conditions (the accident) from a preventative point of view. The basic principle for injury prevention is to control potential exposures and preferably keep them under the human threshold limits. Haddon also built on the, in health sciences well-established, view that preventative measures can be taken in three phases; before, during, and even after an injury occur. Primary preventative measures (before) aim to prevent the exposure as such (the accident), while secondary (during) and tertiary (after) preventions aim to reduce the injury severity, either during the accident sequence (secondary) or afterwards (tertiary) through medical treatment and rehabilitation [5]. One of Haddon's most famous theoretical contributions is the so-called Haddon Matrix, resulting from a cross-tabulation of the epidemiological triad and the three temporal phases of prevention [1, 4].

Haddon's theoretical contributions have influenced safety philosophy in many areas, perhaps most clearly in road traffic where the energy perspective, that injuries ultimately are caused by energies allowed to reach individuals at levels exceeding human thresholds of tolerance and therefore need to be kept under these thresholds, has become a dimensioning principle of vehicle and road environment design [6]. The Haddon Matrix is frequently applied as an analytic tool to a wide spectrum of topics in safety research, as well as in public health research in general [1].

Haddon also contributed with a well-known list of ten preventative alternatives, spanning from primary to tertiary prevention [4].

1. To prevent the creation of the hazard in the first place
2. To reduce the amount of hazard brought into being
3. To prevent the release of the hazard that already exists
4. To modify the rate or spatial distribution of release of the hazard from its source
5. To separate, in time or space, the hazard and that which is to be protected
6. To separate the hazard and that which is to be protected by the interposition of a material barrier
7. To modify relevant basic qualities of the hazard
8. To make what is to be protected more resistant to damage from the hazard
9. To begin to counter the damage already done by the environmental hazard
10. To stabilize, repair, and rehabilitate the object of the damage

Reason [7] contributed with a similar view when arguing for, what he called, the principle of "defense-in-depth", meaning that there is usually a need for several barriers complementing each other. His so-called "Swiss Cheese Model" illustrates how multiple barriers (imaged as cheese slices), each of them with their weaknesses (the holes in the slices), when combined, may complement each other in reducing the likelihood of serious consequences if a harmful event should occur. Thus, one gets access to not just a plan A, but also a plan B, C, D, and so on, in order to reduce the targeted outcome.

The medically anchored approach in injury prevention, as exemplified by Haddon's theoretical contributions, is a fundamental point of departure in all safety management aiming at preventing human consequences such as deaths and injuries. In addition, safety research has contributed with more engineering-oriented frameworks focused on the events as such (as opposed to the consequences) and their causes, plus managerial issues in administration and organizations to advance performance in safety work. It is, of course, not enough to know what should be done; it takes systematics and leadership as well to make things done and ensure intended results in a societal or organizational context. Part II of this book provides examples of effective measures to save lives and prevent injuries from fire, and the final section will highlight issues on how to implement such measures and make things happen at a broader scale.

3 Implications for the Prevention of Fire-Related Deaths and Injuries

The above summarized can be concluded as follows:

It is always the consequences that burden individuals and the community, and therefore, the consequences that need to be prevented and reduced, in this case, deaths and injuries from a fire. A radical way of doing this is to prevent the fires as such. However, since fires remain relatively common, while serious injuries from these are rare, it might be more effective to direct preventative efforts to the contributing factors that mostly determine the negative consequences.

Preventing serious injuries from fire, ultimately deaths, can be accomplished by interventions across the entire process from before to after the fire, see Fig. 7.1. The measures taken can be either individually, technically, and/or organizationally oriented. The principle of "defense-in-depth" is clearly applicable [7].

With reference to Fig. 7.1, the fire-injury process can be described as follows:

1. Ignition may occur through spark, open flame, or hot object.
2. For the fire to grow, it takes dry combustible material in the presence of oxygen.
3. The emissions that harm living organisms in case of fire include toxic gases and heat, primarily. The gases typically attack first by incapacitating the victim. The toxicity depends on the material that is burning, ventilation conditions, and if smouldering or open flame.
4. The degree of exposure, in combination with the lethality of the emissions, determines the speed of the injury process.
5. If the fire continues and escalates, evacuation remains the only option. This can be performed either without assistance or with assistance from cohabitants, neighbours, or professional resources.
6. For those evacuated injured, but still alive, there remains the possibility of avoiding worsening complications and restoring health through adequate treatment and rehabilitation. The result determines the final outcome in terms of deaths and injury severity.

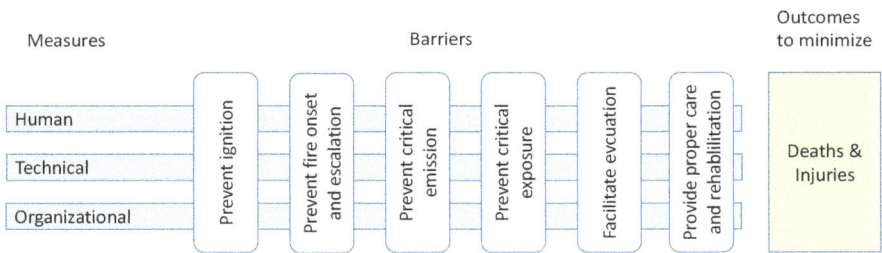

Fig. 7.1 A tentative illustration of the fire-injury process and how deaths and injuries from fires may be counteracted by interventions along the entire process from pre-fire to post-fire conditions

Preventative measures are all those intervening in the implied process and affecting the final outcome. As pointed out, the measures can be individually, technically, or organizationally oriented, separately or in combination. Weaknesses in one respect can be compensated by strengthened measures in other respects. Humans are often considered the least reliable component of so-called sociotechnical systems, and the less one can expect from the individual, the more efforts need to be placed on technology and organization to compensate for human shortcomings. In the context of residential fires and vulnerable groups, the organization can be seen to include actors with the role of supporting the individual, such as social services and medical resources.

Accumulated evidence now demonstrates that serious injury outcomes from fire, including deaths, increasingly are to be seen as a vulnerability problem, at least in richer countries with ageing populations. Vulnerability aspects play roles in several phases of the fire-injury process, such as increasing the risk of ignition and escalation, reducing the capacity to evacuate, and impairing the medical resilience and capacity to respond to care and rehabilitation. Thus, the strategical alternatives to reduce the impact of human vulnerability remain:

1. To try to reduce vulnerabilities, that is, strengthening capacities and resilience among groups at risk
2. To try to compensate for the vulnerabilities by means of technical and organizational arrangements in

    (a) Existing homes, as complementary arrangements
    (b) Alternative homes, meeting higher intrinsic safety standards (e.g. nursing homes)

The first alternative encompasses three perspectives; first, the medical vulnerability following increasing age and illness and resulting in reduced resilience to a fire's physiological injury mechanisms; second, impaired perceptual and cognitive capacities resulting in increased difficulties to perceive and understand what might happen; and third, a reduced physical capacity to act adequately. To address these impairments and reach significant improvements entail considerable challenges, but general efforts to promote health at the population level can be expected to result in long-term positive effects.

Alternative 2a offers certain possibilities in terms of warning systems that are easier to perceive and understand, and extinguishing systems activated automatically. Redirecting warning signals to neighbours or professional first responders ready to assist swiftly is another possibility.

Alternative 2b offers the most radical possibilities to improve the protection for those unable to care for themselves for their safety. The enhanced safety standard may include organizational arrangements as well, such as the continuous presence of staff with sufficient capacities to intervene in case of danger.

7 Implications for Prevention

4 Technical and Organizational Measures for Prevention

As described above, decreasing the vulnerability of the individual is one of the main goals of public health and medical services, but this might be difficult to address from a fire-specific perspective. Therefore, the majority of this anthology is focused

Table 7.1 Haddon matrix of risk factors and prevention inspired by Gielen et al. [8] with references to other chapters in this anthology where more details are provided

		Host	Equipment	Physical environment	Socio/Cultural environment
Pre-event	Prevention of unwanted heat generation	Stop smoking	Safe cigarettes (Chap. 10)	Safe electrical system	Electrical codes
			Childproof lighters		Smoking campaigns (Chap. 16)
					Education not to play with fire (Chap. 16)
	Prevention of ignition	Drug use	Fire-resistant materials (Chap. 10)		Legislation on furniture combustibility (Chap. 10)
		Alcohol	Stove guard (Chap. 11)		
		Disabilities (Chap. 5)	Smoking apron (Chap. 10)		
			Self-extinguishing candles		
Event	Prevention of fire growth	Knowledge of suppression	Fire retardant materials (Chap. 10)	Closed doors (Chap. 9)	Legislation on fire compartmentation
				Residential sprinklers (Chap. 11)	Fire prevention programmes (Chap. 16)
				Detector activated sprinklers (Chap. 11)	
	Initiation of evacuation	Correct appreciation of fire growth rate		Smoke alarms (Chap. 8)	Laws requiring smoke alarms
		Cognitive disability (e.g. hearing) (Chap. 5)			Smoke alarm campaigns (Chap. 16)
	Completion of evacuation	Physical disability (Chap. 5)		Fire resistance of load-bearing structures	Evacuation by the fire service (Chap. 12)
				Door lock easy to open	Evacuation by other actors
Post-event	Recovery	Medical vulnerability (Chap. 4)			Treatment of burns (Chap. 4)

on technical and organizational aspects aiming to compensate for this vulnerability.

Inspired by Gielen et al. [8], a modified Haddon-matrix has been developed and is presented in Table 7.1. In the matrix, the temporal dimension is divided into several subsections adopted from Runefors et al. [9] where it was found to be a generic sequence of events in fatal fires.

For each phase, the opportunities for prevention are divided into four different categories: Host, Equipment, Physical environment, and Socio/Cultural environment. The Host relates to aspects in relation to the victim themselves or other individuals and could be, for example, attitudes, knowledge, and behaviour. The Equipment includes aspects of the specific objects involved in the fire, while the Physical environment includes other objects in the environment. Finally, Socio/Cultural factors are external factors such as legislation, campaigns, and institutions such as the rescue service and hospitals.

The matrix, including a range of different identified measures, is presented in Table 7.1.

As can be seen in the table above, there is a wide range of different measures that can all be a part of a fire safety strategy. The measures are not presented here, but the reader is referred to the chapter in this anthology which is cited in the table.

Due to the variation in both exposure and vulnerability, the effectiveness of different technical measures also varies significantly between different socio-demographic groups in society, and this is also true for who currently have the different measures implemented. This is further discussed in Chap. 14.

5   Conclusions

Section one of this anthology clearly shows that fatalities due to residential fires are strongly related to the vulnerability of the individual. It is of paramount importance for fire safety professionals to acknowledge this fact and let it influence the strategies developed.

Despite this, it is argued that directly influencing the vulnerability of the individual is typically out of reach for fire safety professionals. Instead, fire prevention should focus on compensatory measures from a technical and organizational perspective. A range of such measures that each can play a role in fire safety promotion is presented in the following section of this anthology.

However, even if fire safety professionals typically are not able to affect the vulnerability aspect per se, it is very important to apply the knowledge of risk factors presented in Chap. 1 to target safety promotion activities to individuals with high risk. Since the same risk factors tend to put residents at risk of many other health and safety hazards as well, the fire safety community should join efforts with health and social resources to develop broader programs for safer housing among vulnerable groups, including fire safety.

References

1. Runyan C (2003) Introduction: back to the future – revisiting Haddon's conceptualization of injury epidemiology and prevention. Epidemiol Rev 25:60–64
2. Williams AF (1999) The Haddon matrix: its contribution to injury prevention and control. In: Third national conference on injury prevention and control, pp 1999-05-09–1999-05-12
3. Independent Council for Road Safety International, ICORSI. Dr. William Haddon, Jr. (1926–1985). https://www.icorsi.org/dr-william-haddon-jr-1926-1985. Accessed Sept 2021
4. Haddon W (1980) Advances in the epidemiology of injuries as a basis for public policy. Publ Health Rep 95(5):411–421
5. Gjestland T (1955) The Oslo study of untreated syphilis. Acta Derm Venereol Suppl, p 34
6. Johansson R (2009) Vision Zero – implementing a policy for traffic safety. Saf Sci 47:826–831
7. Reason J (1997) Managing the risks of organizational accidents. Ashgate, Aldershot
8. Gielen AC, Frattaroli S, Pollack KM, Peek-Asa C, Yang JG (2018) How the science of injury prevention contributes to advancing home fire safety in the USA: successes and opportunities. Inj Prev 24:i7–i13. https://doi.org/10.1136/injuryprev-2017-042356
9. Runefors M, Johansson N, van Hees P (2016) How could the fire fatalities have been prevented? An analysis of 144 cases during 2011–2014 in Sweden. J Fire Sci 34(6):515–527. https://doi.org/10.1177/0734904116667962

Prof. Ragnar Andersson is a Senior Professor of Risk Management affiliated to Karlstad University in Sweden where he served as full professor from 2001 until retirement in 2015. His educational background is in engineering and public health. After serving for the Swedish National Board of Occupational Safety and Health in the 1970s and 1980s, he took his PhD in Social Medicine at Karolinska Institutet, Sweden, in 1991 on occupational injury prevention. Dr. Andersson's research is focused on accident and injury analysis and prevention, injury surveillance, and macro-level determinants of risk in broad fields such as occupational, traffic, product, child, senior, and fire safety.

Dr. Marcus Runefors is a lecturer at the Division of Fire Safety Engineering at Lund University in Sweden, where he also finished his PhD in the beginning of 2020. The topic of his PhD was fatal residential fires from both a prevention and response perspective, focusing on the effectiveness of different measures to prevent fatal fires for different groups in the population.

Part II
Preventive Measures for Residential Fires

Chapter 8
Smoke Alarms and the Human Response

Michelle Ball and Kara Dadswell

Abstract Smoke alarms are mandated in all man-made structures designed for human occupancy in most developed nations, and as such, they have become a normal and expected feature of our environment. Most people understand that their purpose is to alert building occupants to the possibility of fire. Despite this, it is wrong to assume that when a smoke alarm sounds the human response will be uniformly predictable. There are many different factors influencing whether or not a person will respond to an alarm, and these vary depending upon whether a person is awake or asleep, and audibility factors within the environment. This chapter will begin with a brief history of smoke alarm use and design and then proceed to a review of recent literature on human response to the smoke alarm signal when people are asleep, and when they are awake.

Keywords Smoke alarms · Human response · Auditory arousal · Cognitive processing during sleep · Alarm signal characteristics

1 Smoke Alarms

1.1 Brief History

Despite their pervasive presence in modern structures, smoke alarms have a relatively brief history compared to other fundamental inventions of modern engineering and architecture. Smoke alarms were not widely used in residential settings until events following Hurricane Agnes in 1971 pointed to their effectiveness. As a part of their disaster relief effort, the US Department of Housing and Urban Development

---

M. Ball (✉) · K. Dadswell
Institute for Health and Sport, Victoria University, Melbourne, VIC, Australia
e-mail: Michelle.Ball@vu.edu.au

© The Author(s), under exclusive license to Springer Nature Switzerland AG 2023
M. Runefors et al. (eds.), *Residential Fire Safety*, The Society of Fire Protection Engineers Series, https://doi.org/10.1007/978-3-031-06325-1_8

purchased 17 000 mobile homes and requested that the National Bureau of Standards (NSB; later to be known as NIST) implement high standard fire safety systems [19]. Consequently, single station smoke alarms were installed outside the bedrooms of each unit. In the ensuing years after the homes were inhabited, the statistically predicted number of fires still occurred, but zero deaths and very few injuries were recorded. From this stunning change in outcomes, it was surmised that smoke alarms were an effective means of alerting occupants to the presence of fire before they could become trapped, and the US mobile housing industry adopted the first smoke alarm regulation, decreeing that one smoke alarm was to be installed outside the bedrooms of every mobile home produced [19].

The mandating of smoke alarms in mobile homes precipitated the NSB to more closely examine their effectiveness, and work commenced to develop standards regarding the optimal number and placement of smoke alarms in residential homes. The Indiana Dunes tests were conducted, involving full scale testing of commercially available smoke alarms that were purposefully installed in homes prior to set demolishment [19]. Over a period of 2 years, 76 separate experiments were conducted using three different homes and involving the burning of real furnishings in varied conditions (e.g., doors/windows open or closed). Results of these experiments led to the conclusion that for optimum safety, smoke alarms should be located on each floor of a home [19]. This recommendation was adopted and laws were enacted across various jurisdictions in the US that required the installation of smoke alarms on each floor in new residential housing. From these promising beginnings, progress was slow. Internationally, laws regarding smoke alarm installation and placement have gradually been implemented, but it took many nations until the first decade of the 2000s for smoke alarms to be made compulsory in residences.

It is important to note that while the reduction in fire deaths following the advancements in smoke alarm legislation is clear, several other coinciding factors may also have lowered the incidence of injury and death. For example, advancements in the engineering of building materials, household furniture and items, and sleeping garments have afforded increased fire protection. Nonetheless, evidence indicates that smoke alarms are a vital component to improved fire safety systems.

Contemporary data continue to support the effectiveness of smoke alarms in the reduction of risk of death in residential fires. When considering the impact of smoke alarms, it is convenient to consider US statistics because the size of the population lends a robustness to the data. US data on home structure fires that were reported to local fire departments spanning the years from 2014 to 2018 indicated that the risk of dying in a home structure fire was 55% lower in homes where there was a working smoke alarm, compared to homes with no smoke alarms present, or none that operated [1]. The power source and method of extinguishment also seem to be important. When automatic extinguishing systems were not present, the death rate per 1000 fires was 35% lower when battery powered smoke alarms were present, 69% lower when the smoke alarms were hard-wired, and 51% lower when smoke alarms with either source of power were present. This climbed to 91%, lower when hard-wired smoke alarms were present with sprinklers [1]. A 2016 meta-analysis using data from US and Australian studies examining the association between smoke alarm presence and injury and death rates reported that the presence of a working smoke alarm halved the death rate in residential fires, but that there was no significant reduction in injuries due to their presence [58].

1.2 Smoke Alarm Types

A smoke alarm consists of two basic components within a single unit, including a smoke detector and an alarm sounding device (signal). Specifications for smoke alarms are generally mandated by local standards. These standards generally dictate aspects of both the detector and the alarm signal that are designed to increase the chance that occupants will be warned of a fire in time to evacuate or extinguish the fire while it is small, thereby decreasing the chance of damage to property, injury, and /or death of occupants. The detector should be designed to be sensitive to small levels of smoke, but at the same time not too sensitive to non-fire-related phenomena in an effort to reduce false alarms, which may cause undesirable behaviors such as the ignoring or disabling of alarms [69].

Smoke alarms vary in how they detect smoke, and how they are powered. New one or two family dwellings across many countries are now required to include smoke alarm units that are hard-wired into the main electricity supply by a professional electrician. These hard-wired units also include a 9 Volt (V) back–up battery in case of power failure. In older dwellings, and by far the most common type of smoke detector, is the independently operating battery powered unit. These devices are installed locally, without the need for professional services, and can be powered by a 9V battery that needs yearly replacement, or by a longer lasting lithium battery (approx. 10 year life). Regardless of power source, both manufacturers and fire services recommended that all smoke alarm units need to be replaced every 10 years to ensure optimal performance. Fire services commonly run public service campaigns to prompt correct maintenance of smoke alarms.

Individual smoke alarms can also be interconnected. Interconnection is an important safety feature that is recommended so that if smoke is detected in the area of one device, they all sound together, thereby increasing the possibility of alerting occupants who may be remote from the smoke alarm closest to the area of fire ignition [49]. Interconnection is mandated in some countries. For example, it has been mandated for new dwellings in the USA since 1989 (NFPA 72; [51]), and in Australia since 2014 [3]. Recently, Scottish legislation in relation to smoke alarms has been updated and has extended the requirement for interconnection to all existing dwellings by 2022 [59].

There are two primary types of detector that are typically used in either hardwired or battery-operated smoke alarm units, including ionization and photoelectric. Smoke alarms are also available that include dual sensors, with one of each type. The two types of detector sense the presence of smoke differently, varying in their response to the visible and invisible properties of smoke [50]. An ionization type of alarm contains a small amount of the radioactive material, Americum-241, situated between two electrically charged plates. The Americum-241 ionizes the air between these plates, causing an electrical current to flow between them. The alarm is activated when smoke enters the chamber of the detector, disrupting the current between the plates. In contrast, photoelectric detectors contain a light source and a light sensor within a sensing chamber. This light source is aimed at an angle away from the sensor, and smoke entering the chamber causes the light to be reflected towards the sensor, causing the alarm to activate [52].

A slowly growing fire that smolders emits more toxic gases and produces larger particles in smoke compared to a flaming fire. This type of fire is commonly associated with burning of household items, for example upholstered furniture that is ignited by a heat source such as a lit cigarette. Conversely, a flaming fire burns faster and hotter and emits smaller particles in smoke. A substantial body of research comparing the performance of different types of smoke detector has reported that upon average, ionization alarms respond fastest in the circumstance of a flaming fire, while photoelectric alarms respond fastest to a smoldering fire (e.g., [20, 24]).

The best type of smoke detector for use in residential settings has emerged as a controversial issue. Public health advocates have argued that photoelectric alarms are superior to ionization alarms for several reasons (e.g., [57]). First, they cite the increased possibility of nuisance alarms that occur with ionization alarms [72], particularly associated with smoke from cooking, leading to decreased functionality because they are more likely to be deliberately disabled by residents. There is certainly evidence in the peer-reviewed literature that ionization alarms are significantly less likely to be functional across time, presumably due to disconnection following repeated nuisance alarms [50]. Second, they also argue that since most residential fires begin as smoldering before transitioning (or not) to flaming, the safest approach is to legislate the use of photoelectric or dual sensor alarms (combination photoelectric/ionization), and have called for a ban on the sale of ionization alarms. There is some evidence that this has occurred in a few regions, for example, a 2007 report for the European Commission on products containing radiation shows that ionization alarms have been prohibited in Switzerland (single, stand-alone units only, with those used as a part of an interconnected system still permitted), Lithuania, and the Netherlands [61]. It is also understood that a small number of states in the USA (Iowa, Massachusetts, and Vermont) may have limited their use by mandating dual sensor alarms (combination photoelectric/ionization). Many other governing bodies have considered this idea, but have not taken it up, primarily because photoelectric and dual sensor alarms are appreciably more expensive than ionization alarms, and it is considered that having an ionization alarm is better than having no alarm at all. Across the world, fire services and fire safety associations widely promote the use of photoelectric or dual sensor alarms as the products of choice for use in residential settings; however, the issue of cost means that ionization alarms remain substantially more prevalent.

Regardless of fire scenario, it is important to note that there is wide variability in the operation of detectors both between and within types, to certain fires. Milarcik et al. [48] statistically compared the performance of different types of residential smoke detection technologies with each other (including ionization, photoelectric, and dual sensor), for differing types of fire (smoldering or flaming) across four published large-scale experimental studies. The findings reported were consistent with the fact that upon average ionization, alarms perform fastest to flaming fires and photoelectric alarms respond fastest to smoldering fires, and when all fires were considered, the dual sensor alarms performed best. However, they also found that overall the difference in response between the technologies was so small as to be statistically equivalent, stating that "…it cannot be determined with confidence which detector technology will alarm first to the next fire" (p. 337). Analysis further showed wide variability between different detectors within each type, regardless of fire scenario. This is compounded by the fact that it is generally unknown which type of fire will next ignite – flaming or smoldering? They concluded that debates about type of detector technology are less instructive and less likely to make a difference to residential fire mortality than efforts to increase the number of detectors present. They argue that increasing the number of detectors in any environment would have the effect of maximizing detection regardless of the circumstances of ignition [48].

Another important factor to be considered is tenability limits. In reference to fire, tenability refers to the ability of an environment to sustain life and is related to things such as heat conditions and toxic gas concentrations. A 2009 study into tenability limits and smoke alarm response reported that flaming fire scenarios produced the most dangerous conditions, with tenability limits exceeded often within just minutes after ignition [47]. Smoldering fires, on the other hand, were found to take much longer to produce untenable conditions, sometimes taking hours to exceed limits. Importantly, it was also reported that alarms of all three types (ionization, photoelectric, and combined) generally provided sufficient time for escape before tenability limits were exceeded for both flaming and smoldering fire scenarios [47]. Although tenability of life is paramount, exposure to smoke poses both acute and chronic threats to health, and therefore, alerting occupants as soon as possible to the presence of fire remains an important consideration beyond survival.

1.3 Standards Governing Smoke Alarms

Standards for smoke alarm signals specify many technical aspects and vary across different countries. Examples in this chapter are provided from the International Standards, the USA, Australia, and the UK only. Additionally, only those in relation to sound pressure level, placement, and signal design (temporal pattern) will be discussed herein. Information about signal pitch is covered in the later section on human response to the smoke alarm, and so, will not be specifically covered in this section.

In relation to sound pressure, although there are subtle variations across nations, the prescribed sound level is commonly not less than 85dBA within a set distance from the sounder (AS 3786 set distance is 3 m; [68]), and no more than 105dBA. The lower threshold is to ensure audibility, and the upper limit is designed to be withstood for short periods without causing hearing damage. This broad rule encapsulates the important notion that an alarm's signal must be loud enough to be heard; however, the same alarm signal may be experienced differently across differing environments. In acknowledgment of this fact, standards usually require that sound pressure be transmitted at a minimum level above the average ambient sound level [e.g., 10dBA above for ISO-8201 [34]; 15dBA above or 5dBA above the maximum sound level having a duration of about 60 seconds for NFPA 72 [51]]. Standards commonly also suggest that the signal should be received at 75dBA at the pillow or bedhead in sleeping areas [9].

Another important specification relates to the placement of alarms. Mandates regarding placement can vary, but the majority of jurisdictions require at least one on each level of a home, with particular emphasis given to placement either within (e.g., USA), or immediately outside the sleeping areas (e.g., UK, Australia). Placement of alarms has a strong influence over the audibility of the alarm signal, as does environmental design. Although the effect is only quite small, a sound will be somewhat amplified in an environment that contains mostly hard surfaces, but somewhat attenuated in an environment in which soft surfaces predominate, such as a bedroom [31]. The same applies to the size of a room, with a sound diminished in a larger space compared to a smaller one [32]. Sound dissipates as it travels, and obviously the further away an operating alarm is from occupants, the less likely it will be heard. Research has shown that the audibility of an alarm signal travelling through walls from a separate room will be substantially decreased regardless of whether the door/s between the alarm and the occupant are closed [32, 43, 49] or open [49]. This attenuation of sound is also affected by the pitch of the alarm signal, with sounds of higher frequency becoming more diminished than those of lower pitch across distances and through barriers [49].

International standards influence some aspects of smoke alarm design and are often drawn upon to inform national standards. For example, International standard 8201 (ISO-8201) titled "Acoustics – Audible and Other Emergency Evacuation Signals" outlines the minimum requirements for aspects relating to the sound emitted by fire alarms and other emergency warning devices that are used across a range of circumstances, including residences and other places where people might be sleeping [34]. It outlines the specifications of the signal that is intended to be used to alert building occupants to the need to immediately evacuate the premises. This standard sets out a repeating three-pulse temporal pattern of 4 seconds duration referred to as the Temporal-Three (T-3). It is comprised of three 0.5 s beeps (on phase), each separated by 0.5 s pause (off phase). Each cluster of three beeps is then separated by a longer 1.5 s pause. The signal should be transmitted at a minimum of 10dBA (decibels; A-weighted sound pressure) above the background noise, and not lower than 65dBA. If it is to be used to awaken sleeping individuals, the minimum sound level is increased to 75dBA at the bedhead, with all doors closed. The standard includes the possibility that a voice alarm can be added with the signal if desired, e.g., Fire! Evacuate! It should be noted that in circumstances where the desired outcome is for occupants to remain in place, then the fire alarm should transmit a distinctly different pattern.

This international standard was designed with the purpose of having a single temporal pattern that would be universally recognizable as signifying the need to evacuate immediately. A standard temporal pattern that is widely recognized by the public is seen as preferable to a voice alarm as it transcends possible misunderstanding that could arise from language barriers. Despite this, historical research has found that signals emitting this temporal pattern are not well-recognized as fire alarm or evacuation signals [27, 56]. Most smoke alarms are now manufactured using the T3 signal, and it is unknown whether recognition has improved in more recent years due to increased familiarity.

2 Human Response to the Smoke Alarm

2.1 Response When People Are Sleeping

Although standards exist to mandate sound pressure and placement of smoke alarms, research examining the best signal to initiate human response was slower to emerge. In fact, early development of smoke alarm technology was focused upon the detection aspects of device design, with little attention paid to signal characteristics beyond the fact that it should be loud enough to be heard [13]. The high frequency beeping noise was used as it was deemed relatively uncommon, and therefore, easy to be distinguished and identified. It was also considered unpleasantly piercing, and therefore, not easy to ignore. From an engineering perspective, it was also cheaper and easier to produce in a small battery-operated device than lower-pitched sounds [9].

By the early 2000s, about 10 years after smoke alarm installation became more widely mandated, accumulated evidence from fire fatality statistics indicated that more residential fire deaths occurred in the presence of an operating smoke alarm than was expected. Examination of these statistics showed that several groups remained at increased risk of death in fire due to individual differences including older (70+) or younger (preschool) age (e.g., [6, 46, 60]), being male, being under the influence of alcohol (e.g., [29, 35, 67, 71]), smoking (e.g., [35, 71]), having a disability (e.g., [1]), and mental health status [70]. The risk becomes compounded when these factors are combined, for example smoking and drinking alcohol (e.g., [5, 54, 70]). A 2015 study comparing outcomes from fatal residential fires to those where all occupants survived further reinforced the importance of human behavior in determining outcomes in residential fire. This study highlighted that taking psychotropic or sedative drugs, living alone, being asleep, and being in the room of fire origin were significant risk factors for death compared to survival [71]. Ahrens [1] also reported that people who died in home fires in the period 2014–2018 where a working smoke alarm was present were more likely to have been in the area of fire origin, have been intimate with ignition, or to have attempted to fight the fire themselves. This highlights the notion that smoke alarms become most important in circumstances when a person would otherwise be unaware that a fire has started, such as while they are sleeping.

It is undeniable that one of the most important risk factors for death in a residential fire is being asleep. The fatality rate in fires is approximately three times greater during the sleeping period than during the waking hours [9]. Recent data from the USA have shown that people who died in home fires where there was no working smoke alarm present were more likely to be asleep than fatalities that occurred in the presence of an operating smoke alarm [1]. Taken together, these facts clearly emphasize the importance of smoke alarms in reducing fire fatalities by alerting sleeping individuals to the possibility of fire.

Factors relating to the environment, the individual, and the alarm signal itself are all important in determining whether a smoke alarm is likely to awaken sleeping individuals. However, as demonstrated above, examination of risk factors for death in fire reveals that individual differences remain an important consideration for smoke alarm design, and different signals have been found to vary in their ability to awaken those most at risk including children, the elderly, people who are hard of hearing, and people impaired by alcohol.

While people sleep their brain remains in an active state, monitoring the external environment for stimuli that may require response [7]. When a signal from the environment is received, it is processed by the brain and examined for significance below the level of conscious awareness. If the signal is processed as lacking in significance, then sleep will be maintained; however, if it is processed as requiring attention, then arousal from sleep will follow. Therefore, it is not simply the loudness of a signal that will predict a response. This is exemplified when we consider that people who live near a railway crossing or airport can very often sleep through the cacophonous sounds that intermittently occur in these environments. The familiarity of the environment renders the sound insignificant.

The significance of a signal can be determined by its novelty, or by learned associations. If an unexpected sound occurs it may signal a situation that needs attention, and wakefulness may follow. Likewise, if a sound is associated with emotional significance such as a person's name, or with a situation signaling danger or provoking action such as the sound of breaking glass, then it is also highly likely that an unimpaired person will awaken very quickly. This is demonstrated by research which showed that people will respond more often to their own name than to a different name in all but the deepest stages of sleep [53]. The importance of learned associations is also highlighted by research demonstrating that people can be motivated or "primed" to respond to specific auditory stimuli while asleep. In 1961 [74], researchers Zung and Wilson conducted a study that attempted to prime participants while awake to respond during sleep to a specific nonthreatening signal (e.g., a doorbell), but not to other similarly benign signals (e.g., a telephone). Their results showed that the response rate to the primed signal increased from 25% to 90% during the deepest stages of sleep.

Along with other work, this has lead psychologists to conclude that the brain appraises the emotional significance of a signal before sleep maintenance or arousal will occur. This has been confirmed by research using brain imaging to show that different areas relating to emotional processing are activated in response to a person's name during sleep, compared to when they are awake [55]. During sleep, emotional stimuli is processed following a different pathway that bypasses the "thinking" part of the brain (cortex) to prompt more immediate arousal, at a lower threshold of sound level, and with a greater chance of causing awakening. The path followed is similar to the one that causes a reflexive fear response when we are awake, and with the same immediacy of readiness to respond. The notion that arousal is affected by signal significance or learned associations can clearly be applied to the design of the smoke alarm signal. It reinforces that the signal should be immediately recognizable and provides support for the use of a standardized signal such as the T-3 pattern when people are asleep, as well as when they are awake.

Given the importance of being asleep as a risk factor for death in fire, research on auditory arousal thresholds (AATs) has been applied to smoke alarm signal design. The term AAT refers to the minimum sound pressure level an auditory signal must reach to be detected by a sleeping individual, causing them to wake. Sleep cycles in stages, moving sequentially from wakefulness through stages 1 to 4, and back again in reverse order before a period of rapid eye movement sleep (REM) is experienced. These cycles recur across the night with about a 90 min periodicity. It can be more difficult or take longer to awaken a person in some stages compared to others. Stages 1, 2, and REM represent lighter sleep, where a person can most easily be roused, and Stages 3 and 4 represent progressively deeper sleep, where a person can be much more difficult to awaken [7]. Most deep sleep occurs in the first third of the night, and after that much more time is spent in lighter sleep stages. As previously explained, standards mandate that a smoke alarm signal should be received at a sound pressure level of at least 75dBA at the pillow, but is this generally loud enough to awaken sleeping individuals? Research using pure sound tones (unrelated to emergency warning signals) has found that the sound pressure necessary to wake one person up may very much vary compared to the next, to the extent that individual differences account for most of the variance in auditory arousal thresholds (AATs; [73]). This study reported that differences in AATs across sleep stages spanning both light (Stages 1, 2, and REM) and heavy sleep (Stages 3 and 4) varied within different adult age groups in the range of 54–82dBA between individuals.

Knowledge from AAT research has been used to inform why sleeping people from the most at-risk groups die despite the presence of a working smoke alarm. Several auditory signals with different spectral complexities have been investigated for their ability to wake people from different vulnerable groups. Spectral complexity refers to the modulation of pitch within a sound, with a pure tone resounding at a single level of pitch, and a square wave resounding across a spectrum of varying pitches. To explain in simple terms, a pure tone might be described as the sound generated when a single key is struck on a piano, whereas a square wave is more closely akin to when a chord combining several notes is played. Other signals including bed and pillow shakers and strobe lights have also been explored. In 2007, Bruck and Ball published a paper summarizing research carried out on the response of sleeping individuals from at-risk groups towards the development of an optimal signal for the smoke alarm. The following section will provide a brief summary of some of the research presented in that paper, adding more contemporary findings where applicable.

As previously highlighted, an important risk factor for death in residential fire is age, with the very young and the very old most vulnerable. It is known that AATs gradually decrease with age across the lifespan, and that it is much harder to rouse a young person from sleep than an older person. Results of a study investigating AATs comparing groups through the childhood years to young adulthood (5–24 years) reported vast differences in average AATs between the youngest group (5–7 years; Mean = 111.6dBA, SD = 12.5dBA) and the oldest group (20–24 years; Mean = 67.8dBA, SD = 21.9dBA). In fact, until early adulthood (20–24 years), the average sound pressure level to provoke a response was considerably above the recommended level of 75dBA to be received at the pillow for a smoke alarm, with the AAT for child groups ranging from 111.6dBA in those aged 5–7 years, to 97dBA for adolescents [22]. These results are in keeping with other sleep studies showing that children experience more deep sleep through the night than adults, and that the deep sleep they experience is qualitatively deeper [2].

When this knowledge is applied to smoke alarm research, studies using different alarm signals have shown fairly consistent results. Early research showed that children aged 6–15 years will not reliably awaken to a high-pitched beeping alarm signal presented at 60dBA [8] or 89dBA [10]. A later study comparing responses of children aged 6–10 years to various alarm signals showed that significantly fewer children responded to the high-pitched (4000 Hz) pure tone alarm compared to a lower-pitched (520 Hz) square wave (modulating 500–2500 Hz) signal. It further showed that voice alarms (including the child's mother's voice using the child's own name, and an actress's voice spoken in urgent tones) were both more successful in terms of the number of children awakened and timeliness of awakenings, compared to the high-pitched alarm signal. However, no advantage was apparent for these two signals when compared to the lower-pitched (520 Hz) signal [15]. These results have been confirmed in recent large-scale studies with children investigating a range of different signals presented at 85dBA at the pillow including maternal voice alarms using the child's name, a female stranger's voice, a male stranger's voice, a hybrid alarm (combining the female stranger's voice and the 520 Hz signal), the lower-pitched 520 Hz square wave, and the conventional high-pitched (approx. 3200 Hz) signal. Regardless of comparative signal, these studies consistently report that the conventional high-pitched alarm performs significantly worse in arousing children from sleep [63–65]. It was further reported that the 520 Hz signal and the female stranger's voice outperformed the signal with the mother's voice using the child's name, confirming the earlier findings of Bruck et al. [15] that personalizing the signal did not improve effectiveness [64].

Although these studies were conducted in the child's own home while they were sleeping in their own beds, all used somewhat contrived methods since sounds were delivered using externally provided audio equipment. Additionally, most delivered sounds using the modified method of limits (i.e., presenting sounds at gradually increasing volumes) in order to determine which signal would prompt awakening at the lowest sound level (i.e., to investigate AATs). A separate project took a novel approach to investigate the response of children to smoke alarms using more naturalistic methods. Bruck and Thomas [14] recruited a community sample of parents of children aged 5–15 years and asked them to set off the home smoke alarm closest to their child's bed, 1–3 h after sleep onset. Home smoke alarms at this time still emitted the high-pitched pure tone (as do alarms in most homes today), and it was reported that 78% of children aged 5–15 years slept through 30 s of alarm presentation (ages 5–10 years 87% slept through, and for 11–15 years 56%).

Age can affect the response to smoke alarms in older adults differently to children. Humans experience less deep sleep as they age, so it seems intuitive that elderly people would have little trouble in responding to a smoke alarm signal. However, as we age, we are also more likely to experience hearing loss, especially regarding sensitivity to higher pitched signals. Cruickshanks et al. [25] studied hearing in the right ear of men aged 48–92 years who were awake and demonstrated that the threshold for being able to detect a tone presented at 3000 Hz was considerably higher than for a 500 Hz tone. From their data, it can be seen that a 3000 Hz signal would need to be presented on average at least 30dBA louder than a 500 Hz signal in order for a 70 year old man from the study cohort to detect it. In 2006 [11], Bruck and Thomas conducted a study investigating the response of sleeping older adults (aged 65–85 years) to different signals including a 3000 Hz high-pitched pure tone T-3, a 520 Hz square wave T-3, a 500 Hz pure tone, and a male voice. Consistent with the findings for children reported earlier, they found that the high-pitched 3000 Hz signal was the least effective of all presented. This signal needed to be transmitted at 20dBA higher volume on average to initiate a response compared to the best signal, which was once again the 520 Hz square wave (T-3). They reported that people aged over 75 were particularly vulnerable to sleeping through the high-pitched alarm, and that the minimum pillow volume of 75dBA was insufficient for this age group if the 3000 Hz signal was used.

Further research investigating the optimal signal to awaken people who are hard of hearing was conducted by Bruck and Thomas [12] for the US Fire Protection Research Foundation. These researchers investigated three auditory signals using the T-3 pattern including a 400 Hz square wave, a 520 Hz square wave, and a 3000 Hz pure tone (high-pitched smoke alarm signal), together with an under mattress bed shaker, a pillow shaker, and strobe lights. They used the modified method of limits (with signals gradually increasing in intensity across time) to determine waking thresholds and found that the 520 Hz square wave was the singular most effective signal, successfully awakening 92% of their hard of hearing participants when presented at 75dBA for 30 s, increasing to 100% when the sound pressure level reached 95dBA. They further reported that 80–83% responded to the bed or pillow shaker (respectively) at the intensity of purchase, and that the bed shaker specifically was significantly less likely to awaken people aged over 60 compared to people from younger age groups. Finally, they reported that strobe lights were not an effective means to awaken participants from any group. They concluded that the best alarm for alerting people who are hard of hearing should likely combine the 520 Hz signal with a vibrating alerting device such as a pillow or bed shaker, based upon the signals they tested.

Finally, the most widely reported risk factor for death in fire is alcohol intoxication. Examination of 17 studies published prior to 2011 showed that where data are collected about blood alcohol concentration (BAC), about half of all fire fatalities tested positive, and about one fifth to one quarter of these were highly intoxicated (defined as BAC .20 mg/dl; [18]). A study comparing demographic, behavioral, and environmental factors for 95 victims of fire from Australian coronial records showed that 58% of fatalities tested positive for alcohol, and 95% of these showed BAC of .10 mg/dl or greater. This study showed that being aged 18–60, the involvement of smoking materials in ignition, having no pre-existing conditions preventing escape, and being male were all significantly associated with fatalities who had consumed alcohol, compared to those who had not [18].

Two studies are known to have used the modified method of limits to examine AATs to different alarm signals when participants were under the influence of alcohol. First, Ball and Bruck [4] reported results of a small pilot study comparing the effectiveness of different auditory signals in awakening self-reported deep sleeping young adults under sober, .05 mg/dl BAC, and .08 mg/dl BAC alcohol conditions. They compared a female voice alarm with the high-pitched 3000 Hz smoke alarm signal, and a 520 HZ square wave T-3 and found that the female voice alarm and the 520 Hz square wave T-3 were significantly more likely to awaken individuals under the influence of both alcohol conditions. Most importantly, analyses also showed that it was significantly more difficult to awaken participants under the influence of alcohol compared to when they were sober, even at the lower level of intoxication [4]. Stochastic modelling using these same data subsequently showed that the probability and estimated waking up threshold for the various alarm signals were different between males and females, with males proving less sensitive (and therefore harder to awaken) than females across all conditions, including under the influence of alcohol [33].

The Ball and Bruck [4] study was a pilot investigation with a small number of participants only; however, their findings lead the US Fire Protection Research Foundation to fund a larger scale project. This larger study compared the response of sleeping young adults (aged 18–26 years) at .05 mg/dl BAC to several different signals, including a 400 Hz square wave, a 520 Hz, a 500 Hz pure tone, a 3100 Hz, a bed shaker, a pillow shaker, and a strobe light, all presented using the T3 pattern [16]. They reported that the 400 Hz and 520 Hz square waves were significantly more effective than the other auditory signals, and woke participants at the AAT of 75dBA or less for 93–100% of participants, respectively. They also reported that bed shakers, pillow shakers, and strobe lights were all found to be ineffective in awakening young people under the influence of alcohol.

In response to the assumption that this is due solely to the pitch of the signal, a study compared signals of different pattern, pitch, and spectral complexity (pure tone vs. square wave). The study tested alarms including beeping signals in the low- to-mid frequency range (400, 520, 800 and 1600 Hz square waves), whooping white noise signals (spanning 400–1600 Hz and 400–800 Hz), and two signals combining square wave (520, 800 and 1200 Hz) and pure tones (400, 800 and 1600 Hz) presented consecutively in order of ascending pitch [17]. All signals were presented using the T-3 pattern to match international standard ISO-8201 [34]. Results showed that the lower-pitched 400 and 520 Hz square wave signals produced significantly lower AATs compared to the other signals. The researchers concurred with previous work to conclude that the 520 Hz square wave signal would be their recommended sound for the smoke alarm signal [17].

Across all studies reported here comparing the effectiveness of different signals in awakening people who are most at risk of death in fire, a remarkably consistent finding is that the 520 HZ square wave T-3 has been found to be the most successful. However, it is important to note that unimpaired adults generally respond very well, regardless of signal. Although statistical differences are found between AATs for different alarm sounds, for unimpaired adults these differences are in the magnitude of 1–2 s [66] and are so small as to be unlikely to alter outcomes in the case of a home fire. However, as has been demonstrated, the same cannot be said for vulnerable groups. When considering this body of work, it is important to note that these studies necessarily contained an element of priming, in that participants were usually aware that the intention of the study was to wake them up with a signal after sleep onset. Nonetheless, there was also an attempt to preserve ecological validity by carrying out the procedures in a person's own home while they were sleeping in their own bed. Furthermore, the priming effect was equal for all signals. A pleasing result from the extensive body of work presented within this chapter is that local standards in several countries now mandate a 520 Hz signal for new smoke alarms (e.g., Australia) or for all smoke alarms to be used in areas where people are sleeping (e.g., USA). This progress acknowledges the elevated risk for death in fire that is associated with a raft of individual human characteristics and behaviors.

2.2 Response When People Are Awake

Despite the historic intention of smoke alarms in residential homes to wake people up during fire emergency, they were originally used in large and public buildings to alert people to the presence of fire when they are generally awake, but possibly unaware. Beyond the design and technical features of smoke alarms, *people* play an integral role in their effectiveness as a fire safety measure. Hence, it is pertinent to consider how people might respond to a smoke alarm signal they become aware of. Ideally, when an alarm signal sounds, awake people should respond immediately by ceasing all prior activity and moving quickly to the closest building exit for evacuation, unless directed otherwise. Despite general knowledge of this protocol, it is remarkably common for people to not respond in this way, but rather to continue with their prior activities, delaying evacuation and decreasing the time available for safe retreat [44]. As a result, pre-emergency activity has become a point of interest for human behavior in fire research and has provided some surprising results. For example, information from 375 evacuees of a 32-story high-rise office building fire in the US revealed that 65% of people either continued with their prefire activity and/or waited for clear instructions for action before responding to the alarm

[40] - But why is it that people do not respond to smoke alarms as intended? A number of underlying psychosocial factors can explain this lack of response to emergency signals, including the smoke alarm.

First, a necessary precursor for action is attention. If a person does not pay conscious attention to sensory information (i.e., smoke alarm signal), then that information is unable to be cognitively processed any further, and therefore is unable to be acted upon [21]. Attention directed towards prior activities can hinder the recognition of, and response to, smoke alarms. When a person is immersed in an activity at the time a smoke alarm sounds, even when that activity seems unimportant (e.g., watching TV, working on a computer, playing video games), they may fail to pay attention to the auditory sensory cue and continue with their activity as normal. In a similar way to someone who may be asleep, this unintentional ignorance is the result of attentional bias towards the prior activity impeding the taking in of new, unrelated (fire cue) information [38].

However, even when people are aware of and pay attention to a smoke alarm signal, this does not guarantee action. Even when smoke alarms are noticed, the absence of other obvious cues may make the signal ambiguous, and people may continue with their preexisting activity until a cue that is more explicit and/or intense is perceived [45]. The frequency, intensity, consistency, and credibility of cues all inform a person's perception of fire threat [26, 41]. The credibility of smoke alarms can be compromised by previous exposure to false alarms as people draw on their past experiences to inform decision-making in new situations [38]. Hence, a history of previous false alarms can result in a biased and incorrect interpretation of real alarms [37]. The way a person perceives the nature and intensity of a smoke alarm and their analysis of their own personal risk will influence their subsequent action or inaction [23]. More specifically, a person who interprets a significant fire threat (e.g., fire in close proximity) is likely to respond more readily than a person who perceives the risk to be low (e.g., fire on another floor of a building) ([41, 62]). A study by Gerges et al. [28] found that 74% of people reported they would ignore a fire alarm completely, yet "getting the kids and leaving" and "leaving immediately" were the top two ranked actions reported if visual fire cues were observed (i.e., flames and smoke).

In addition to drawing on our past experiences for information to guide our behavior in a similar situation, people also seek information from their social context. Irrespective of individual personality differences, our behavior in social settings is largely determined by a set of social scripts, known as schemas, which we develop over the course of our lives. These scripts help us to function effectively in social settings because they provide us with a set of norms, or rules of how to behave and predictions of what to expect from other people. These schemas provide us with knowledge regarding protocols for expected behavior in familiar situations (e.g., cooking dinner at home, ordering a coffee at the café, or attending a football match). Even in unexpected emergency events people adhere to social expectations relevant to the (non-emergency) context they are in [39]. For example, people eating dinner in a restaurant may be reluctant to evacuate immediately because social rules require them to pay for their meal before leaving. Likewise, people living in an apartment complex may not consider fire safety as their responsibility unless they are designated a role, e.g., as a fire warden. In addition, when faced with a somewhat ambiguous or novel situation where our schemas are not particularly strong, people may seek guidance by observing the behavior of others.

The presence and behavior of other people in social situations influences our own behavior significantly. In fire emergencies, people can be leaders or followers, but most commonly take on the follower role when others are present. This means they may not immediately respond, but will wait to be guided by the actions of others [39]. Over 50 years ago, Latane and Darley [42] conducted a pivotal study on social influence, or the 'Bystander Effect' in fire emergencies. Participants were seated in a waiting room that subsequently began to fill with smoke and were exposed to one of three conditions including alone, accompanied by other naïve people, or accompanied by deliberately passive study confederates. Findings revealed that participants were most likely to report the smoke when alone (75%), and to do so more swiftly. Alarmingly, when people were with others, only 10% of those seated with the passive confederates and 38% of those with naïve people reported the smoke. Three underlying psychological mechanisms are proposed to mediate the influence of passive bystanders. These include diffusion of responsibility (i.e., the belief that someone else will speak up/act when in the presence of others); evaluation apprehension (i.e., the fear of making an inaccurate interpretation of a situation and taking subsequent socially incorrect actions that will be observed by other people); and pluralistic ignorance (i.e., the assumption that others "know better" when the situation is ambiguous; [42]). Evidence from a recent replication study supports the negative influence of passive occupants on the inaction of others [36]. However, this study also found a positive influence of proactive bystanders, whose evacuation behavior was followed. It appears that when a fire cue is ambiguous, people seek guidance about behavior by observing others. If other people remain passive, this leads to a reduction in threat perception.

Presumably, fire drills will alter human behavior by reinforcing a schema of the best way to respond. However, research on egress has focused very much on collecting data to be input into evacuation models used by fire engineers, and much less focus has been on how people actually perform in a real fire emergency as a result of taking part in fire drills. Furthermore, exposure to repeated fire drills can have the reverse of the desired effect by creating a contempt of false alarms [30]. This does not mean that fire drills are not important, or that they do not change human behavior, but rather that more work needs to be done to investigate their real-world impact.

3 Conclusion

The body of research on human response to smoke alarms has provided important information that has been used to improve their effectiveness in the decades since their first inception. However, this research also shows that their effectiveness should not be naively considered as a safety guarantee. As described above, there are many factors involved in the smoke alarm-human response interaction. The reality is there are times when people will not respond to fire alarms – regardless of whether they are awake or asleep. The research presented in this chapter clearly demonstrates that smoke alarms save lives in residential settings. It has also clearly shown that different types of smoke detector are best suited to sensing different types of fire. There are segments of the community that strongly advocate for the use of the more costly photoelectric smoke alarms over the less expensive ionization units, but the research clearly supports that it is better to have any type of smoke alarm, than to have none at all.

There is also a substantial body of research that has investigated the optimal pitch for the smoke alarm signal when it is to be used to awaken people who are sleeping. This research has overwhelmingly supported the use of a 520 Hz square wave signal as superior in waking vulnerable groups compared to other signals tested. This includes the much used high-pitched alarm that until recently was universally used in commercially available smoke alarms. Pleasingly, engineering standards in many jurisdictions now specify the use of the 520 Hz signal, especially when the alarm is to be used to alert sleeping individuals.

References

1. Ahrens M (2021) Smoke alarms in U.S. home fires. National Fire Protection Association website: https://www.nfpa.org//-/media/Files/News-and-Research/Fire-statistics-and-reports/Detection-and-signaling/ossmokealarms.pdf
2. Aström C, Trojaborg W (1992) Relationship of age to power spectrum analysis of EEG during sleep. J Clin Neurophysiol 9(3):424–430. https://doi.org/10.1097/00004691-199207010-00010
3. Australian Government Department of the Prime Minister and Cabinet (2015) Interconnection of smoke alarms – COAG decision regulation impact statement-Australia Building Codes Board. Interconnection of Smoke Alarms – COAG Decision Regulation Impact Statement – Australian Building Codes Board | Regulation Impact Statement Updates (pmc.gov.au)
4. Ball M, Bruck D (2004) The effect of alcohol upon response to different fire alarm signals in sleeping young adults. In: Paper presentation, 3rd human behaviour in fire conference, Belfast, Ulster
5. Ballard JE, Koepsell TD, Rivara FP, Van Belle G (1992) Descriptive epidemiology of unintentional residential fire injuries in King County, WA, 1984 and 1985. Public Health Rep 107(4):402–408
6. Barillo DJ, Goode R (1996) Fire fatality study: demographics of fire victims. Burns 22(2):85–88. https://doi.org/10.1016/S0379-7112(98)00035-6
7. Bonnet M (1982) Performance during sleep. In: Webb WB (ed) Biological rhythms, sleep and performance. Wiley, pp 205–237
8. Bruck D (1999) Non-awakening in children in response to a smoke detector alarm. Fire Saf J 32(4):369–376. https://doi.org/10.1016/S0379-7112(98)00035-6
9. Bruck D, Ball M (2007) Optimizing emergency awakening to audible smoke alarms: an update. Human Factors 49(4):585–601. https://doi.org/10.1518/001872007X215674
10. Bruck D, Bliss A (2000) Sleeping children and smoke alarms. In: Paper presentation, 4th Asia-Oceania symposium on fire science and technology, Tokyo, Japan
11. Bruck D, Thomas I (2006) Reducing fire deaths in older adults: investigation of auditory arousal with different alarm signals in sleeping older adults. Fire Protection Research Foundation

12. Bruck D, Thomas I (2007) Waking effectiveness of alarm (auditory, visual and tactile) for adults who are hard of hearing. The Fire Protection Research Foundation
13. Bruck D, Thomas I (2008) Towards a better smoke alarm signal – an evidence based approach. In: Paper presentation, Fire Safety Science – Proceedings of the ninth international symposium, Karlsruhe, Germany. https://doi.org/10.3801/IAFSS.FSS.9-403
14. Bruck D, Thomas IR (2012) Community-based research on the effectiveness of the home smoke alarm in waking up children. Fire Mater 36(5-6):339–348. https://doi.org/10.1002/fam.1081
15. Bruck D, Reid S, Kouzma J, Ball M (2004) The effectiveness of different alarms in waking sleeping children. In: Paper presentation, 3rd human behaviour in fire conference, Belfast, Ulster
16. Bruck D, Thomas I, Ball M (2007) Waking effectiveness of alarms (auditory, visual and tactile) for the alcohol impaired. Fire Protection Research Foundation
17. Bruck D, Ball M, Thomas I, Rouillard V (2009) How does the pitch and pattern of a signal affect auditory arousal thresholds? J Sleep Res 18:196–203. https://doi.org/10.1111/j.1365-2869.2008.00710.x
18. Bruck D, Ball M, Thomas IR (2011) Fire fatality and alcohol intake: analysis of key risk factors. J Stud Alcohol Drugs 72(5):731–736. https://doi.org/10.15288/jsad.2011.72.731
19. Bukowski RW (2001) A history of NBS/NIST research on fire detectors. In: Paper presentation, 12th international conference on automatic fire detection, Gaithersberg, MD
20. Bukowski RW, Peacock RD, Averill JD, Cleary TG, Bryner NP, Walton WD, Reneke PA, Kuligowski ED (2008) Performance of home smoke alarms: analysis of the response of several available technologies in residential fire settings, NIST technical Note 1455-1. National Institute of Standards and Technology, Washington, DC
21. Burns CG, Fairclough SH (2015) Use of auditory event-related potentials to measure immersion during a computer game. Int J Human-Comput Stud 73:107–114. https://doi.org/10.1016/j.ijhcs.2014.09.002
22. Busby KA, Mercier L, Pivik RT (1994) Ontogenetic variations in auditory arousal threshold during sleep. Psychophysiology 31(2):182–188. https://doi.org/10.1111/j.1469-8986.1994.tb01038.x
23. Choi M, Lee S, Park M, Lee H-S (2018) Effect of dynamic emergency cues on fire evacuation performance in public buildings. J Infrastruct Syst 24(4). https://doi.org/10.1061/(ASCE)IS.1943-555X.0000449
24. Cleary T (2010) Results from a full-scale smoke alarm sensitivity study. Fire Technol 50:775–790. https://doi.org/10.1007/s10694-010-0152-2
25. Cruickshanks KJ, Wiley TL, Tweed TS, Klein BE, Klein R, Mares-Perlman JA, Nondahl DM (1998) Prevalence of hearing loss in older adults in Beaver Dam, Wisconsin. The Epidemiology of Hearing Loss Study. Am J Epidemiol 148(9):879–886. https://doi.org/10.1093/oxfordjournals.aje.a009713
26. Day RC, Hulse LM, Galea ER (2013) Response phase behaviours and response time predictors of the 9/11 World Trade Center evacuation. Fire Technol 49:657–678. https://doi.org/10.1007/s10694-012-0282-9
27. Farley T, Ball M (2012) Identification, recollection and perceived urgency of the temporal-three evacuation signal in an Australian sample. In: Paper presentation, 5th human behaviour in fire conference, Cambridge, UK
28. Gerges M, Mayouf M, Rumley P, Moore D (2017) Human behaviour under fire situations in high-rise residential building. Int J Build Pathol Adapt 35(1):90–106. https://doi.org/10.1108/IJBPA-09-2016-0022
29. Giebultowicz J, Ruzycka M, Wroczynski P, Purser D, Stec A (2017) Analysis of fire deaths in Poland and influence of smoke toxicity. Forensic Sci Int 277:77–87. https://doi.org/10.1016/j.forsciint.2017.05.018

30. Gwynne S, Boyce K, Kuligowski E, Nilsson D, Robbins A, Lovreglio R (2016) Pros and cons of egress drills. In: Paper presentation, Interflam 2016, 14th international conference on fire science and engineering, London, UK
31. Halliwell RE, Sultan MA (1986a) Guide to the most effective locations for smoke detectors in residential buildings (Note on construction; No. 62F). National Research Council Canada, Institute for Research in Construction. https://doi.org/10.4224/21273267
32. Halliwell RE, Sultan MA (1986b) Attenuation of smoke detector alarm signals in residential buildings. In: Paper presentation, Fire safety science 1st international symposium, Berkeley, CA. https://iafss.org/publications/fss/8/507
33. Hasofer AM, Thomas IR, Ball M, Bruck D (2005) Statistical modelling of the effect of alcohol and sound intensity on response to fire alarms. In: Paper presentation, Fire safety science – 8th international symposium, Beijing, China. https://iafss.org/publications/fss/8/507
34. International Organization for Standardization (ISO) (2017) Alarm systems – audible emergency evacuation signal – Requirements (ISO 8201 – 2017). https://www.iso.org/standard/67046.html
35. Jonsson A, Bonander C, Nilson F, Huss F (2017) The state of the residential fire fatality problem in Sweden: epidemiology, risk factors, and event typologies. J Fire Saf Res 62:89–100. https://doi.org/10.1016/j.jsr.2017.06.008
36. Kinateder M, Warren WH (2016) Social influence on evacuation behavior in real and virtual environments. Front Robot AI 3:Article e43. https://doi.org/10.3389/frobt.2016.00043
37. Kinateder MT, Kuligowski ED, Reneke PA, Peacock RD (2015) Risk perception in fire evacuation behavior revisited: definitions, related concepts, and empirical evidence. Fire Sci Rev 4:Article e1. https://doi.org/10.1186/s40038-014-0005-z
38. Kinsey MJ, Gwynne SMV, Kuligowski ED, Kinateder M (2019) Cognitive biases within decision making during fire evacuations. Fire Technol 55:465–485. https://doi.org/10.1007/s10694-018-0708-0
39. Kobes M, Helsloot I, de Vries B, Post JG (2010) Building safety and human behaviour in fire: a literature review. Fire Saf J 45(1):1–11. https://doi.org/10.1016/j.firesaf.2009.08.005
40. Kuligowski E, Hoskins B (2010) Occupant behavior in a high-rise office building fire, NIST technical note 1664. National Institue of Standards and Technology
41. Kuligowski ED, Mileti DS (2009) Modeling pre-evacuation delay by occupants in World Trade Center Towers 1 and 2 on September 11, 2001. Fire Saf J 44(4):487–496. https://doi.org/10.1016/j.firesaf.2008.10.001
42. Latane B, Darley JM (1968) Group inhibition of bystander intervention in emergencies. J Pers Soc Psychol 10(3):215–221. https://doi.org/10.1037/h0026570
43. Lee A (2005) The audibility of smoke alarms in residential homes (CPSC-ES-0503). U.S. Consumer Product Safety Commission. https://www.cpsc.gov/s3fs-public/audibility%20(1).pdf
44. Lin J, Zhu R, Li N, Becerik-Gerber B (2021) How occupants respond to building emergencies: a systematic review of behavioral characteristics and behavioral theories. Saf Sci 137:Article e105171. https://doi.org/10.1016/j.ssci.2019.104540
45. Lo Y, Mendell NR, Rubin DB (2001) Testing the number of components in a normal mixture. Biometrika 88(3):767–778. https://doi.org/10.1093/biomet/88.3.767
46. Marshall SW, Runyan CW, Bangdiwala SI, Linzer MA, Sacks JJ, Butts JD (1998) Fatal residential fires: who dies and who survives? JAMA 279(20):1633–1637. https://doi.org/10.1001/jama.279.20.1633
47. Mealy CL, Wolfe A, Gottuk DT (2009) Smoke alarm response and tenability. In: Paper presentation, 14th international conference on automatic fire detection AUBE '09, Duisberg, Germany
48. Milarcik EL, Olenick SM, Roby RJ (2008) A relative time analysis of the performance of residential smoke detection technologies. Fire Technol 44:337–349. https://doi.org/10.1007/s10694-008-0046-8

49. Moinuddin KAM, Bruck D, Shi L (2017) An experimental study on timely activation of smoke alarms and their effective notification in typical residential buildings. Fire Saf J 93:1–11. https://doi.org/10.1016/j.firesaf.2017.07.003
50. Mueller BA, Sidman EA, Alter H, Perkins R, Grossman DC (2008) Randomized controlled trial of ionization and photoelectric smoke alarm functionality. Injury Prev 14(2):80–86. https://doi.org/10.1136/ip.2007.016725
51. National Fire Protection Association (2019) National fire alarm signaling code (NFPA 72)
52. National Fire Protection Association (2021) Ionization vs photoelectric. https://www.nfpa.org/Public-Education/Staying-safe/Safety-equipment/Smoke-alarms/Ionization-vs-photoelectric
53. Oswald I, Taylor AM, Treisman M (1960) Discriminative responses to stimulation during human sleep. Brain 83(3):440–453. https://doi.org/10.1093/brain/83.3.440
54. Patetta MJ, Cole TB (1990) A population-based descriptive study of housefire deaths in North Carolina. Am J Public Health 80(9):1116–1117. https://doi.org/10.2105/ajph.80.9.1116
55. Portas C, Krakow K, Allen P, Josephs O, Armony JL, Frith CD (2000) Auditory processing across the sleep-wake cycle: simultaneous EEG and fMRI monitoring in humans. Neuron 28(3):991–999. https://doi.org/10.1016/s0896-6273(00)00169-0
56. Proulx G, Laroche C (2003) Recollection, identification and perceived urgency of the temporal-three evacuation signal. J Fire Prot Eng 13(1):67–82. https://doi.org/10.1177/2F1042391503013001004
57. Public Health Australia Association (2014) Public Health Association of Australia: policy-at-a-glance – Smoke Alarms in Residential Housing Policy. https://www.phaa.net.au/documents/item/267
58. Rohde D, Corcoran J, Sydes M, Higginson A (2016) The association between smoke alarm presence and death rates: a systematic review and meta-analysis. Fire Saf J 81:58–63. https://doi.org/10.1016/j.firesaf.2016.01.008
59. Scottish Government (2020) Fire and smoke alarms: changes to the law. https://www.gov.scot/publications/fire-and-smoke-alarms-in-scottish-homes/
60. Sekizawa A (1991) Statistical analyses on fatalities characteristics of residential fires. In: Paper presentation, Fire Safety Science—3rd international symposium, Edinburgh, Scotland
61. Shaw J, Dunderdale J, Paynter RA (2007) Radiation Protection 146: a review of consumer products containing radioactive substances in the European Union. European Commission. http://www.thewfsf.org/legislation_eu_files/EuropeanCommissionRadiationProtection146.pdf
62. Sherman MF, Peyrot M, Magda LA, Gershon RRM (2011) Modeling pre-evacuation delay by evacuees in World Trade Center Towers 1 and 2 on September 11, 2001: a revisit using regression analysis. Fire Saf J 46(7):414–424. https://doi.org/10.1016/j.firesaf.2011.07.001
63. Smith GA, Chounthirath T, Splaingard M (2019) Effectiveness of a voice smoke alarm using the child's name for sleeping children: A randomized trial. J Pediatr 205:250–256. https://doi.org/10.1016/j.jpeds.2018.09.027
64. Smith GA, Chounthirath T, Splaingard M (2020a) Comparison of the effectiveness of female voice, male voice, and hybrid voice-tone smoke alarms for sleeping children. Pediatr Res 88(5):769–775. https://doi.org/10.1038/s41390-020-0838-1
65. Smith GA, Chounthirath T, Splaingard M (2020b) Do sleeping children respond better to a smoke alarm that uses their mother's voice? Acad Pediatr 20:319–326
66. Smith GA, Kistamgari S, Splaingard M (2020c) Optimizing smoke alarm signals: Testing the effectiveness of children's smoke alarms for sleeping adults. Injury Epidemiol 7:Article e51. https://doi.org/10.1186/s40621-020-00279-6
67. Squires T, Busuttil A (1997) Alcohol and house fire fatalities in Scotland, 1980–1990. Med Sci Law 37(4):321–325. https://doi.org/10.1177/002580249703700407
68. Standards Australia (2014) Smoke alarms using scattered light, transmitted light or ionization. AS 3786:2014; Incorporating Amendment Nos 1 and 2
69. Thomas I, Bruck D (2010) Awakening of sleeping people: a decade of research. Fire Technol 46:743–761. https://doi.org/10.1007/s10694-008-0065-5

70. Watts-Hampton T, Bruck D, Ball M (2007) Examination of risk factors and mental health status in an accidental fire death population. In: Paper presentation, 7th Asia-Oceania Symposium on Fire Science and Technology, Hong Kong. https://iafss.org/publications/aofst/7/86/view/aofst_7-86.pdf
71. Xiong L, Bruck D, Ball M (2015) Comparative investigation of 'survival' and fatality factors in accidental residential fires. Fire Saf J 73:37–47. https://doi.org/10.1016/j.firesaf.2015.02.003
72. Yang J, Jones MP, Cheng G, Ramirez M, Taylor C, Peek-Asa C (2011) Do nuisance alarms decrease functionality of smoke alarms near the kitchen? Findings from a randomised controlled trial. Injury Prev 17(3):160–165. https://doi.org/10.1136/ip.2010.027805
73. Zepelin H, McDonald CS, Zammit GK (1984) Effects of age on auditory awakening thresholds. J Gerontol 39(3):294–300. https://doi.org/10.1093/geronj/39.3.294
74. Zung WK, Wilson WP (1961) Response to auditory stimulation during sleep. Arch Gen Psychiatry 4(6):548–552. https://doi.org/10.1001/archpsyc.1961.01710120018002

Associate Professor Michelle Ball is the Deputy Head of Psychology and the Leader of the Clinical and Community Health and Wellbeing research program within the Institute for Health and Sport at Victoria University. Michelle is an expert in human behavior in fire, and her past research includes investigating the best smoke alarm signal to awaken sleeping individuals. She has also extensively investigated why some people die in accidental residential fires, while others survive. More recently, her work has focused on conducting research with local Australian fire services to assist their Firelighting Consequence Awareness Program to identify young people who are at risk of repeated firelighting behavior.

Dr. Kara Dadswell is a Lecturer in Psychology in the College of Health and Biomedicine and Research Fellow in the Institute for Health and Sport at Victoria University. Kara's PhD research, "Predicting Recidivism in Young People who Light Fire: Finalisation, Implementation and Evaluation of a Screening Tool," completed in 2019 was a collaborative project with Fire Risk Victoria's Firelighting Consequence Awareness Program. For the past 7 years, Kara has lectured to fire engineering students about human behavior in fire, including evacuation and the human response to the smoke alarm signal, helping them to bring a psychological perspective to engineering solutions for fire safety systems in residential and commercial buildings.

Chapter 9
Impact of Interior Doors on Residential Fire Safety

Victoria N. Hutchison and Simo Hostikka

Abstract Doors play an important role in residential fire safety. Research has documented that doors can be an effective means to slow the spread of fire and smoke in home fires and have the potential to increase the available egress time for home occupants. While doors can be used as valuable barriers to the effects of fire, they can also serve as obstacles for detection, occupant notification, and evacuation. The impact of doors in residential fires can be influenced by both human and fire behaviors. Additionally, there may be a risk of pressure peaks during the early stage of the fire that may make it difficult to open doors that do not open outwards. This chapter provides an overview of the role interior doors play in residential fires, including the benefits, inhibiting factors, and unknowns.

Keywords Interior doors · Smoke alarm · Audibility · Evacuation · Compartment fires · Pressure effects

1 Introduction

Doors are a fundamental element in residential dwellings and apartments worldwide. Interior doors define and compartmentalize a home, providing physical, visual, and acoustical privacy. However, interior residential doors have undergone a dramatic change over the last several years. Doors have historically been constructed from solid pieces of wood. But the global shift toward environmentally sustainable products has caused a shift in priorities, including the more efficient use of material and financial resources. To optimize materials resources, the construction materials for interior doors have changed from solid-core wood doors to hollow-core

V. N. Hutchison (✉)
Fire Protection Research Foundation, Quincy, MA, USA
e-mail: vhutchison@nfpa.org

S. Hostikka
Aalto University, Espoo, Finland
e-mail: simo.hostikka@aalto.fi

composite doors. While doors can act as a physical barrier to fire and smoke, interior residential doors are generally not viewed as strong fire-resistive elements.

2 Doors in Residential Dwellings

While the global residential building stock is diverse, the most common type of residential units can be classified into two categories: single and multifamily dwellings. To quantify the impact of interior doors on residential fires, it is first important to understand the types of doors, their characteristics, and locations within residences.

2.1 Types of Residential Interior Doors

A vast array of doors may be found in residential dwellings, including hinged privacy doors, sliding doors, pocket doors, and folding doors. Interior doors are often characterized by their design, such as flush doors, paneled doors, sash doors, or louvered doors and their construction type – either hollow-core or solid. Today, hollow-core, flush panel doors are becoming increasingly common in interior residential applications. Due to their use of engineered materials, these doors are low-cost, lightweight, and easy to install [18].

Hollow-Core doors

Hollow-core doors consist of a solid wood or composite frame with an essentially hollow interior, which is often constructed of cardboard, arranged in a honeycomb pattern. The specific material, pattern, and density of the core can vary. The outside of the door typically consists of some type of paneling or timber veneer. Hollow-core doors are intended to act as a low-cost, lightweight, and environmentally friendly alternative to solid wood doors. These doors can be styled to replicate the look of solid wood doors, while using less materials. These doors are most commonly used as interior residential doors, due to their reduced strength, insulation, and security as compared to solid doors; however, they can be used as exterior doors under certain circumstances [17].

Solid-Core doors

Solid-core doors utilize an engineered construction method to provide a door that is a hybrid of hollow-core and solid wood doors. This door type uses a solid core that is constructed of engineered or composite wood, like Masonite or Fiberboard. A fine-grade surface wood veneer or engineered wood that is made to give the appearance of a frame and panel door is then glued on top of the solid core.

Solid-core doors that are at least 44.45 mm (1 ¾ inches) thick can offer more fire resistance than other interior doors [17].

Solid-Wood doors

Solid wood doors are constructed entirely of natural woods, such as pine, oak, and maple, among others. While they can be made of a single, unified slab of wood, this is rather rare. They are most often built using the frame-and-panel method of construction, which creates a classic six-panel door that has been used for centuries around the world. While these paneled doors appear to be one piece of contoured wood, these doors consist of a conglomerate of individual panels, mullions, stiles, and rails that secure the six panels together [18].

Fire-Rated doors

A fire door is a door that acts as part of a passive fire protection system to delay the spread of fire and smoke between compartments within a home or structure. Fire doors are classified by their fire-resistance rating, which determines the duration in which the fire door, or passive fire protection system, is designed to withstand the conditions of a standard fire resistance test.

2.2 General Placement of Doors in Residences

In a traditional residential dwelling, there will be a combination of interior and exterior doors.

While any requirement for fire resistance barriers or door sets is dependent on local regulations, most one- and two-family dwellings are not required to have fire-resistant doors. The most common door type in one- and two-family homes today is hollow-core doors, although solid wood and solid-core doors are still used. However, some regions, like the UK, recommend that single-family dwellings with at least one story exceeding 4.5 m have a fire-resisted, protected stairway. For the stairwell to be protected, all doors leading into the protected stair or hall area would need to have a rated fire resistance per the relevant standard [4].

In an apartment setting, multiple dwelling units typically share a common hall or exit way. In this type of multifamily dwelling, the hallway needs to be a protected exit corridor, therefore the doors leading out of each individual dwelling unit and the exit doors are generally required to be self-closing and have a rated fire resistance per the applicable standards, such as by Boverket's Building Regulations (BBR), NFPA 101®, *Life Safety Code*, or other local or regional standards.

3 Residential Fire Scenarios and Occupant Behaviors

3.1 Residential Fire Scenarios

When examining residential fires from various countries including the United States, Norway, Estonia, Denmark, Sweden, and the Netherlands, living room fires appear to be the leading area of origin for residential fire fatalities, followed by the bedroom [1, 3]. While kitchen or cooking area fires continue to be a leading area of origin in home fires around the world, these fires are less likely to result in fatalities than those in living rooms and bedrooms. Across the board, the largest percentage of fire fatalities occur during sleeping hours. In most countries examined, smoking was a leading cause of residential fire fatalities. Data indicates that single-family dwellings and apartments are the dwelling types that account for the large share of fire-related fatalities. While the overall number of victims per dwelling type is fairly evenly split, data indicate that occupants in apartments may be at higher risk of dying in a fire, particularly in Europe [3].

3.2 Occupant Door Position Habits

When assessing residential fire risks, occupant habits with regard to door position must be understood. A survey was conducted on 304 occupants, predominately located in the United Kingdom, to study door closing habits in their own residential dwellings. While it does not provide an international perspective, it does provide insight into common door positions and the reasoning for one position or the other. Overall, there was found to be a 60% probability of the occupant's bedroom door being closed while sleeping and a 45% probability of the living room door being closed, if present [5]. Occupants having children or pets were more likely to sleep with the bedroom door open. However, the probability of door closure varies significantly with the property type. Hopkin et al. found apartment residents to be 19% more likely to close bedroom doors than those living in one- or two-family dwellings [5].

4 Fundamentals: Role of Interior Doors in Residential Fires

Whether the interior residential doors are used to compartmentalize different areas of a residence or separate a residential unit from a common corridor, they impact several aspects of residential fire safety, with both positive and negative attributes. Doors can influence fire dynamics, detection of smoke, occupant notification, pressure effects in the home, and safe egress. Beyond the physical aspects, human behavior and the decision to close an interior door impacts the role interior doors can play in residential fire safety.

4.1 Fire Performance of Interior Doors

Interior residential doors are typically intended to act as a partition separating rooms and corridors in a residence, rather than as a passive, rated fire barrier. This is particularly true in single-family dwellings. Larger residential complexes may be subject to additional regulations to provide a protected exit corridor, but nevertheless, the interior doors within each individual apartment unit will likely not be made of fire-resistive construction, but rather act as a partition between rooms. Although fire and smoke separations are required in commercial building codes to minimize the impacts of fire, there are limited requirements for residential dwellings [10]. Interior doors can, however, act as a temporary barrier to fire and smoke.

The performance of a fire door or interior partition door assembly can be characterized by the ability of the door to retard the passage of fire and its effects (heat and smoke) into an adjacent compartment. There are several testing standards available that establish the methodology for evaluating the fire performance of door assemblies, including UL 10(B), *Standard for Fire Tests of Door Assemblies,* UL 10(C), *Standard for* Positive Pressure *Fire Tests of Door Assemblies,* NFPA 252, *Standard Methods of Fire Tests of Door Assemblies,* NFPA 80, *Standard for Fire Doors and Other Opening Protectives,* the *British Standard Specification for Fire Tests on Building Materials, and Structures, B.S. 476 Part 1,* EN 1634, *Fire resistance and smoke control tests for door and shutter assemblies, openable windows, and elements of building hardware,* among others. The temperatures within the furnace during the testing are required to comply with the standard temperature-time curve as specified in ASTM E-119 and NFPA 252.

An interior residential door's impact on slowing fire spread from one compartment to another was examined in a study conducted by Gross and Shoub [9] through a series of conventional standard furnace fire tests of 16 interior doors [9]. It was found that a traditional, solid wood, paneled door and frame only acts as a fire barrier for approximately 5 minutes. Since one of the objectives of this study was to assess alternative methods to improve fire performance of wood doors utilized in homes, the study also found that conventional or fire-retardant paints did not appear to have a noticeable impact on fire performance; however, a fire-retardant paint with fiberglass reinforcement extended a wood-paneled doors' ability to act as a fire barrier for an additional 11 minutes.

Similarly, a study by Kerber tested three different types of doors that are reflective of the doors found in residential dwellings today [2]. This study examined a hollow-core oak door, a hollow-core composite door, and a solid wood 6-panel door. Interestingly, the type of wood or material used on the door had little impact on its fire performance. The time to failure for all three doors was approximately 300 seconds, or 5 minutes, which is consistent with the results of the Gross and

Shoub study from 1966. The two hollow-core doors showed similar fire behavior, with relatively rapid fire spread to the unexposed side of the door. Surprisingly, the solid wood-paneled door also failed within approximately the same time frame, with the points of failure being on the paneled sections of the door. Since the relative thickness of the panel was significantly thinner than the rest of the wooden door, the panel areas failed quickly while the remainder of the door stayed in tack. These fire test results show the overall thickness of the door as the primary driver of their respective failure times – where failure is qualified as when the unexposed side of the door sustained burning.

4.2 Notification: Doors as a Barrier to Sound

In any fire scenario, early and effective detection and notification of the fire is essential for safe occupant egress. A closed interior door can be an effective barrier to fire, heat, and smoke; however, it has the potential to impair the alerting of sleeping occupants to fire, particularly if the alarm is located outside of the sleeping room. The risk presented by a closed, interior residential door with regard to notification is two-fold. First, the door could delay activation of a smoke alarm if an alarm is not present in the room of origin. And second, the door could delay occupant notification of the fire due to the audible attenuation by the door. With high-risk fire scenarios likely to occur when occupants are assumed to be asleep, it is essential to minimize delays in detection and occupant notification. Thus, the impact of an interior residential door on detection and notification is important to quantify by an assessment of the passage of smoke through closed doors and sound transmission through doors and other building materials.

4.2.1 Smoke Alarm Activation Delays from a Closed Door

One of the most important performance metrics for residential fire safety is the calculation of the time between alarm activation and the onset of untenable conditions for occupants in the home. Detection can be adversely impacted by closed doors since the barrier has the potential to delay or prevent activation of the smoke alarm, when it is located outside the room of origin. Studies, including Bukowski et al. (2008) and Thomas et al. (2010), have shown that alarm activation and the delay in activation time are strongly related to door position [23, 26].

The quantitative assessment of the potential time delay is dependent on a number of factors, including the location of the fire, the smoke alarm presence and location, distance from the source of the fire to the alarm, the air tightness of the home, sensitivity of the detector, type of door and position, among other variables.

Experiments conducted by Thomas and Bruck on four bedroom fires found that when the door in the fire compartment was closed, the amount of smoke that escaped around the cracks of the door was too low of a concentration to activate the alarms in the hallway [23]. Similarly, experiments by Bukowski showed that the time to untenability was reached before alarm activation in 50% of the closed bedroom door experiments, when no alarm was present in the room of origin [7, 26].

If smoke alarms are not placed inside and outside the bedroom or the residence does not have interconnected alarms, the delay or lack of smoke alarm activation from a closed interior door can substantially impact the available safe egress time for occupants and compromise safety.

4.2.2 Delays to Occupant Notification by Sound Attenuation

When no obstacles are present, sound travels uniformly in a direct path from the sounder to the receiver, where the observed sound pressure level decreases proportional to 1/distance. But when a barrier is put in its path, the sound is diffracted; some of the sound is transmitted through the barrier and some is reflected. The value by which doors reduce sound pressure levels is dependent on the type of door and its corresponding characteristics. According to Schifiliti et al. (2016), hollow-core flush panel doors with an air gap, hollow-core flush panel doors hung with edge sealing, and solid hardwood doors hung with edge sealing attenuate sound by 14 dBA, 20 dBA, and 26 dBA, respectively [8]. A common stud wall is also estimated to reduce the sound pressure level received on the other side of the wall by approximately 35 dBA [11]. Alternative construction methods and materials can influence the attenuation of sound through respective barriers.

To determine the sound received at a specific point in an enclosed space, the calculation methods outlined by Schifiliti can be applied [8]. This calculation accounts for factors such as the emitted sound pressure level, distance from the source, and the characteristics of the compartment, including the type and quality of the finishes and furnishings. When the alarm is located outside the area of concern, additional factors such as directional considerations, distance from the alarm to the partition (e.g., door), the sound attenuation through the wall or door, and the distance to the receiver on the other side of the partition (e.g., at the pillow in the bedroom) need to be considered.

The audibility of an alarm signal by occupants is dependent on a few variables: alarm characteristics, sound pressure level of the alarm, location of the alarm with respect to occupant location, and the sound transmission loss through building elements such as doors and walls, and occupant characteristics. Regulations like NFPA 72, *Fire Alarm and Signaling Code,* and the British Standard, *BS 5839-Part 1* require a minimum sound pressure level of 75 dBA to be received at the pillow when a smoke alarm is sounding. However, research has found 72.5 dBA (±17.7 dBA) to be the average awakening threshold of sober, normal hearing adults in response to a high frequency alarm [7].

Several studies [7, 10, 24, 25] have examined the impact of the position of a hollow-core door on the received sound pressure level inside a bedroom from 85dBA and 90 dBA alarms outside the bedroom. Some analyzed an alarm placed directly outside the bedroom door, while others examined the impact of an alarm

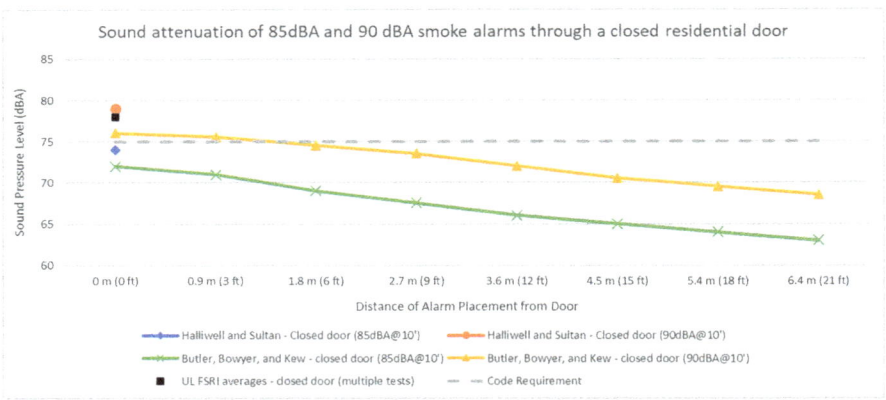

Fig. 9.1 Sound attenuation of 85dBA and 90dBA smoke alarms through a closed interior door

being placed at varying distances down a hallway. These results are depicted in Fig. 9.1. As shown, when the door is closed, an 85 dBA smoke alarm directly outside the bedroom will generally not meet the 75 dBA requirement at the pillow; a 90 dBA alarm may be acceptable for up to 1.5 m (5 ft) from the bedroom door. The Butler et al. [24] study showed that the sound pressure level received at the pillow could be 10–15 dBA lower than the required 75 dBA sound pressure level, as the distance of the smoke alarm from the closed bedroom door exceeds 6 m (~20 ft).

Through further alarm audibility testing by Thomas and Bruck, five unique residential geometries were studied with representative alarm frequencies. In the results, they found that an 85 dBA alarm located in the hallway resulted in audibility that ranged between 40.0 and 74.8 dBA in a bedroom with an open door and 37.4 dBA and 55.9 dBA when the bedroom door was closed[1] [23]. While the percentage by which the door reduces the sound level received in the bedroom will depend on a number of characteristics, research indicates that the value can be significant in some cases.

Given that only about 55.6% of occupants wake to a sound pressure level of 75 dBA, and only 33% wake to 64 dBA, a closed door can present significant risks in terms of achieving adequate notification [7]. Although requirements for bedroom alarms and the interconnection of alarms are increasing, this is currently not common practice. Most of the residential housing stock where alarms are installed likely only have an alarm in the hallway, thus the impact of a closed bedroom door on the received sound levels does introduce risks that can delay occupant notification, and in turn, egress.

---

[1] Note: This study took measurements inside the bedroom, diagonal from the bedroom door, at pillow height. This additional distance could correlate to lower sound pressure levels than some other referenced studies.

4.3 Occupant Tenability: Doors' Impact on Temperature, Smoke Spread, and Gas Exposure

Once occupants are notified of the fire, whether from an alarm or by other means, there is a limited amount of time in a residential fire before the conditions become untenable. The time and severity of the conditions are dependent on the fire scenario, layout of the home, the vulnerability of the occupants, the location of the occupants in relation to the fire, and the occupant's ability for self-rescue or reliance on the fire brigade.

Occupant tenability, defined as an occupant's ability to survive in a fire setting, is a critical parameter in residential fire scenarios. Occupants are exposed to numerous airborne contaminants and physical hazards in a fire environment and during egress, namely, thermal effects and toxic gas exposures, like carbon monoxide (CO), carbon dioxide (CO_2), hydrogen cyanide (HCN), among others [29]. Exposure to adequate doses of these toxic by-products can cause incapacitation and death through narcosis and irritancy. These fire products can impede egress by causing painful stimuli to the eyes, nose, throat, and lungs, which can lead to inflammation of the lungs, ultimately restricting breathing and leading to death. Additionally, escape can be slowed or hindered by smoke, visually obscuring the egress path, or by thermal barriers such as skin pain, burns, or hyperthermia that may result in death during or after exposure [29].

The effects of sensory irritation, visual obscuration by smoke, and thermal exposure are generally present immediately upon exposure and the ultimate hazard is dependent on and proportional to the concentration. Recommended tenability limits for visibility through smoke is OD/m 0.2 for small enclosures and 0.08 for large enclosures [31]. The widely accepted tenability limit for skin exposure to radiant heat is approximately 2.5 kW/m². This exposure corresponds to a 200 °C hot gas layer and can be tolerated for a few minutes by most occupants [31]. Threshold exposure concentrations of common asphyxiant gases at which serious impacts to occupant health and safety are expected have been defined in various studies [29–31] and are summarized in Table 9.1.

Over the years, research on occupant tenability in residential applications has highlighted the important role interior doors can play in protecting or slowing occupants' exposure to the toxic by-products of fire, and in turn, lowering their

Table 9.1 Tenability limits for incapacitation or death from exposures to common asphyxiant gases [31]

	5-min exposure		30-min exposure	
	Incapacitation	Death	Incapacitation	Death
CO	6000–8000 ppm	12,000–16,000 ppm	1400–1700 ppm	2500–4000 ppm
CO_2	7–8%	>10%	6–7%	>9%
HCN	150–200 ppm	250–400 ppm	90–120 ppm	170–230 ppm
Low O_2	10–13%	<5%	<12%	6–7%

probability of experiencing an incapacitating dose prior to escape or fire department rescue [19–22, 27, 28].

Madrzykowski and Weinschenk conducted a series of twelve experiments where a fire was ignited on the basement level, and measurements on compartment temperature and concentrations of oxygen and carbon monoxide were captured in bedrooms with an open and closed door on the first story of a single-family dwelling [27]. Through these experiments, it was found that the oxygen concentrations behind the closed interior doors remained at acceptable levels (above 20%), while the open-door scenarios had oxygen concentrations ranging between 0.3% and 19.5%, which created negative health implications in the majority of the tests [27]. The experimental data also suggest a strong correlation between a closed interior residential door and the ability to keep the CO concentrations to survivable levels in the room behind the closed door. With a closed interior door, the CO levels were consistently around 0.1% (1000 ppm), which has an effect of slight heart palpitations, whereas when the door was open the CO concentrations ranged from 0.2% (2000 ppm) to 3.3% (33,000 ppm). A 0.2% CO exposure for 30 min can cause slight heart palpitations, while concentrations between 0.32% and 3.3% can result in death, for short periods of exposure. In most of the experiments, the open bedrooms experienced elevated temperatures and reached fatal CO exposures and oxygen concentrations below survivable levels, while the rooms protected by a close door maintained tenable conditions [27].

Similarly, the benefits of a closed door inside the premises of the fire compartment with respect to occupant tenability were confirmed by Kerber [28]. Given a living room fire in a single-family one-story dwelling, measurements were captured in two side-by-side bedrooms where one door was closed and the other was open. The oxygen level never dropped below 19.5% in the room with a closed door, whereas it dropped below 10% in the open bedroom [28]. Similarly, the temperature in the hallway outside the bedroom was 900 °C, while the temperature in the room with the closed door was only 125 °C, over seven times lower.

It should be noted that when an occupant is exposed to toxic gases in a fire atmosphere, they inhale and are exposed to a mixture of toxic products of varying concentrations; therefore, the exposures are normalized by the concept of fractional effective concentration (FEC) or fractional effective dose (FED), where the exposure concentration of any by-product during a fire is quantified as a fraction of the dose predicted to give a negative effect (e.g., incapacitation, loss of consciousness, etc.). The ultimate impact on the occupant is dependent on the sum of the received dose of each toxic gas exposure.

ISO 13571 [6] specifies a methodology to estimate the fractional effective dose (FED) – the time to incapacitation from either thermal or gaseous effects of fire. A FED value of 1 is intended to indicate that a healthy adult has obtained a sufficient dose of fire-related toxicants and exposures to cause incapacitation. However, there is wide variation in occupant's susceptibility. For instance, young children, the elderly, and unhealthy adults are significantly more susceptible to the impact of fire effluents than healthy young adults. So, to ensure the majority of the population will be able to escape, a safety factor is commonly applied by setting the acceptable FED at 0.3 [21].

Trainia et al. (2017) conducted a series of seventeen experiments in a one- and two-story single-family dwelling that investigated the impact of structural geometry, fire location, and door position on occupant tenability [10]. The results of the one-story experiments indicated that in both living room origin and bedroom origin fires, the time to untenability (FED = 0.3) in the bedroom with a closed door was approximately 2.5 times longer than the other rooms in the home, and a FED exposure of nearly 46 times less than other areas of the home. With fire department intervention occurring within approximately 6 min in the one-story home and approximately 10 min in the two-story home, all rooms had exceeded the FED for susceptible populations prior to fire department intervention, except for the bedroom with the door closed. The average time to untenability in all open rooms was 5 min and 32 s in the one-story home and 9 min 36 s in the two-story home experiments. In the various experiments, occupants in the room behind closed doors had between 11 min and 22 min to escape prior to the room becoming untenable, depending on the scenario. Crewe et al. found similar results for time to untenability in rooms with closed doors [21]. When considering that egress time from residential structures can range between 2 and 16 min, according to a study by the National Resource Council of Canada, a closed door can significantly increase an occupant's probability for safe egress.

While Bukowski found that a closed door can extend available egress time by approximately 10 times [26], it should be recognized that tenability in areas of the home not protected by closed doors will likely be poor [27, 28] and may require the occupant to depend on fire department rescue.

4.4 Pressure Peaks: Doors' Impact on Egress

Beyond the concerns of detection, notification, and tenability, we must also consider the potential for the door to act as a barrier to egress. In an egress situation, occupants must be able to open the doors that are on their way to safety. In addition to the behavioral and smoke-induced physiological challenges, fire-induced pressure may prevent the door's use if the door opens inwards and is relatively air-tight. Interior doors are usually not airtight and are therefore unlikely to face the pressure-related opening problems.

The possibility of pressure-related door opening challenges has long been recognized in the context of smoke control. The design standards for pressurization systems, such as NFPA 92, *Standard for Smoke Control Systems,* and EN 12101–6, *Smoke and Heat Control Systems,* calculate the critical force by balancing the moments of pressure and handle pulling forces: $F = \Delta P \times A \times (W/2)/(W-d)$, where ΔP is the pressure difference, A is the door leaf area, W is the door width, and d is the distance from the doorknob center to the edge of the door nearest to the knob. Possible door closers would increase this force. For typical measurements of

$A = 1.8$ m^2, $W = 0.9$ m, and $d = 7.5$ cm, we get an approximate formula for the required opening force: $F \approx \Delta P$, when ΔP is in Pa and F in N. Most standards seem to propose a critical force in the range of 110 to 130 Pa. This means that the critical overpressure of the fire compartment is somewhere between 100 and 200 Pa.

A key event that made researchers and fire authorities aware of the fire-induced pressure problem took place in Cologne, Germany, in 2013. The fire ignited in the living room of a 'Passivhaus' in the night. The occupant woke up, tried to extinguish the fire but failed, and decided to escape, just to notice he could not pull the door open. After a moment, he managed to open a balcony door and survived to report about the event. The doors were later tested and found to be in good working conditions. In their investigation of the incident, Brohez and Duhamel carried out CFAST simulations of the fire, showing peak pressures of 500 Pa [12].

Soon after the Cologne fire, Finnish firefighters observed a similar situation in their training, where they tried to attack an apartment fire but could not open the inwards-opening exterior door due to the high internal pressure. Likewise, occupants inside the apartment also would not have bee able to overcome the high pressure forces on the door to egress either. This conclusion was later confirmed by Kallada, Janardhan, and Hostikka in a scientific experiment where a fireman with a breathing apparatus ignited a polyurethane mattress inside a 58.5 m^2 flat and 16 s later tried to open the inwards-opening door leading into the stairway. Opening the door was found to be impossible due to the excessive overpressure conditions [14]. According to the measurements 26 s from ignition, the internal overpressure was 800 Pa.

The dynamics of the pressure development inside a closed house or apartment seem to be quite different from the temperature development, which usually follows the HRR with some delay. Figure 9.2 illustrates the HRR and pressure behaviors in a heptane pool fire inside a closed apartment with three different settings of the mechanical exhaust ventilation [14]. Although the HRR reached its peak 70 s from ignition, the pressure peaks were reached already at about 30 s, after which the pressure difference decreased and approached zero despite the continuously burning fire. Sudden extinction of the fire due to the fuel burnout caused another, negative

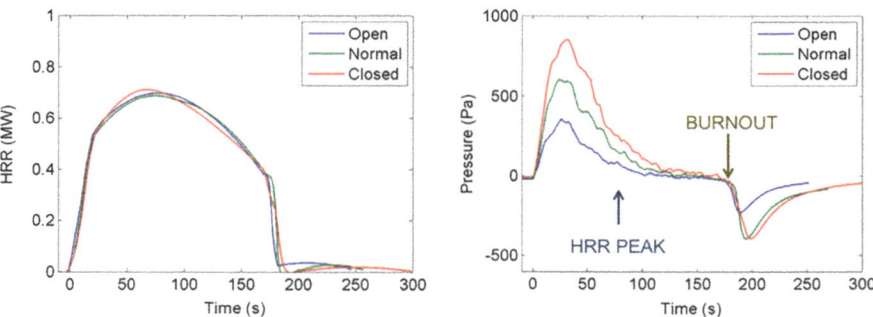

Fig. 9.2 Experimentally measured heat release rate (left) and apartment pressure (right) in the experiments of Kallada Janardhan and Hostikka (2017)

peak in pressure. The magnitude of the pressure peaks showed a clear dependence on the ventilation system condition: using the ventilation system as it was built and used led to a peak overpressure of 600 Pa. Closing the system tightly increased the peak pressure to almost 900 Pa, and opening the ventilation ducts by removing the room dampers decreased it to 300 Pa.

But why was this, rather obvious risk of egress impairment, not noticed until now, after about 50 years of modern fire science? There appears to be two main reasons. First, most of the experimental fire research has focused on temperature as a main fire consequence, and high temperatures are only achieved if the fire is well-ventilated. In most cases, this means open enclosure, where pressure differences cannot be observed. Much fewer studies have been done in closed enclosures, and they have mainly focused on the effects of vitiation. The second reason seems to be the fact that the problem is actually new; it has been created by the increasing airtightness of the modern buildings, driven by the energy efficiency requirements. In Nordic countries, for instance, the change has been quite dramatic, with air permeability values q_{50} of reducing from the order of 10 m^3/hm^2 for 1970s and 80s buildings [15] to less than 3 m^3/hm^2 in the twenty-first century [16], and now approaching a value well below 1 m^3/hm^2 due to the current building regulations.

The influence of the building's airtightness on the pressure peak has been studied by numerical simulations. Hostikka et al. [13] used a validated CFD fire model using the data shown in Fig. 9.2 and then used the model to quantify the effects of the apartment envelope airtightness, ventilation configuration, and fire growth rate [13]. The building envelopes were classified based on their q_{50}-values as Traditional (q_{50} = 3 m^3/hm^2), Modern (q_{50} = 1.5 m^3/hm^2), or Near-Zero (q_{50} = 0.75 m^3/hm^2). The ventilation system had a mechanical inlet and outlet and small-diameter (120 mm) ductwork with dampers (closing systems). The three investigated damper configurations represent the situations where (1) there are no dampers, (2) only the inlet branch is closed by a damper, and (3) there are dampers on both branches. Figure 9.3 shows the simulated peak pressures for a 50 m^2 apartment with medium, fast, and ultrafast t^2-fire growth rates. The results indicate that in medium-growth rate fires, the critical pressure would not be exceeded with certainty in traditional buildings and possibly in modern buildings when dampers are not used for both branches. For all the other scenarios, peak pressure could prevent door opening, at least momentarily. The time frames when this occurs for the fast fires were determined by choosing a critical pressure of 100 Pa. With more airtight envelope, the pressure criterion is exceeded earlier, and the duration of the egress impairment is longer. In general, the dangerous period starts between 20 and 80 s from the ignition and ends between 220 and 240 s. Unfortunately, these are the moments when typical home fires develop life-threatening conditions.

In addition to the possible prevention of door opening, high pressure differentials can also open doors that are initially closed if they lack sufficient locking mechanism. This could lead to smoke spread and reduced tenability beyond the room of fire origin. However, little to no research has focused on the pressure resistance of residential doors, to date.

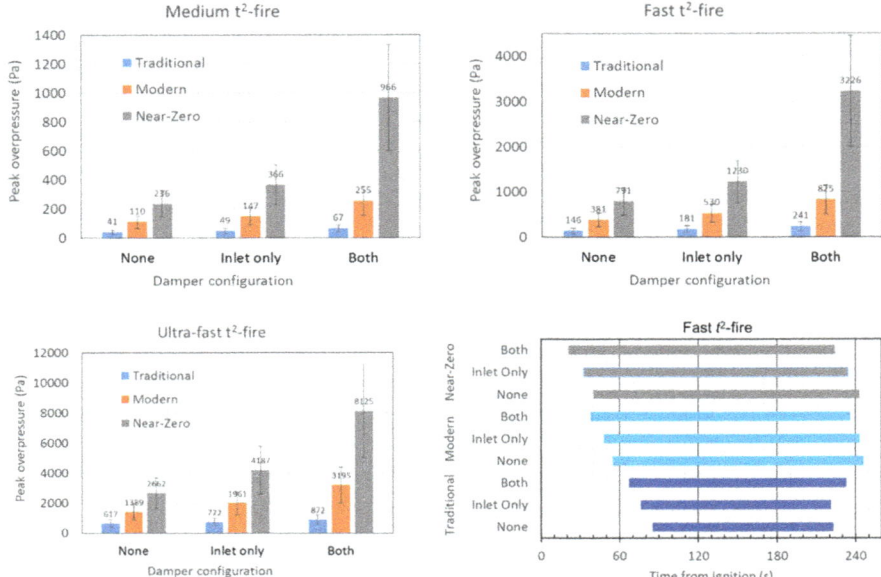

Fig. 9.3 Simulated peak pressures for medium, fast, and ultrafast fires, and no-escape time frames for a fast t^2-fire inside a 50 m^2 apartment with different levels of the envelope airtightness and damper configurations

5 Conclusions

Any closed door, whether hollow-core, solid-core, solid-wood, or fire-rated, can provide protection against the effects of fire, such as heat and smoke, for occupants outside the room of origin. A closed door can extend the tenability time, providing occupants more time to escape and buying time for the fire service to arrive and act on the fire. However, the barrier of a closed door can adversely affect alarm activation and received audibility. The development of the building envelopes and ventilation systems through the modern energy-efficiency norms has also increased the probability of escape impairment through pressure increase, which may prevent occupants from opening an inwards-opening door during the first minutes of a residential fire. The risks and rewards of door position must be taken into account for residential fire safety.

References

1. Ahrens M, Maheshwari R (2020) Home structure fires. NFPA, Quincy
2. Kerber S (2012) Analysis of changing residential fire dynamics and its implications on firefighter operational timeframes. Fire Technol 48:865–891. https://doi.org/10.1007/s10694-011-0249-2

3. Fire Service Academy (2018) Fatal residential fires in Europe: a preliminary assessment of risk profiles in nine European countries. European Fire Safety Alliance, Arnhem. Retrieved from https://europeanfiresafetyalliance.org/wp-content/uploads/2018/11/20181120-Fatal-residential-fires-in-Europe.pdf
4. HM Government (2013) The building regulations 2010, approved document B (fire safety), volume 1: dwelling houses
5. Hopkin C, Spearpoint M, Wang Y (2019) Internal door closing habits in domestic premises: results of a survey and the potential implications on fire safety. Saf Sci:44–56
6. ISO 13571 (2012) Life threatening components of fire – guidelines for the estimation of time to compromised tenability in fires. ISO
7. Olenick S, Boehmer H, Klassen M (2019) Door messaging strategies – implications for detection and notification. Fire Protection Research Foundation, Quincy
8. Schifiliti R (2016) Design of detection systems. In: Hurley MJ (ed) SFPE handbook of fire protection engineering. Springer, pp 1314–1377
9. Shoub H, Gross D (1966) Doors as barriers to fire and smoke. National Bureau of Standards, District of Columbia
10. Traina N, Kerber S, Kyritsis DC, Horn GP (2017) Occupant tenability in single family homes: part I – impact of structure type, fire location and interior doors prior to fire department arrival. Fire Technol:1589–1610
11. US Deperatment of Housing and Urban Development. (2009) Sound transmission classification guidance - noise attenuation. HUD
12. Brohez S, Duhamel P (2018) Inwards doors blocked by fire induced overpressure in airtight apartment: a real case in Germany. Chemical Eng Trans 67:25–30
13. Hostikka S, Kallada Janardhan R, Riaz U, Sikanen T (2017) Fire-induced pressure and smoke spreading in mechanically ventilated buildings with air-tight envelopes. Fire Saf J 91:380–388. https://doi.org/10.1016/j.firesaf.2017.04.006
14. Kallada Janardhan R, Hostikka S (2017) Experiments and numerical simulations of pressure effects in apartment fires. Fire Technol 53:1353–1377
15. Mortensen LH, Bergsøe NC (2017) Air tightness measurements in older Danish single-family houses. Energy Procedia 132:825–830
16. Vinha J, Manelius E, Korpi M, Salminen K, Kurnitski J, Kiviste M, Laukkarinen A (2015) Airtightness of residential buildings in Finland. Building and Environment 93(Part 2):128–140. https://doi.org/10.1016/j.buildenv.2015.06.011
17. Build (2019, December 13) Hollow core doors. Australia. Retrieved from: https://build.com.au/hollow-core-doors
18. The Spruce (2020, December 17) Wood door comparison: solid wood, solid-core, and hollow-Core. United States
19. Peacock RD, Averill JD, Reneke PA, Jones WW (2004) Characteristics of fire scenarios in which sublethal effects of smoke are important. Fire Technol 40(2):127–147
20. Guillaume E, Didieux F, Thiry A, Bellivier A (2014) Real-scale fire tests of one bedroom apartments with regard to tenability assessment. Fire Saf J 70:81–97
21. Crewe RJ, Stec AA, Walker RG, Shaw JE, Hull TR, Rhodes J, Garcia-Sorribes T (2014) Experimental results of a residential house fire test on tenability: temperature, smoke, and gas analyses. J Forensic Sci 59(1):139–154
22. Su JZ, Benichou N, Bwalya AC, Lougheed GD, Taber BC, Leroux P (2010) Tenability analysis for fire experiments conducted in a full-scale test house with basement fire scenarios. National Research Council of Canada, Ottawa
23. Thomas I, Bruck D (2010) The time of activation of smoke alarms in houses - the effect of location, smoke source, alarm type and manufacturer, and other factors. Victoria University, Melbourne
24. Butler H, Bowyer A, Kew J. Locating fire alarm sounders for audibility. Building Services Research and Information Association. Application Guide 1/81, 1981

25. Halliwell RE, Sultan MA. Attenuation of smoke detector alarm signals in residential buildings. Proceedings of the First International Symposium of Fire Safety Science (IAFSS), 1986
26. Bukowski RW, Peacock RD, Averill JD, Cleary TG, Bryner NP, Walton WD, Reneke PA, Kuligowski ED. Performance of Home Smoke Alarms: Analysis of the Response of Several Available Technologies in Residential Fire Settings. NIST Technical Note 1455–1, February 2008 revision
27. Madrzykowski D, Weinschenk C (2018) Understanding and fighting basement fires. UL Firefighter Safety Research Institute, Columbia
28. Kerber S (2010) Impact of ventilation on fire behavior in legacy and contemporary residential construction. Underwriters Laboratories, Northbrook
29. Purser DA (1989) Modelling toxic and physical Hazard in fire. Second international symposium of fire safety science. Hemisphere Publishing Corporation, Washington, pp 391–400
30. Purser DA (2010) Toxic hazard calculation models for use with fire effluent data. In: Stec A, Hull R (eds) Fire toxicity. Woodhead Publishing Limited, Cambridge, pp 619–636
31. Purser DA, McAllister JL (2016) Assessment of hazards to occupants from smoke, toxic gases, and heat. In: Hurley MJ (ed) SFPE handbook of fire protection engineering. Society of Fire Protection Engineers, New York, pp 2308–2428

Ms. Victoria N. Hutchison is a Research Project Manager at the Fire Protection Research Foundation (FPRF), the research affiliate of the National Fire Protection Association (NFPA) in the United States, where she plans, manages, and facilitates fire and life safety research in support of the NFPA mission. Victoria holds a MSc in Fire Protection Engineering from Worcester Polytechnic Institute, a BSc in Fire Protection and Safety Engineering Technology from Oklahoma State University and serves as the Deputy Editor for the SFPE Handbook of Fire Protection Engineering. Prior to joining FPRF, her experience focused on fire protection system design and engineering analyses for commercial and residential properties.

Prof Simo Hostikka received his MSc in 1997 from Helsinki University of Technology, and DSc (Tech) from the same university in 2008. Since 1997 he worked as a researcher, principal scientist and team leader at VTT Technical Research Centre of Finland, where he led projects on the fire risk analyses and engineering. His main fields of research have been the numerical fire simulation and probabilistic risk analyses. He has served as a principal developer of the thermal radiation and solid pyrolysis sub-models of the Fire Dynamics Simulator (FDS) software. Since 2014 he works at Aalto University, leading a team of about 10 doctoral students and post-doctoral researchers. He has served as Building Technology MSc program director and teaches two courses in fire dynamics and risk analysis.

Chapter 10
Prevention of Ignition and Limitation of Fire Development in Furnishing and Home Environment

Anne Steen-Hansen and Karolina Storesund

Abstract Some fire safety measures will benefit all types of homes and occupants, while other measures may not be helpful for people who are considered as especially vulnerable in a fire situation. Fire safety should therefore be planned and designed with a holistic perspective, taking both the specific building and individual into account.

One important factor in residential fire safety is the furnishing. The furnishing may be easily ignited and may represent large amounts of fuel that can lead to a rapid fire development with high heat release and large amounts of toxic smoke.

Fire statistics has shown that the most typical ignition sources in dwelling fires are open flames, smoking materials and electrical apparatuses and installations. Upholstered furniture and mattresses are often involved in residential fires, both as the first items ignited and as objects responsible for fire development. This chapter describes the problem connected to soft furnishing and proposes ways of solving it. Other types of furnishing, their role in fire development and possible solutions to the problem are also described.

1 Strategies for a Holistic Assessment of Residential Fire Safety

Fire safety in private homes should be regarded as an obvious quality, just as personal safety in cars, trains and aircrafts has become the standard. Therefore, the chosen fire safety measures should be simple, easy to implement, aesthetically

---

A. Steen-Hansen (✉)
Department of Civil and Environmental Engineering, Norwegian University of Science and Technology, Trondheim, Norway

RISE Fire Research, Trondheim, Norway
e-mail: anne.steen-hansen@ntnu.no

K. Storesund
RISE Fire Research, Trondheim, Norway

© The Author(s), under exclusive license to Springer Nature Switzerland AG 2023
M. Runefors et al. (eds.), *Residential Fire Safety*, The Society of Fire Protection Engineers Series, https://doi.org/10.1007/978-3-031-06325-1_10

pleasing and cost-effective. They should also be durable, with a long life-time and require a minimum of maintenance.

The assessment should as far as possible include environmental and sustainability considerations; e.g. does the intended safety measure represent any obvious negative effects on health or environment? Which raw materials are required, and will the solution be recyclable? Could another measure give the same level of safety?

The probability of ignition can be reduced by simple measures, like by:

- Avoiding that combustible items are placed in the close vicinity of ovens and other heat producing units (e.g. sofas and beds close to wood stoves, electric heaters placed below curtains).
- Avoiding the use of extension leads.
- Avoiding the use of flaming candles, and instead using battery-powered candles.
- Controlling that electrical equipment has no obvious faults like loose connections, hot parts or irregular behaviour.
- Using timers on kettles and coffee makers.
- Allowing smoking only in safe areas, or under supervision if necessary.

In the context of fire safety in dwellings, Arvidsson et al. [1] defined the term *forgiving system* as a "System or product that allows an individual to make mistakes without being injured or killed by fire". Technical measures that may be implemented and may target different needs with regard to prevent fires or make the fires hard to arise and thereby work as a "forgiving" solution include:

- Stove guards.
- RIP cigarettes and different measures aimed at reducing the fire risk from smoking.
- Self-extinguishing candles and candle extinguishers.
- Fire protection of electronic equipment.
- Fire safe furnishing.
- Measures aimed at reducing the risk from open flame.
- Detection and alarms.
- Automatic extinguishing systems.

Although many of these measures could be helpful for all on a general basis, individuals who experience an increased vulnerability to fire will, depending on their specific challenges, be helped by targeting the preventive measures to their specific needs. Targeting and adjusting technical preventive measures to specific challenges is just a part of a necessary holistic view of the circumstances that influence the probability and consequences of fires in dwellings, as is described in [2–4] and it includes recognizing the physical, social and organizational surroundings of the individual, as illustrated in Fig. 10.1.

The prevention of fatal fires for vulnerable groups of people is an issue that requires attention and cooperation from several public sectors as well as cooperation between different fields of science. Having identified the fire safety challenges for an individual, it is important to select suitable measures to target these specific challenges. Changing attitudes, raising the awareness and teaching fire safety are all

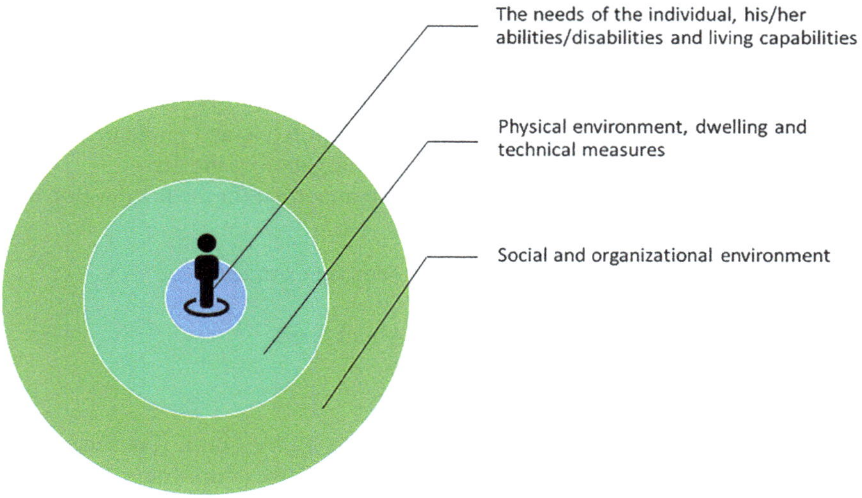

Fig. 10.1 Circumstances that influence the risk of fatal dwelling fires [2, 5]

Labels (outer to inner):
- The needs of the individual, his/her abilities/disabilities and living capabilities
- Physical environment, dwelling and technical measures
- Social and organizational environment

important measures in all of these situations. Fire safety for vulnerable groups is further described in Chap. 17.

New products and solutions for fire prevention are continuously being developed and made available on the market. Not all technical solutions are clearly defined with respect to performance requirements, properly documented or certified. However, clear and defined requirements for function and documentation will strengthen the availability and the quality of fire preventive technical solutions and thereby help improving the fire safety for people in general, and for people who experience an increased fire risk in particular.

This chapter is focusing on fire safety in connection to the content of a home, especially the furnishing. However, in a holistic view the combination of products with good fire properties and other types of fire safety measures is important to obtain the desired fire safety level. Such measures can, e.g., be fire detectors, stove guards, automatic extinguishing systems and manual extinguishing equipment, which are described in other chapters of this anthology. Implementation of organizational measures may also be important.

2 Fire Development and the Role of the Content of the Dwelling

The furnishing of homes – or more specifically the amount and types of materials in items like sofas, mattresses, carpets and curtains – is of great importance for residential fire safety. Materials that are easily ignitable, spread fire fast and release large amounts of heat and toxic smoke can lead to a rapid fire development and result in too little available time for safe egress (ASET) [6]. This period of time can be increased by introduction of barriers that prevent heat development, prevent ignition or mitigate the fire development [7]. Examples of such barriers could be choice of materials with good fire properties in furnishing items, and implementation of fire safety measures that efficiently can lead to mitigation of the fire.

The following factors related to the room are important for the fire development:

- Size and location of the ignition source.
- Furnishing: type, amounts, location, geometry and surface area.
- Reaction to fire properties of the furnishing.
- Reaction to fire properties of walls, ceiling and floor.
- Ventilation conditions.
- Room geometry.

To be able to design and apply efficient fire safety measures, it is necessary to know how, where and why residential fires start, how these fires may develop and how fires pose a threat to people in the dwelling.

2.1 Fire Development in a Compartment

A fire can be described by a series of stages: First, a material is ignited by an ignition source; e.g. an open flame, a spark or a smouldering cigarette. The fire then develops in the ignited object, and the development may be slow or fast dependent on factors like ignition source, material, geometry, ventilation, etc. Some fires start as smouldering fires, i.e. as a low temperature combustion with no flames, but with considerable smoke production. Smouldering combustion takes place on the interior surface (e.g. in pores and cavities) of a material. Upholstery foam, combustible insulation materials and porous wood products are examples of materials in which smouldering combustion may occur [8]. A smouldering fire may transform into a flaming fire when the conditions are changed, which can happen when the combustion front reaches the material surface and the access to air is increased.

When a flaming fire is established the development may escalate, the fire can spread to other objects in the room. This may lead to flashover, which is when the room is completely involved in the fire. Flashover is a very critical point in the fire development, as it enables the fire to spread out of the room to other parts of the building. The chances to survive in a room after flashover are minimal. After flashover, the fire is fully developed and will continue to burn until either all combustible materials are consumed, there is too little oxygen to support the combustion, or until the fire is extinguished by manual or automatic firefighting equipment. A schematic presentation of fire development in a compartment is shown in Fig. 10.2.

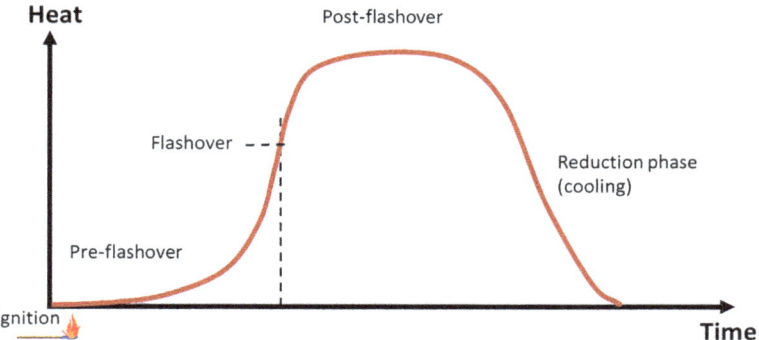

Fig. 10.2 Schematic presentation of fire development in a compartment

2.2 How and Where Residential Fires Start

There are many potential ignition sources in a regular dwelling, but the most common according to, for example, Norwegian fire statistics are electricity and open flame [9]. In this context, *open flame* includes smoking materials, like matches, lighters and cigarettes. Fires starting on the cooking top are, in the case of Norwegian statistics, included in the number of fires with electric start. For example, in 2018 as much as 55% of all fire brigade call-outs to Norwegian dwelling fires started on the cooking top, including incidents where the fire service reported that they avoided that a dangerous situation developed into a flaming fire [9]. The number of cooking incidents that actually do develop into a fire is considerably lower and was estimated to be just below 8% of all dwelling fires in the period 1998–2007 [10, 11]. Cooking fires caused about 10% of the fire fatalities in Norway in this period. Smoking is the most common cause of ignition of upholstered furniture, the ignition source being either a smouldering cigarette, or a match, or lighter [12, 13].

As concerns the cause and origin of fire, fatal fires do not reflect the average residential fire. It is, e.g., reported that the bulk of all residential fires start in connection with cooking in the kitchen, but that the leading cause of fatal fires is smoking. The majority of fatal fires occurring in Norway, Sweden and Denmark start in the living room, followed by the bedroom as a common point of origin [9, 14, 15]. In the USA, it is most common that fatal fires start in the bedroom, followed by the living room [16]. The bed and furniture are usually the first ignited objects in fatal fires, often related to ignition caused by cigarette smoking or use of open flames. A Swedish study showed that 17% of fires starting in a bed were fatal [15]. Electrical appliances are involved in many fires, both those resulting in fatalities and those without. During the 1998–2007 period, stoves stand out in the Norwegian fatal fire statistics as the most common appliance when the cause of fire is faulty electrical equipment, or incorrect use of such equipment [10, 11].

It is being maintained that a large proportion of residential fires start as smouldering fires [17]. This is, however, hard to document, because the majority of fires develop into flaming fires, which makes it hard or impossible to identify the smouldering afterwards. The majority of fatal fires have grown large when the fire brigade arrives and have spread out of the room in which the fire started [15]. However, it is a well-known fact that fires may start through smoldering in a number of materials, e.g., when upholstered furniture and mattresses are exposed to a smouldering cigarette, or through overheating in electrical installations near combustible insulation or wood.

2.3 Role of Furnishing in Fatal Fires

Furnishings, such as upholstered furniture, mattresses and textiles, are very important for the fire development in the early stages. Some of these products can be easily ignited, contribute to rapid spread of fire and produce a lot of smoke and heat when they burn. This limits the time available for safe egress, rescue and firefighting.

US statistics shows that more people die in residential fires that start in upholstered furniture, mattresses and bedding than in any other items. It is estimated that about 1% of the fire services' responses to home fires in the period 2013–2017 comprised fires that started in furnishings of these types, while as much as 17% of the fire fatalities could be related to these fires [12].

The picture is quite similar in other countries. Fire statistics from England for the period April 2019 to March 2020 shows that close to 5% of fires in dwellings started in soft furnishings. These fires led to 26% of the fatalities in dwelling fires [18]. Fires that started in all kinds of furniture and textiles in interior in the same period comprised 22% of all dwelling fires and 37% of related fatalities. Furnishing and textiles (clothing not included) were assessed to be the items mainly responsible for the fire development in 20% of these fires. These fires resulted in close to 47% of the dwelling fire fatalities [19]. This implies that fires involving such furniture items are more hazardous for people than other fires.

One of the conclusions from a Swedish study of residential fatal fires in the period 1999–2013 was that fires starting in the living room or bedroom more often result in fatalities than fires starting in other rooms [15]. Twenty-seven percent of fatal fires started in the living room, while 22% in the bedroom. Of the two thirds of the fatal fires where the first ignited object was known, 57% fires started in upholstered furniture, bed or other types of furnishing.

In a Norwegian study of fatal fires in the period 2005–2014, 37% of the fires started in the living room and nearly 13% in the bedroom. The first ignited material was not registered in the Norwegian statistics; however, it is reasonable to believe that soft furnishing contributed to a high degree in the start and development in many of these fires [20].

It is quite obvious that it is of crucial importance for residential fire safety to prevent these fires from starting and to mitigate or delay the fire development if an ignition should occur.

3 Regulation and Documentation of Fire Properties of Furnishing

3.1 Regulations

The probably most efficient way to control fire safety in residential buildings is to give mandatory requirements in regulations. Other requirements may be of more voluntary nature, e.g. directives given by insurance companies, by building owners, or by organizations. Different possibilities for regulation of the contents of residential buildings are shown in Fig. 10.3.

Fire safety of the construction elements and building products in a residential building is normally regulated through building codes and will not be discussed here.

Regulation of fire properties of interior textiles, armchairs, sofas and mattresses has been discussed nationally and internationally for many years, without resulting in more stringent requirements for such products, at least not on a harmonized level. All products sold on the European market, including loose furnishings, shall fulfil the General Product Safety Directive (GPSD) 2001/95/EC [21]. Although fire safety is not explicitly stated in the directive, it must be regarded as an important safety property of a product.

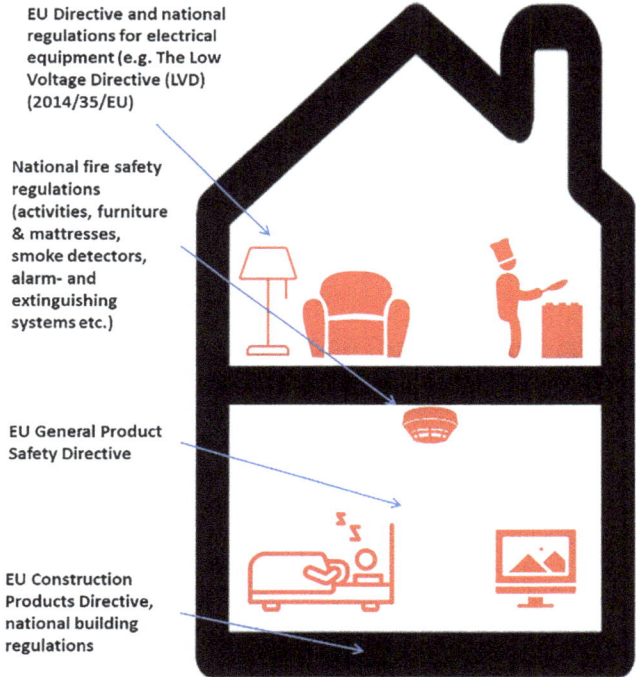

Fig. 10.3 Regulations on different levels can affect the fire safety level of the content in a home

Some European countries have regulations on this area, and there is a spread in where the regulations are applied (e.g. public buildings, private homes, hospitals etc.) and also in the level of required fire properties. Different ignition sources are used in the required tests for soft furnishing and span from a smouldering cigarette to a larger flaming source [22].

The European countries UK, Ireland, Germany, France, Portugal, Spain, Italy, Norway, Sweden and Finland have introduced fire requirements for loose furnishings. These requirements mainly cover public areas such as hospitals, prisons, hotels, theatres, etc. However, for the domestic environment, most countries lack fire requirements. In Europe, only UK, Ireland and the Nordic countries have fire requirements for private homes [23]. Both Norway and Sweden require that mattresses and upholstered furniture shall resist ignition by a smouldering cigarette.

Outside Europe, USA stands out as a country in the world with stringent requirements on loose furnishings, especially on mattresses where federal requirements apply in all states, and where a larger flaming ignition source is used in the testing for approval. For upholstered furniture, there are no federal requirements and each state is free to determine their own requirements. California is the state that places the most stringent requirements on upholstered furniture, and the ignition source applied in testing is a smouldering cigarette [24]. Ignition resistance against a smouldering cigarette is, however, the lowest level of fire requirements. This qualification gives no information about fire behaviour of the furniture item when exposed to a flaming ignition source.

The fire safety regulations on upholstered furniture and mattresses in UK were imposed in 1988 and are regarded to be rather strict, demanding that the products can withstand a relatively large flaming ignition source called *crib 5* [25]. Crib 5 is a flaming ignition source that gives a heat output approximately corresponding to half of that of a folded double-sheet of 22 g newspaper [26].

3.2 Documentation

In Europe, the fire safety properties of furnishing products are regulated by the Product Safety Directive. There are no requirements on CE marking of textiles and furniture.

For some types of buildings, like prisons, hotels and hospitals, there may be specific requirements describing fire properties of, e.g., mattresses and upholstered furniture, and do therefore also require that the products they purchase have sufficient fire safety documentation. Such documentation includes normally reports from fire testing according to recognized standards. The reports describe which standard was used, which ignition source the product was exposed to and the results from the test. Such information will also be relevant for private consumers who request fire rated furnishing products to increase the residential fire safety.

Fire safety measures do also need documentation. This is relevant for, e.g., extinguishing equipment, flame retardant chemicals, smoke alarms, fire detection systems, stove guards, etc. The documentation shall contain information about possibly applied test methods or standards and obtained test results, any classification, applied assessment methods, scope and limitations of the product, instructions for application, mounting and use, efficiency, etc. For some products, information in a safety data sheet may also be of relevance.

4 Fire Safety of Furnishing Items

4.1 Fire Properties of Interior Textiles

Choosing textiles with good fire properties for furnishing items like curtains, blankets and pillows may be a simple way of improving the residential fire safety. In the initial phase of a fire, the fibre type and the textile construction are important factors for the fire behaviour of a textile. A denser and heavier woven textile will burn slower than a more loosely woven textile of the same material. The surface structure is also of importance; a textile with a fluffy surface will ignite more easily than the same material with a smooth surface. Factors that may have importance for the fire behaviour of textiles are:

- Chemical composition of textile fibres.
- Fibre density.
- Textile structure and surface.
- Thickness.
- Fire retardant treatment.
- Dirt (grease, dust).
- Fire properties of accessories such as ribands and tufts.

These factors may each affect the fire properties in different ways, some will have positive effect on fire behaviour, while others have negative. The fire behaviour will depend on the end-use application of the textile, e.g. if the textile is used as a curtain, carpet, or as cover textile on a sofa. The combination of materials in the interior product will also be important for the resulting fire properties, e.g. the combination of textile and upholstery foam in a piece of furniture. Different fire retardant treatments may have effect in different phases of the fire and could, for example, either prevent ignition or limit the combustion rate. Some fire retardants will act against smouldering ignition, while others are active against a flaming ignition source. A fluffy surface will generally be more easily ignitable than a smooth, dense surface, and the rate of flame spread in the textile will also be influenced by the surface structure.

This means that documentation of fire properties must be relevant for the textile product in its final use. If a textile is to be used as a curtain, the documentation must assess the fire properties in a configuration that is relevant for curtains, for example, by use of a recognized fire test method for free hanging textiles. If the textile is

Table 10.1 Fire behaviour of different furnishing textiles [27–30]

Fibre type		Fire behaviour
Natural fibres	Cotton, linen (cellulosic fibres)	Easily ignitable. A char layer is formed during combustion. May initiate and support smouldering combustion.
	Wool, silk (protein fibres)	Less ignitable than cellulosic fibres. Contain nitrogen and can produce hydrogen cyanide during combustion.
Regenerated fibres	Viscose	Easily ignitable, burns quickly.
	Acetate, triacetate	Easily ignitable, burns quickly, melts and drips.
Synthetic fibres	Polyester	Shrinks away from the ignition source, melts and drips after ignition. Upward flame spread is often slow. Melted material increases horizontal and downwards flame spread.
	Polyamide (nylon)	As polyester, but contains nitrogen and can produce hydrogen cyanide during combustion.
	Acrylic fibre	Easily ignitable. High heat release during combustion, charring material. Contains nitrogen and can produce hydrogen cyanide during combustion.
	Modacrylic fibre	Less ignitable than acrylic fibre. Melts and withdraws from the flame. Regarded as flame-resistant fibre.
	Polyvinyl chloride (PVC)	Difficult to ignite. Melts and withdraws from the flame. Regarded as flame-resistant fibre. Contains chlorine and produces hydrochloric acid during combustion.
Inorganic fibres	Glass fibre	Non-combustible. Limited range of application since the fibre normally is brittle.

applied in upholstered furniture, the documentation must be based on a fire test method for this type of product, taking into account the other materials in that product with which a potential fire would interact.

Fire properties of some common furnishing textiles are listed in Table 10.1. All materials produce toxic smoke gases during combustion, and the type and concentration of gases and the amount of smoke will be of importance. A textile that is difficult to ignite and that burns slowly, giving off small amounts of smoke with a high degree of toxicity, may therefore be a better option than a textile that burns quickly with a high heat release and a fast flame spread.

4.2 Flame Retardants

Flame retardants are chemicals that are added to materials and products to reduce the risk of ignition and may further prevent or delay the fire development. Some flame retardants may provide a protective physical barrier between the flame and combustible material, by, e.g., formation of a char layer when exposed to heat. Other flame retardants may slow down or inhibit the combustion process by limiting the available oxygen for the combustion or by interacting with the chemical combustion reactions.

In recent years, there has been increasing awareness about the fact that some flame retardants affect health and the environment negatively, and this has caused concern about the consequences of fire safety regulations for interior products. It is feared that strict requirements to obtain a certain level of fire safety implicitly mean that harmful flame retardant chemicals need to be applied to the products in question to be able to pass the tests. Some flame retardants are no longer allowed to be used in many countries, e.g. brominated fire retardants. It is important to be aware of harmful effects and avoid use of unwanted products. However, there is also a request for fire retardant additives and chemicals that are environmentally friendly and that pose no health risk.

Most flame retardant textiles can be washed or cleaned as untreated textiles. The instructions for cleaning or washing must then be followed. The flame retardant effect can be reduced over time, through washing and wear-and-tear. There are also alternatives where the flame retardancy is built into the fibre matrix (e.g. the polyester-based Trevira CS) which make them inherently flame retardant.

Some flame retardants are added to the final material or product through impregnation or surface treatment. There are also products on the market intended to spray onto the object to increase the ignition resistance. It is important to follow the instruction manual thoroughly when such products are used and to assess if the intended application area is within the scope of the flame retardant chemical. This type of products can often not document a certain fire classification, but may improve the fire safety of highly combustible furnishing objects, textiles and decorations. The user instructions must be based on facts and relevant tests, and the manufacturers must be able to provide documentation of the efficiency of their products. It may, however, be difficult for non-fire-experts to assess the quality of the product if the fire documentation is not provided by a recognized organization (e.g. fire laboratory, research institution, university, certification body, etc.).

It should, however, be noted that fire retardant chemicals often are targeted against one type of achievement, most commonly to prevent or delay ignition. A flame retardant preventing ignition by a match flame may have little or no effect in decreasing the fire development with respect to flame spread and heat release when the object has been ignited. A flame retardant effective against flaming ignition may show no effect against smouldering ignition. Research projects indicate that there are no correlation between the ability to ignite by a smouldering cigarette and by a flaming source, and also that resistance to these small ignition sources does not reflect the fire growth properties of a furniture item [31, 32].

4.3 Upholstered Furniture and Mattresses

As mentioned in Sect. 2.2, one of the most common ignition sources in combination with upholstered furniture is a smouldering cigarette. However, other ignition sources are also possible, as a lit candle or a lamp that falls over in a sofa, sparks from a fireplace, radiant heat from an electric oven, etc.

It is a well-known fact that upholstered furniture and mattresses may ignite easily and burn rapidly with a very high heat release and a large production of toxic smoke [23, 32, 35, 36]. These fires lead to a larger percentage of fire fatalities than their percentage of fire causes would imply [12]. Fire in a single upholstered armchair may easily release enough heat energy to lead to a rapid flashover in an ordinary living room. Fire development in armchair is illustrated in Fig. 10.4.

Upholstered furniture is common as the first object ignited in residential fires, but does also have an important role as the object responsible for further fire development [19, 32, 37]. The largest part of the fire load is normally contained in the filling material and therefore it is important to prevent that a fire spreads from the cover fabric to the filling material. One way of improving the fire properties of soft furnishing is to add chemical flame retardants to the cover fabric or to the filling material or both. This could both improve the ignitability of the products and slow down the fire development. However, as described in Sect. 10.5.2, there is a large concern about flame retardants today, as many of these products may lead to harmful health and environmental effects.

However, to avoid any fire performance requirements as a means to reduce the use of flame retardants is not a good idea. As a minimum, there should be a small flame ignition resistance requirement, to ensure that furniture is not easily ignitable. Although there may still be a conflict between fire performance and the use of chemical flame retardants, it is better to have low fire safety requirements, than no requirements at all. In that way, a focus is maintained upon reaching a certain fire performance level. Fire performance requirements on individual furniture components (e.g. foam, cover) should be avoided since this may force unnecessary use of chemical flame retardants.

Considerable research has been performed to solve the fire safety problem connected to soft furnishing products over the years, and lately, the development of sustainable and environmentally friendly fire safe upholstered furniture has been

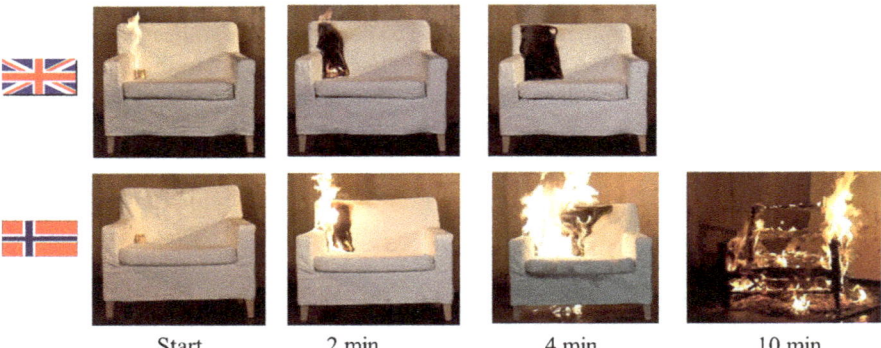

Fig. 10.4 Comparison of fire development in upholstered armchairs with identical design. The chair in the upper photos satisfies the UK fire safety requirements (resist exposure to ignition source crib 5). The chair in the lower photos satisfies the Norwegian requirements (resist ignition by a smouldering cigarette). (Photos: Thor Kr. Adolfsen, Norwegian Fire Protection Association)

brought into focus [15, 26]. Research shows that it could be possible to increase the fire safety level of such products considerably through smart combinations of materials and clever design [23, 35, 39–41]. A correct use of materials will constitute an adequate barrier against ignition in many cases, also without using flame retardant chemicals. There is promising work showing that introducing a textile as a barrier material between the upholstery foam and the cover material is efficient in reducing the fire hazard from burning upholstered furniture [31, 32, 38, 39] and that the interaction between the barrier and cover material is important for the fire growth [36].

For mattresses, the requirements might be different, since a weak ignition protection in a mattress will not be adequate if the duvet and pillow are ignited first, which represents a large start fire.

One of the challenges with fire safety of upholstered furniture and mattresses is that such products may have a long lifetime in a home and it is often not an option, or not even wanted, to replace them with new products with the required fire properties. It is therefore a need for simple, efficient safety measures that can be applied on existing furniture, with the aim of protecting the highly combustible filling material from heat and flame. There exist spray-on flame retardant chemicals on the market that could be a solution in that it prevents the cover material from ignition and further flame spread. Another solution with this effect is to cover the furniture or even replace the cover material with fabrics of better fire protective properties (e.g. a dense wool fabric). If the furniture has a detachable cover fabric, a fire barrier material could be introduced between the cover and the foam.

4.4 Curtains and Draperies

Curtains are manufactured in many different types of fibres, both natural, regenerated and synthetic. The fire load (i.e. the energy content) of a curtain is normally not very large (depending on the size of the curtain) compared to other elements of the furnishing. However, fires often start in curtains and may spread rapidly in the material itself or when the burning curtain falls down and ignites another object, like an upholstered sofa.

Larger draperies and door curtains may, however, release large amounts of heat in a fire and may lead to flashover in a smaller room [33].

4.5 Bedding Items

Duvets and pillows are composite products consisting of a cover material and a filling material. The cover material is normally a textile of cotton, polyester, a mixture of these fibres, or can be made of other types of fibres. Common filling materials are down, mixtures of feathers and down, and polyester fibres [27, 28].

Duvets and pillows will normally resist ignition from a smouldering cigarette in a standardized test, but often not ignition from a match flame.

The bedding items in use are covered with quilt covers and pillow cases, often made of cotton, linen, polyester or blends.

The combination of the cover materials and the filling materials is determining for how a fire may develop in the bedding items. A fire that starts in a duvet can become a large ignition source that would expose the mattress and other combustible objects in the vicinity. Some mattresses on the market are tested for resistance to larger fire sources and will probably resist ignition from a burning duvet. Documentation of fire properties shall then be available for these mattresses.

There are bedding items on the market that contain flame retardant chemicals or fibres. These products may be good alternatives when fire start in the bed is regarded as a risk. Flame retardant products are described briefly in Sect. 10.3.2.

4.6 Carpets

A fire may start in a carpet or it may spread to the carpet from other burning objects, like curtains, upholstered furniture or a mattress. The fire spread in the flooring material will normally be of importance at some stage after the initial phase in the fire. There may be exceptions, for example, if the initial fire exposure is larger than the type of ignition source the flooring is intended to resist, the flooring may contribute considerably to the fire development [34]. As for textiles in general, the ignition and fire spread ability of the carpet will depend on factors like fibre type, density, surface structure (fluffy or smooth), backing material, adhesives, etc. A dense wool carpet with short pile is an example of a carpet that would be expected to have relatively good fire properties. A fluffy carpet made of easily ignitable textile fibres will probably show a poor fire behaviour.

5 Other Methods for Prevention of Ignition in Dwellings

5.1 Reduced Ignition Propensity Cigarettes (RIP)

As already mentioned, a smouldering cigarette is the most common ignition source for ignition of upholstered furniture and mattresses. Seventeen percent of all fatal fires with known fire cause in Norway in the periods 1997–2008 and 2005–2014 were due to smoking [20, 42]. Likewise, smoking material is identified as the leading cause of fatal fires in many countries worldwide [12, 14, 15, 43, 44]. In November 2011, a regulation on self-extinguishing cigarettes was introduced in the EU and EC. Such cigarettes are designed so that they do not burn in all their length but self-extinguish if they are left unattended. The purpose of the requirement was to reduce the number of fires caused by cigarettes [45].

However, it is unclear whether the regulatory requirements for self-extinguishing cigarettes have had the desired effect on fire statistics. US Consumer Product Safety Commission reported in 2012 that it was premature to conclude that use of the RIP cigarette alone will greatly reduce the threat of unintentional fires ignited by cigarettes involving mattresses or soft furnishings [46]. A Swedish study performed 3 years after the introduction of the requirement for self-extinguishing cigarettes on the market was not been able to demonstrate any effect either on the fire statistics or on the fatal fire statistics [47]. Furthermore, small-scale tests were performed on models of upholstered furniture, where it was observed that the cigarettes mainly smouldered in their full length without extinguishing. The solution with introducing RIP cigarettes must therefore be viewed with caution, as it cannot be said to be an efficient or reliable fire safety measure on its own.

5.2 Smoking Apron and Smoking Blanket

Smoking aprons and smoking blankets are made of fire-resistant textile and are used for covering the clothing of persons when they are smoking tobacco. These measures are mostly used when the smokers themselves are not able to deal with situations where embers fall from the cigarette and where they need help to be able to smoke. As it has not been demonstrated that the requirement for self-extinguishing cigarettes works as expected, one should not solely rely on these types of cigarettes, but rather use a smoking apron or smoking blanket where this type of measure is practical [5].

5.3 Protection of Electric Components

Electrical components can pose an increased risk of ignition due to negligent use or because of faulty devices, either through their heat generating function or loose currents leading to over-heating, e.g. in sockets. Electric ovens, dishwashers, washing machines and dryers are examples of electrical equipment that can generate heat and cause ignition. This type of ignition can be prevented by component protection that causes the power to such equipment to be turned off when a dangerous situation is detected. Protection can be achieved by integrating an electronic switch between the frame and the outlet or integrated as part of the fixed electrical installation. This protection technology is being used in electrical equipment in homes. On one hand, it is intended to control and monitor the parameters of electrical devices, household appliances, heating and lighting. On the other hand, it is used to disconnect the power supply when a dangerous situation is detected [5].

There are also possibilities of installing specific extinguishing systems that are integrated into the electrical installation (e.g. socket) or electronic device. The integration of component protection in electrical appliances can also relate to smoke and heat detectors and other sensors such as people presence. The integration allows the adjusting of the logic of the control unit. If, for example, these sensors detect smoke in a laundry room, the power can be disconnected from all appliances in that area [5].

In addition, these control systems can communicate via the internet and send an alarm signal to an external monitoring service. A challenge for component protection is the time required for disconnection of devices when overheating is detected. A fire may start before the network connection is cut off and fire spread may not be able to be prevented.

6 Concluding Remarks

This chapter is dealing with different ways to prevent fire from starting in dwellings and methods that will prevent a small fire from developing into a large and uncontrollable fire. The chapter's main focus is on fire properties of materials in the furnishing.

However, a key word is holistic thinking in order to obtain an optimal fire safety solution. The fire safety measures mentioned here should be used in combination with active measures for detection and mitigation, and there should also be organizational measures that ensure that the right measures are implemented for the person in question, and that the fire safety is maintained and revised regularly.

References

1. Arvidson M, Larsson I, Bergstrand A, Franzon J (2015) Förlåtande system och produkter: Kartläggning av funktion och effektivitet vid bostadsbränder. SP Sveriges Tekniska Forskningsinstitut, Borås
2. Gjøsund G, Almklov PG, Halvorsen K, Storesund K (2016) Vulnerability and prevention of fatal fires. In: Walls L, Revie M, Bedford T (eds) Risk, Reliability and Safety: Innovating Theory and Practice: Proceedings of ESREL 2016. Taylor & Francis Group, CRC Press, Glasgow
3. Storesund K (2015) Managing fire risk for vulnerable people – accessibility of targeted fire preventive measures. In: 1st SFPE Europe Conference on Fire Safety Engineering, Copenhagen
4. Storesund K, Steen-Hansen A (2016) Preventing fatal fires involving vulnerable people. SFPE FPEeXTRA:8
5. Storesund K, Sesseng C, Steen-Hansen A et al (2015) Rett tiltak på rett sted – Forebyggende og målrettede tekniske og organisatoriske tiltak mot dødsbranner i risikogrupper. SP Fire Research AS, Trondheim
6. Society of Fire Protection Engineers (2019) SFPE guide to human behavior in fire, 2nd edn. Springer, Cham

7. Runefors M, Johansson N, Van Hees P (2016) How could the fire fatalities have been prevented? An analysis of 144 cases during 2011–2014 in Sweden: an analysis. Journal of Fire Sciences 34:515–527
8. Piechnik K, Mikalsen RF (2020) Fire without flames – 13 amazing facts about smouldering fires. Trondheim, Norway
9. DSB (2019) Brannstatistikk 2018 – Tall fra rapporteringsløsningen (BRIS) fra brann- og redningsvesenet til DSB. Direktoratet for samfunnssikkerhet og beredskap, Tønsberg
10. Stølen R, Steen-Hansen AE, Stensaas JP, Sesseng C (2011) Brann til middag? Undersøkelse av sikringstiltak mot branner på komfyr, SINTEF NBL, Trondheim
11. Steen-Hansen AE, Stensaas JP, Sesseng C, Stølen R (2010) Analysis of cooking fires in Norway. In: Interflam 2010: proceedings of the Twelfth International Conference. Interscience Communications Ltd, Nottingham, pp 1353–1364
12. Ahrens M (2020) Soft furnishing fires: They're still a problem. Fire and Materials fam.2874. https://doi.org/10.1002/fam.2874
13. Gann RG (2020) Solving the soft furnishings fire problem (without incurring collateral damage). Fire Mater https://doi.org/https://doi.org/10.1002/fam.2936
14. Gummesen P (2017) Residential fires in Denmark – a background analysis. Diploma engineer, Technical University of Denmark
15. Andersson P, Johansson N, Strömgren M (2015) Characteristics of fatal residential fires in Sweden. SP Swedish National Testing and Research Institute, Borås
16. DHS (2016) Civilian fire fatalities in residential buildings (2012–2014). U.S. Department of Homeland Security, U.S. Fire Administration, Emmetsburg, Maryland, USA
17. Ahrens M (2016) Home structure fires. National Fire Protection Association, Quincy
18. Home Office UK (2020) Fire Statistics Table 0603: primary fires, fatalities and non-fatal casualties in dwellings ad other buildings by material or item first ignited, England
19. Home Office UK (2020) Fire Statistics Table 0604: primary fire fatalities and casualties by material responsible for development of fire, England
20. Sesseng C, Storesund K, Steen-Hansen A (2017) Analysis of fatal fires in Norway in the 2005 – 2014 period. RISE Fire Research, Trondheim
21. (2002) DIRECTIVE 2001/95/EC OF THE EUROPEAN PARLIAMENT AND OF THE COUNCIL of 3 December 2001 on general product safety (Text with EEA relevance)
22. Guillaume E, de Feijter R, van Gelderen L (2020) An overview and experimental analysis of furniture fire safety regulations in Europe. Fire Mater 44:624–639. https://doi.org/10.1002/fam.2826
23. Storesund K, Amon F, Haghighatpanah S et al (2019) Fire safe furniture in a sustainable perspective. RISE Fire Research/Brandforsk, Trondheim
24. State of California, Department of Consumer Affairs (2014) Technical Bulletin 117–2013: Requirements, Test Procedure and Apparatus for Testing the Smolder Resistance of Materials Used in Upholstered Furniture. Frequently asked questions (FAQs)
25. UK Department for Business, Innovation and Skills (2010) The Furniture and Furnishings (Fire) (Safety) (Amendment) Regulations 2010
26. Krasny J, Parker W, Babrauskas V (2001) Fire behavior of upholstered furniture and mattresses. William Andrew Publishing, Norwich
27. Storesund AK, Steinbakk SH, Steen-Hansen A (2012) Brannsikkerhet og helse- og miljøeffekter i forbindelse med stoppete møbler, madrasser og innredningstekstiler. SINTEF NBL, Trondheim
28. SINTEF (2013) 321.052 Brannsikkerhet og løs innredning. SINTEF Byggforsk, Trondheim, Norway
29. Stull JO (2008) Fibers and textiles. In: Fire protection handbook, 20th ed. National Fire Protection Association, Quincy, pp 6–75 to 6–102
30. Hatch KL (1993) Textile Science. West Publishing, New York
31. Harris D, Davis A, Ryan PB et al (2021) Chemical exposure and flammability risks of upholstered furniture. Fire Mater 45:167–180. https://doi.org/10.1002/fam.2907

32. Sundström B (2021) Combustion behavior of upholstered furniture. Important findings, practical use, and implications. Fire Mater 45:97–113. https://doi.org/10.1002/fam.2920
33. Sundström B, Bengtsson S, Olander M, et al (2009) Brandskydd och lös inredning – En vägledning. SP Fire Research
34. Hertzberg T, Blomquist P, Tuovinen H (2007) Reconstruction of an arson hospital fire. Fire Mater 31:225–240. https://doi.org/https://doi.org/10.1002/fam.935
35. Sundström B (1995) Fire Safety of Upholstered Furniture: the final report on the CBUF research programme. Interscience Communications Ltd, London
36. Pitts WM, Werrel M, Fernandez M et al (2021) Effects of upholstery materials on the burning behavior of real-scale residential upholstered furniture mock-ups. Fire Mater 45:127–154. https://doi.org/10.1002/fam.2915
37. Steen-Hansen AE, Kristoffersen B (2007) Hvor brannsikre er stoppete møbler og madrasser? SINTEF NBL, Trondheim
38. Storesund K, Steen-Hansen A (2013) Fire safety level of interior textiles and upholstered furnishing in Norway–Considering health and environmental effects from changes in product safety regulations. In: Conference Proceedings Interflam 2013, London, UK, 24-26th June 2013. Interscience Communications, London, pp 535–540
39. Nazare S, Pitts WM, Shields J et al (2019) Assessing fire-blocking effectiveness of barrier fabrics in the cone calorimeter. J Fire Sci 37:340–376. https://doi.org/10.1177/0734904119863011
40. Storesund K, Steen-Hansen A, Bergstrand A (2015) Fire safe upholstered furniture – alternative strategies to the use of chemical flame retardants. SP Fire Research AS, Trondheim
41. Storesund K, Amon F, Steen-Hansen A et al (2021) Fire safe, sustainable loose furnishing. Fire Mater 45:181–190. https://doi.org/10.1002/fam.2859
42. Skaar TE (2013) Alkohol og brann. Rapport fra kartlegging og sammenhenger mellom alkoholbruk og dødsfall i boliger. Norsk brannvernforening, Oslo
43. Rodgers KM, Swetschinski LR, Dodson RE et al (2019) Health toll from open flame and cigarette-started fires on flame-retardant furniture in Massachusetts, 2003–2016. Am J Public Health 109:1205–1211
44. (2020) Detailed analysis of fires attended by fire and rescue services, England, April 2019 to March 2020. Home Office, Office for National Statistics, London, UK
45. WHO (2014) Fact sheet on reduced ignition propensity (RIP) cigarettes
46. Mehta S (2012) Cigarette ignition risk project. U.S. Consumer Product Safety Commission, Bethesda, Maryland, USA
47. Larsson I, Bergstrand A (2016) Study: reduced ignition propensity (RIP) cigarettes–theory and reality. In: Proceedings of the 14th International Conference and Exhibition on Fire Science and Engineering (Interflam 2016). Interscience Communications Ltd, Windsor, UK, pp 235–246

Prof. Anne Steen-Hansen has been working as a professor in Fire Safety Engineering at the Norwegian University of Science and Technology (NTNU) since August 2019, and has also a part-time engagement as a Chief Scientist at RISE Fire Research in Trondheim. She holds a MSc in physics and mathematics from 1986 and received her PhD on the topic smoke production in 2002. Her field of interests includes materials' reaction to fire, fire investigation, fire statistics, domestic fire safety, industrial fire safety and fire terminology. Anne is the Director of the Fire Research and Innovation Centre (FRIC) in Norway, and has been President of EGOLF (European Group of Organisations for Fire Testing, Inspection and Certification) from 2016 to 2022.

Mrs. Karolina Storesund has been working as a senior scientist at RISE Fire Research in Trondheim, with particular focus on reaction-to-fire properties and fire safety for vulnerable groups. She holds an MSc in Textiles from University of Leeds. Karolina was Director of the Fire Research and Innovation Centre and is now coordinator at the Norwegian Research Center for AI Innovation at the Norwegian University of Science and Technology (NTNU).

Chapter 11
Active Fire Protection Systems for Residential Applications

Magnus Arvidson

Abstract Residential sprinkler systems and associated design and installation standards were developed in the USA during the 1970s and 1980s. In contrast to traditional automatic sprinkler systems, the objective is to provide improved protection against injury and life loss rather than property protection. Field experience from USA indicate that the death rate is in the order of 90% lower where sprinklers and hardwired smoke alarms are present. Water mist fire protection systems can provide similar protection to residential sprinklers, using lower discharge densities. There are recognized fire test procedures as well as design and installation standards, but the market share is currently relatively low. Fixed-installed or mobile pre-engineered fire protection systems may also result in reduced water flow rates, as they are typically activated by a smoke and heat, or flame detector, which result in earlier activation. The systems are intended to be used as an alternative, or complement, to residential sprinklers for a particular part or parts of a dwelling. Many fires start in the kitchen in connection with cooking on the stove. A stove guard is a technical device that monitors the stove. When there is a risk of fire, it alarms and disconnects the power supply to the stove.

Keywords Residential sprinkler systems · Water mist systems · Stove guards · Residential fires · Kitchen fires

1 Introduction

Automatic fire protection systems require, per definition, no human intervention to operate and the most common type of system in residential area applications is probably residential sprinkler systems. Automatic sprinklers are located at ceiling level and are connected to a water source, most commonly the public water main. The sprinklers operate by the heat from the fire to prevent flashover (total involvement) in the room of fire origin and thereby give residents the time to safely escape and the fire department time to respond. Water mist fire protection systems can

---

M. Arvidson (✉)
RISE Research Institutes of Sweden, Borås, Sweden
e-mail: magnus.arvidson@ri.se

© The Author(s), under exclusive license to Springer Nature Switzerland AG 2023
M. Runefors et al. (eds.), *Residential Fire Safety*, The Society of Fire Protection Engineers Series, https://doi.org/10.1007/978-3-031-06325-1_11

provide similar protection to residential sprinklers, using lower discharge densities. Approved automatic nozzles are available in the marketplace.

Fixed-installed or mobile pre-engineered systems may also result in reduced water flow rates when compared to a traditional residential sprinkler or even a traditional water mist system, making them suitable where the water supply or storage is limited. Typical applications include care homes and permanent or temporary accommodation for elderly, social housing, or simply private dwellings with extensions. The systems are typically activated by a smoke and heat, or flame detector, which result in earlier activation compared to residential sprinklers.

Many fires start in the kitchen in connection with cooking on the stove. A stove guard is a technical device that monitors the stove. When there is a risk of fire, it alarms and/or disconnects the power supply to the stove. The device can have detectors that respond to smoke, heat, movement, or a combination of these. The detector unit may be integrated in the cooker or it can be installed afterwards under the hood or on the wall behind the stove.

This chapter describes these technologies, installation requirements, test procedures as well as any field experience and studies.

2 Residential Sprinkler Systems

This section describes the background and development of residential sprinklers, how systems are designed and installed, the adoption and use, and field experience and summarizes some of the studies that have been conducted.

2.1 The Background and Development of Residential Sprinklers

Automatic sprinkler systems as known today have been used since the late 1800s. The systems were primarily developed for property protection of industrial and commercial properties. In 1973, the National Commission on Fire Prevention and Control issued the report America Burning [1]. The report evaluates the fire loss in the USA and provides recommendations to reduce loss and increase safety of citizens and fire service personnel. Among 90 recommendations were a proposal that the US Fire Administration (USFA) should support the development of the necessary technology for improved automatic extinguishing systems for dwellings.

At the same time that the America Burning report was issued, the National Fire Protection Association (NFPA) initiated the development of NFPA 13D, which when released in its first edition in 1975 had the title "Installation of Sprinkler Systems in One- and Two-family Dwellings and Manufactured Homes." In contrast to the NFPA 13 standard on traditional automatic sprinkler systems, the objective was life safety rather than property protection [2].

Between 1975 and 1980, several research projects and field tests were conducted [3, 4]. A crucial question during the development work was that the sprinkler system needed to be affordable and that it could function with the existing water supply of a building [5]. Based on the outcome from the testing and development work, NFPA 13D was rewritten and published in its second edition in 1980. It was not until 1981 that the first commercial residential sprinklers were approved [6]. A residential sprinkler is characterized by early activation and a high, flat, and wide water distribution pattern. The sprinkler must be able to distribute water over sofas, drapes, curtains, and the like in the outer edges of a room and prevent the spread of fire along walls and ceilings.

NFPA 13D had a major impact and began also to be applied in apartment buildings and NFPA realized that the time was ready for a new, national standard for residential sprinklers in apartment buildings and other types of housing. The result was NFPA 13R (R stands for Residential) published in 1989 where the sprinkler concept was expanded to include residential buildings up to and including four stories in height. The concept also included hotels, motels, and certain types of care homes.

2.2 Installation Requirements in NFPA 13D and 13R

The overall performance objective of NFPA 13D [7], "Standard for Installation of Sprinkler Systems in One- and Two-Family Dwellings and Manufactured Homes," is to provide improved protection against injury and life loss. A sprinkler system shall be designed and installed to the standard to prevent flashover (total involvement) in the room of fire origin and thereby give residents the time to safely escape and the fire department time to respond. Sprinklers are only required to be installed in living areas. Sprinklers in smaller bathrooms or closets, pantries, garages, or carports, attached open structures, attics, and other concealed non-living spaces are not required. The sprinkler system shall be hydraulically designed to provide at least the water flow for a minimum discharge density of 2.05 mm/min or the sprinkler listing, whichever is greater, to all the sprinklers within a compartment, up to a maximum of two sprinklers.

Where stored water is used as the sole supply of water, the standard requires that the quantity should correspond to at least 10 min of discharge. For a single-storey building that is less than 185 m^2 in area, the quantity of water can be reduced to equal a 7 min discharge.

Two common types of fire sprinkler layouts are acceptable under NFPA 13D, a regular stand-alone and a multipurpose system. A stand-alone sprinkler system serves only the fire sprinklers. A multipurpose system combines the domestic cold-water system with the residential sprinkler system. This solution could provide increased reliability as any impairment to the water supply would be more rapidly recognized. If correctly designed, it may also eliminate the need for any back flow prevention device as water is not stagnant in the piping.

NFPA 13R [8], "Standard for the Installation of Sprinkler Systems in Low-Rise Residential Occupancies," covers the design and installation of automatic sprinkler systems in residential occupancies up to and including four stories in height in buildings not exceeding 18 m. The intent of the standard is to provide a sprinkler system for improved protection against injury, life loss, and property damage in multi-family dwellings.

Sprinklers should be installed throughout a building, but are permitted to be omitted in smaller bathrooms or clothes closets, linen closets, and pantries within dwelling units. In addition, sprinklers are not required for many exterior attached open structures such as stairs, carports and certain balconies, or in attics, elevator machine rooms, and similar spaces that are not intended for living purposes or storage. The sprinkler system shall be hydraulically designed to provide at least the water flow for a minimum discharge density of 2.05 mm/min or the sprinkler listing, whichever is greater, to all the sprinklers within a compartment, up to a maximum of four sprinklers. The water supply shall be capable of supplying the system demand for at least 30 min.

Where buildings are greater than four stories in height, the residential parts of such buildings should be protected with residential or quick-response sprinklers in accordance with NFPA 13. There were four main reasons why four stories were chosen as the limit [9]:

1. The concept was intended for multi-dwelling houses with a wooden frame, the use of which is limited to a maximum of four floors in most building regulations.
2. The rescue service's efforts in the event of fire are an important part of the concept and in lower buildings they use extendable ladders and need not to rely on machine ladders.
3. In higher buildings, more people are at risk of being exposed to a fire and it was judged that buildings over four floors require a sprinkler concept with the higher reliability associated with the recommendations in NFPA 13.
4. Buildings with more than four floors normally require riser pipes or indoor fire hydrants with a water requirement sufficient to supply a sprinkler system in accordance with NFPA 13.

2.3 Residential Sprinkler Requirements in the USA

Currently (2020), all US model building codes contain requirements for fire sprinklers to be installed in all new, one- and two-family homes and all multifamily residences [10]. The International Residential Code (IRC) is a model code used as a basis for the locally adopted regulations for the construction of single-family homes in almost all jurisdictions. As a model code, the IRC requires sprinklers to be installed in all new homes. However, each state or local jurisdiction can reject specific parts of the model code for their particular jurisdiction during their adoption process, and most reject the sprinkler requirement. The only states or regions that currently require sprinklers in new, one- and two-family homes are California, Maryland, and the District of Columbia [10].

Home and building industry groups have actively organized efforts to prevent sprinkler mandates in at least 25 states. Several other states have agreed to let local jurisdictions decide whether to adopt the sprinkler requirement, and many have. For example, in Illinois, more than 100 communities have adopted requirements for sprinklers [10].

Several organizations advocate sprinkler protection for all new homes and provide information about residential sprinkler systems for the public, like the Home Fire Sprinkler Coalition, the National Fire Protection Association, and the International Residential Code Fire Sprinkler Coalition.

2.4 Adoption and Use of Residential Sprinklers Outside of USA

Residential sprinklers gradually started to be used outside of USA in the late 1990s. The adoption and use in some European countries are discussed below.

The Swedish Fire Protection Association published design and installation recommendations for residential sprinkler systems in 1997 [11]. These recommendations were to a large extent based on NFPA 13D and 13R. The awareness and use of residential sprinklers were enhanced in Sweden during the beginning of 2000s as a result of the national research project, "Residential sprinklers save lives". The project resulted in several sprinkler model installations, a handbook [12], revised design and installation recommendations [13], and a video illustrating the performance of a residential sprinkler [14]. Figure 11.1 shows two photos from the video. In 2009, a Nordic standard, INSTA 900-1 [15], was published that was implemented in Sweden and Norway as a national standard. The second part of the standard, INSTA 900-2 [16], covers fire test procedures for residential sprinklers and was adopted from UL 1626 [17]. The third part, INSTA 900-3 [18], contains fire test procedures for water mist fire protection nozzles. In 2019, almost 40,000 residential sprinklers were installed in Sweden, which corresponded to about 5% of all installed sprinklers [19].

Since July 2010, the Norwegian building code has required sprinklers in almost all new buildings, with the exception of single-family houses and some small buildings in which people do not sleep. This opened a market for residential sprinklers installed per INSTA 900-1. In 2019, approximately 190,000 residential sprinklers were installed in Norway, which corresponded to almost 24% of all installed sprinklers. The water mist market totalled 29,213 nozzles and 73% of them were residential nozzles [20].

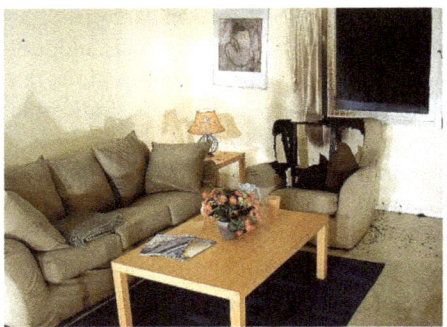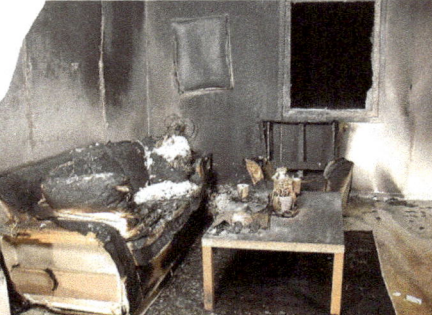

Fig. 11.1 The performance of a residential sprinkler (left) with limited fire damage as compared to the fire damage caused by flashover (right). (Photos from the video "Residential sprinkler saves lives" from 2001 [14])

In the United Kingdom, British Standard BS 9251:2014 [21] gives recommendations for the design, installation, maintenance, and testing of fire sprinkler systems in domestic and residential occupancies. This British Standard superseded BS 9251:2005. A series of regulatory changes have led to dramatic growth in the market. First, the Rose Park care home fire in Glasgow in 2004, which killed 14 elderly residents, led Scotland a year later to mandate the installation of sprinklers in all new care homes and in apartment buildings higher than 18 m. In 2007, England and Wales introduced requirements to fit sprinklers in new built apartment buildings higher than 30 m, along with a number of incentives to fit sprinklers in new three-storey and four-storey houses (a four-storey house needs sprinklers or a second staircase). The publication in 2011 of BS 9991 [22], a code of practice for fire safety in residential buildings, introduced further incentives for sprinklers in apartments in the UK. In 2016, Wales became the first country to require sprinklers in all new housing. The Grenfell Tower disaster in London in 2017 killed 72 residents and led many local government authorities voluntarily to fit sprinklers in existing high-rise social housing. As part of its response to this disaster, late in 2020 the government introduced a requirement to fit sprinklers in new built apartment buildings in England higher than 11 m [23]. Meanwhile, the Scottish government announced that in 2021 it would introduce requirements to fit sprinklers in all new built flats and shared multi-occupied residential buildings [24]. The British residential sprinkler market in 2020 is estimated to be over 500,000 sprinklers and expected to grow further with the new requirements.

Elsewhere in Europe, there are regulatory requirements to fit sprinklers in large care homes in Denmark and in most new care homes in Finland. In Finland, the requirements were retrospective and led to over half of all existing care homes being retrofitted with sprinklers. While their markets are still small, some care homes have been protected with residential sprinklers in Belgium, France, Germany, and The Netherlands. In 2020, an increasing number of projects, including for apartment buildings, were reported to be specifying sprinklers in France and The Netherlands. Looking ahead, the French government is encouraging the use of wood in residential buildings and this is expected to lead to greater use of residential sprinklers in France.

In 2018, a European standard on the design, installation, and maintenance of residential sprinkler systems, EN 16925:2018 [25], was published. The standard includes three system types, 1, 2, and 3, dependent on the application. System type 1 is intended to be used in one- or two-family dwellings and requires the lowest discharge densities and fewest number of sprinklers in the design. System type 3, intended for apartment buildings, care homes as well as small hotels and hostels, requires more stringent design criteria. Some countries may have a national informative annex with guidance on the minimum design discharge density and on the number of design sprinklers for each system type. In 2020, a European standard for testing of residential sprinklers, EN 12259-14:2020, was published [26]. The fire tests of this standard are identical with those of UL 1626 [17].

2.5 Residential Sprinkler Field Experience

Several communities in USA have documented field experience with residential sprinklers. Given below are two examples.

In 1992, Prince George's County in Maryland introduced a regulation requiring the installation of residential sprinklers in all new single- and multi-family homes [27]. Since 1992, more than 45,285 building permits have been granted for single- and multi-dwelling houses. For 15 years, from 1992 to 2007, a total of 13,494 fires occurred in single-family houses or townhouses. At 245 of these fires, residential sprinklers were installed. No person perished in the fires and only six cases of personal injury have been reported. In the 13,249 fires that occurred in homes without sprinklers, a total of 101 people lost their lives and 328 were injured. Home fires accounted for a total of 89% of all Prince George's County fire fatalities during this time. The average direct fire damage cost for a fire in a single-family house or townhouse without sprinklers was $9983, compared to $4883 if sprinklers were installed. The fire damage cost was thus about half as high. The average direct fire damage cost for a fire (without sprinklers) that resulted in fatalities was $49,503, i.e. just over 10 times higher than if sprinklers were installed.

Scottsdale, Arizona, is a suburb of Phoenix with approximately 258,000 residents (2019). The city has long experience of sprinkler systems [28–30]. In January 1986, sprinkler requirements were introduced in all types of new buildings, including single-family dwellings. Ten years later, on January 1, 1996, sprinklers were installed in 19,649, or 35% of all single-family homes and in 13,938, or 49% of all multi-family homes in Scottsdale. A further 5 years later, on January 1, 2001, the number of single-family dwellings with sprinklers had increased to 39,258 (51%) and the number of multi-dwelling houses with sprinklers to 19,422 (57%), i.e. almost 60,000 dwellings. In a total of 97 fires, it is estimated that 13 lives were saved by residential sprinklers. The statistics also show a significant reduction in the average fire damage cost with residential sprinklers.

2.6 Residential Sprinkler Studies

Ahrens [31] has analyzed data from the National Fire Incident Reporting System (NFIRS) in the USA regarding sprinkler reliability and efficiency. The analysis is based on data from the years 2010 to 2014. Some form of sprinkler was installed at 49,840 of all fires in buildings that were reported. This represented an average of 10% of all reported fires. Sprinklers were mostly found in institutional buildings such as nursing homes, hospitals, and prisons. Most fires and deaths occurred in residential buildings, but sprinklers were found in only 8% of the residential fires. Sprinklers operated and controlled the fire in 91% of the residential fires where the fire was large enough to activate the sprinklers. Only one sprinkler operated in 88% of these fires and in 98% of the fires, five or fewer sprinklers operated. Compared to reported residential fires with no smoke alarms or any sprinklers, the death rate per 1000 reported fires was 88% lower where hardwired smoke alarms and any automatic extinguishing systems (AES) were present and 90% lower where sprinklers and hardwired smoke alarms were present. When sprinklers were present, the average loss per fire was less than half the average compared to properties with no AES. In three out of five (62%) of fires in which sprinklers failed to operate, the system was shut off.

Optimal Economics Ltd. [32] provides a detailed analysis of data on fires in premises in the UK, during the years 2011 to 2016, where sprinkler systems were installed. The analysis included 2294 incidents of which 1725 (75%) were in non-residential buildings and 414 (18%) in dwellings. In total, sprinkler systems operated in 945 of the 2294 incidents. Of these, 276 (29.2%) of the cases were in dwellings and 42 (4.4%) in other types of residential buildings. Sprinklers in dwellings controlled or extinguished the fire in 99.5% of the cases and in all the other residential building fires. However, the latter performance effectiveness figure was, as mentioned, based on few incidents. Fires in dwellings where the sprinkler system operated had an average area of fire damage of under 4 m^2, as compared to approximately 18 m^2–21 m^2 for all dwelling fires in England during a similar period of time.

Gritzo et al. [33] have analyzed the contribution of fire on the total lifecycle carbon emissions of one- and two-family dwellings and the reduction to that contribution achieved with residential sprinkler systems. It is concluded that the contribution of fire to the total lifecycle carbon emissions of homes without sprinklers is between 0.4% and 3.7%. The contribution of fire risk to the total lifecycle carbon emissions of a home is reduced to 0.2% when sprinklers are used, as all large fires are eliminated. In support of this analysis, fire tests [34] were conducted to measure the reduction in the environmental impact by residential sprinklers.

Hall et al. [35] have analyzed the reduction of the cost of personal injury in fires with residential sprinklers. The hypothesis was that a fire that is reduced by residential sprinklers not only reduces the frequency of injuries, but also the severity of the personal injuries when they occurred. A calculation model was used to investigate the impact on the number of personal injuries and the cost of personal injury per 100 residential fires. Cost data were available for (a) medical costs, (b) legal and liability costs, which are usually relatively low, (c) costs associated with lost work time, and (d) pain and suffering costs. The latter tended to dominate the total cost. Sprinkler effect was estimated for total injury costs and for medical costs alone. Four types of injuries were studies; burns only, smoke inhalation only, both burns and smoke inhalation, and other injury. The main results of the study show that residential sprinklers reduce the number of injuries in the event of a residential fire by 29%, medical costs by 53%, and total costs of injuries by 41%.

Butry [36] has conducted a benefit-cost analysis to measure the expected present value net benefits (PVNB) of a residential fire sprinkler system in a newly constructed, single-family house. Three typical single-family house types were investigated. The sprinkler designs vary by installation cost and require annual maintenance, but all were designed to meet the NFPA 13D standard. The estimated benefits of fire sprinklers include reductions in the following: the risk of civilian fatalities and injuries, homeowner insurance premiums, uninsured direct property losses, and uninsured indirect costs. The results show that residential sprinkler systems not requiring expensive annual maintenance are economical.

BRE Global has undertaken a cost benefit analysis of residential sprinklers installed in the UK [37]. The study shows that residential sprinklers are cost-effective in all residential care homes for elderly people, children, and disabled people (including care homes with single bedrooms). Residential sprinklers are also cost-effective in most blocks of purpose built flats, larger blocks of converted flats, and traditional bedsit type HMOs where there are at least six bedsit units per building. Note: A house in multiple occupation (HMO) is a British English term which refers to residential properties where 'common areas' exist and are shared by more than one household.

3 Water Mist Fire Protection Systems

Water mist fire protection systems typically use less water than sprinkler systems but higher operating pressures. The fire protection performance of such systems for residential area applications has been investigated in several research projects.

In the mid-1990s, the US Fire Administration (USFA) funded two projects to explore the possibilities of using water mist systems as an alternative to residential sprinklers. Primarily, it was the opportunity to reduce the water demand that was the most interesting to investigate as there are many areas in the USA where the availability of water reduces the possibilities of using residential sprinklers. The first study [38] investigated the possibilities of using water mist for the type of fire scenarios that are relevant in residential areas. The tested systems included a low-pressure system, three different high-pressure, and a "dual-fluid" system. The latter system generated mist by air impingement as opposed to small orifices. Only two of the systems tested showed reasonably good results. For these systems, it was possible to draft preliminary installation instructions. The installation cost for these two systems was estimated and concluded higher than that for residential sprinklers, mainly due to the higher material cost. Based on the first study, USFA went on to a second study [39, 40]. The intention was, among other things, to further study the use of water mist in a residential environment, to develop a test method, and to make a recommendation for installation standards. Since the first study showed that the cost of high-pressure systems was too high, low-pressure systems were studied. These systems are likely to use plastic pipes and do not require additional piping for air or other media for the atomization of water. Additional fire tests were conducted using two commercial and two prototype nozzles. The operating pressures were between 7.7 and 11 bar. It was concluded that the level of performance was comparable to that of residential sprinklers, using lower total water flow demand. However, the higher operating pressure means that the systems cannot be connected directly to the public water supply and a pressure pump is required. Therefore, a lower reliability due to the increased number of components is expected. A calculation shows that the increased probability of malfunction may be 0.03 per year. This means that if 100 systems are used for 1 year, one can expect that three more systems will malfunction compared to residential sprinkler systems directly connected to the public water supply. Sprinkler statistics (industry) show that the malfunction of a properly sized sprinkler system is 0.02–0.03 [41], which gives an idea of the order of magnitude of the increase. The main contribution to the lower reliability is the probability that the valve required to "isolate" the pump is closed. The contribution from other components such as the pump and the pressure switch is low. Regarding nozzle clogging, practical tests show that this cannot be expected to be a problem for the nozzles used in the test series.

RISE Research Institutes of Sweden have conducted a more recent series of residential sprinkler and water mist nozzle fire tests [42] in a test compartment sized 3.66 m by 3.66 m (12 ft. by 12 ft.). The fire test source consisted of either a simulated or an authentic upholstered chair. Benchmark residential sprinkler tests were conducted using a water flow rate of 30.3 l/min. This was the minimum listed flow rate given by the manufacturer for the compartment size. Additional tests were conducted using 60.6 l/min, corresponding to the relevant design density of 4.1 mm/min in NFPA 13. The performance of several commercial, automatic low- and high-pressure water mist nozzles was determined. The flow rates of the water mist nozzles ranged from about 17 to 37 l/min. Generally, it could be concluded that the performance of these nozzles was comparable or better than the residential sprinklers using approximately half to one-quarter of the water flow rate. Figure 11.2 exemplifies the performance with the measured mean gas temperature inside the test compartment. The gas temperature was measured at eye-level (1.6 m above floor) at the centre point of each of the four quadrants of the test compartment, except for the quadrant with the fire test source. The data are for the tests with the simulated upholstered chair.

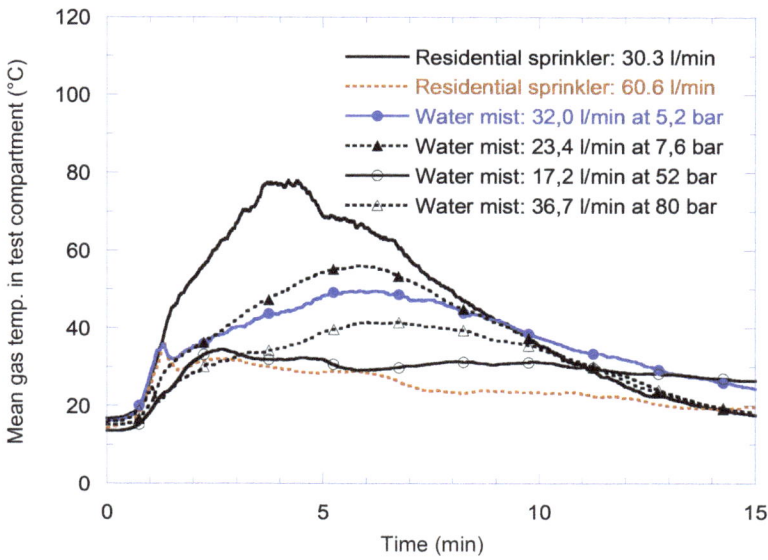

Fig. 11.2 The mean gas temperature at eye-level (1.6 m above floor) inside the fire test compartment when testing residential sprinklers and water mist fire protection system nozzles [43]

The high-pressure water mist nozzles provided the best cooling. This observation supports the assumption that smaller water droplets provide efficient gas phase cooling. The combustible foam cushion that was used for the fire test source was completely or almost completely consumed in all tests. The lowest measured mean gas temperature inside the test compartment was recorded in the test with the residential sprinkler flowing 60.6 l/min.

Underwriters Laboratories Inc. (UL) has developed a fire test procedure for automatic water mist nozzles intended for residential area applications, UL 2167 [43]. The method resembles that used for residential sprinklers; however, the application is limited to one- and two-family dwellings and manufactured homes. If a single nozzle activates during the tests, an actual system should be designed using two nozzles. If two or three nozzles activated, four nozzles should be included in the design.

British Standard BS 8458:2015 [44] provides recommendations for the design, installation, water supplies, commissioning, maintenance, and testing of water mist fire protection systems with automatic nozzles. The field of application includes systems installed in residential and domestic occupancies up to a maximum ceiling height of 5.5 m. The document primarily covers water mist fire protection systems used for life safety, but the systems may also provide property protection.

4 Pre-engineered Fixed-Installed or Mobile Area Fire Protection Systems

Pre-engineered systems are systems which have the number of nozzles and the piping calculations for the system pre-defined by the manufacturer. This results in less work and responsibility to the designer/installer to ensure that the water supply will be enough for the application. This also means that the application may be specific to a hazard, room, location, or property. Determining whether the solution is fit-for-purpose is still the responsibility of the installer. Pre-engineered systems may also result in reduced water flow rate when compared to a traditional residential sprinkler or even a traditional water mist system where the water supply has to include a safety margin for a maximum number of nozzles. This makes the systems more suitable for retrofit or temporary use, where water supply or storage is limited.

There are several pre-engineered fire protection systems in the marketplace that are either fixed-installed or mobile and are intended to be used as an alternative, or complement, to residential sprinklers for a particular part or parts of a dwelling. Typical applications include care homes and permanent or temporary accommodation for elderly, social housing, or simply private dwellings with extensions.

4.1 Fixed Pre-engineered Water Mist Systems

Fixed pre-engineered systems are primarily used as an alternative to a traditional sprinkler system (also fixed) and therefore are most frequently used to meet building code requirements. These systems are optimized to minimize the flow of water, which is usually limited in a single home, or because there is usually much less space available for a tank. The specific design flows allow for a single type of pipe diameter which has a maximum length (maximum acceptable pressure loss) for the whole installation. Given these are domestic systems intended to protect one or two dwellings, pipe lengths do not need to be significant. A multi-dwelling building would have a system on every dwelling, connected directly to the existing water drinking supply of that home as opposed to a central system with tanks and booster pumps for the exclusive use of fire fighting. Such systems must meet the same fire performance requirements of traditional sprinklers or traditional water mist systems, and the installation is intended to remain as part of the structure of the building with the intention of meeting building code requirements.

Such systems have also, more recently, been used to upgrade the fire safety of existing buildings, either to voluntarily bring them up to existing code or because occupants are found to be more vulnerable than the code at the time of construction assumed. Once again, the reduced water flow makes them easier (and less costly) to retrofit than traditional systems.

4.2 Mobile Pre-engineered Water Mist Systems

A mobile water mist unit is intended to be used as a safety-enhancement device, not to meet building code requirements. It is most frequently used for those with limited mobility or high-risk behaviour who might be a victim of a fire while intimate to the fire itself. As a result, these units are most frequently designed to cover a single room or only a limited area of a room, such as a couch, bed, or chair, where the source of the fire might take place.

A mobile system may consist of a unit containing a smaller sized water tank, a pump, a fire alarm panel, and an integrated water mist nozzle. The unit should be strategically positioned inside the room to be protected and is connected to an electric power supply. The system may be activated by a separate smoke and heat, or flame detector positioned at the ceiling or only to the area of protection (in the case of flame detector). The choice of detection method is the result of the vulnerability of the occupant and therefore the need of quick activation. The amount of water in the tank is sufficient for a care giver to respond to where the activation has occurred and may include up to 10–15 min duration. Additional nozzles, for example above specific fire hazard areas, the bed, or in adjacent rooms, can be connected to the unit if the pre-engineered design supports this functionality. Because the system will most probably wet the occupant and there is limited run time on the system, it is assumed that this system is used in applications where help can arrive in short notice. These systems, therefore, usually have an output signal facility to indicate that they have been activated so that attention of the care giver can be summoned.

The system must be positioned, installed, and maintained by an authorized installer. Periodical inspection includes a verification that the system and the nozzles are not being obstructed. These systems do not have to meet the fire performance tests of existing national and international standards used to meet building code. Performance may be assessed in a case by case basis based on the occupation and risk.

In 2007, Sweden and Norway issued a common guidance for the installation and fire testing of mobile pre-engineered water mist systems. The stated objective is that the system should provide an early alarm and control a fire such that gas temperatures and toxic gases are limited during the time required for the fire service to rescue and fight a fire. The manufacturer should verify and declare that the product meets the requirements of the guidelines and guarantee the function of the system; no approvals are issued [45].

4.3 Fire Tests and Field Experience

RISE Research Institutes of Sweden have conducted a series of residential sprinkler and automatic water mist nozzle fire tests that included a commercial pre-engineered mobile high-pressure water mist system [42]. The system was activated by a combined heat and smoke detector which provides for earlier activation compared to a frangible glass bulb used for residential sprinklers. The flow rate of 8 l/min was significantly less than that of the other systems. The performance was comparable to that of the fixed-installed automatic water mist nozzles in the study. However, the results suggest that the position of the fire test source relative to the position of the unit is a crucial factor and underlines the importance of a thoughtful positioning in practical applications.

Field experiences indicate that life has been saved by these types of systems. In a pilot project in 2012, the City of Copenhagen installed 50 mobile systems in homes with residents judged having an increased probability of fire. The project was immediately successful and an additional 220 units were purchased in 2013 and 2014. After 3 years, the project was evaluated, and it turned out that nine lives were probably saved, and the cost of fire damage was reduced [46].

Runefors and Frantzich have conducted a cost-benefit analysis of mobile pre-engineered water mist systems in Sweden [47]. The advantage of mobile systems is that they can be arranged in a room without major intervention in the home. Some of the systems are also possible to reassemble in new dwellings. If the analysis includes mobile systems for the entire elderly population, the societal benefit does not exceed the overall cost. But for particularly vulnerable groups, it is concluded that the benefit outweighs the cost of the installation. This is especially true for older people who are smokers. For this group, the measure is highly socio-economically profitable with a benefit ratio of 1.57–4.92 depending on age group and whether the system is reused in other homes or not.

5 Stove Top Protection Systems

Many fires start in the kitchen in connection with cooking on the stove. A stove guard is a technical device that monitors the stove. When there is a risk of fire, it alarms and (if no one responds) disconnects the power supply to the stove. The device can have detectors that respond to smoke, heat, movement, or a combination of these. The detector unit may be integrated in the cooker or it can be installed afterwards under the hood or on the wall behind the stove. The device is usually discreetly designed and does not require much space. In addition, a stove guard can be supplemented with a fire extinguishing module. The stove guard may be connected to the Wi-Fi and send a remote warning to the user's mobile phone, or to another receiver that is able to respond on the alarm.

All stove guards marketed in the EU and ESS must be designed and manufactured in accordance with EN 50615:2015 [48], be type tested, and CE marked. The standard divides the stove guards into three classes:

- Category A: The stove guard should be capable of extinguishing a fire. When the extinguishing agent is applied, the power supply to the stove is disconnected.

- Category B: The stove guard disconnects the power supply to the stove when there is a risk that a fire may occur.
- Category AB: The stove guard disconnects the power supply to the stove when there is a risk that a fire may occur, and it can also extinguish a possible fire.

The extinguishing ability (Category A) is tested with a pan with sunflower oil. The stove guard must detect the fire within 45 s and the fire must be extinguished without splashing oil. The fire must not reignite within 10 min. In addition, a fire in a roll of kitchen paper must be extinguished. The ability to prevent a fire from occurring (Category B) is tested with a pan with sunflower oil. The oil is heated on the highest power position and the voltage to the stove must be disconnected before the oil reaches 330 °C. Thereafter, the temperature of the oil must not exceed 350 °C during the following 10 min. A challenge for manufacturers is that the stove guard must be able to distinguish an incipient dangerous situation, for example when a pan with hot oil approaches the self-ignition temperature, from normal cooking. If the stove guard often disconnects the stove during normal operation, the user may lose confidence in the technology, which becomes an annoyance. If the stove guard does not disconnect the power supply before or when a fire occurs, an incident can in the worst case lead to a fully developed kitchen fire. Therefore, a false alarm test is also included with three pans filled with boiling water and a pan with oil. It is only when the oil gets too hot that the stove guard disconnects the power. Some stove guards therefore have several types of detectors, such as Infra-Red (IR), heat, and motion detectors as well as built-in logic to reduce the probability that the power supply is accidentally disconnected.

The most common type of stove guard in the marketplace is of Category B, although the other categories can be found in the market.

5.1 Fire Tests and Field Experience

There are some documented experiments with stove guards, but since technological development has progressed rapidly in recent years, the results are not certainly relevant to today's technology. In 2010, the fire test laboratory at SINTEF in Norway conducted tests with stove fires [49]. A total of 76 tests were performed, of which 23 were initial tests without stove guards. In addition to using different types of stoves, the plate used, the type of cookware, and the type of oil or cooking fat were varied. Seven different stove guards were tested. Based on the tests, only three stove guards could be considered to perform satisfactorily. The major challenge for them was to distinguish an incipient dangerous situation, for example when a pan with hot oil approaches the self-ignition temperature, from normal cooking. It was only one stove guard which managed to reduce the probability of false activation in combination with a high probability of reacting to an initial dangerous situation. This stove guard was the most advanced of those tested and had an IR detector to measure the infrared heat radiation, an optical flame detector, and a temperature sensor. The detector unit was also mounted directly above the cooker top, which means that the function is less affected (no shielding of the view) by the design of the pans and where they are placed on the top. Since 2010, stove guards meeting the requirements in EN 50615 are required to be installed in all new dwellings in Norway [50], but there are currently no available studies whether or not they have reduced the number of kitchen fires.

In 2011, RISE Research Institutes of Sweden tested some of the stove guards in the marketplace [51]. Since at that time there was no standardized test method, a methodology was developed. The objective was to test the stove guards in as real an environment as possible and they were judged to work if they disconnected the power supply early enough to prevent a fire or before the food developed very heavy smoke. Four different stove guards were tested and two different stoves, one with a ceramic cooker top and one with cast iron plates. A total of 74 different tests were conducted. In cases where the stove guard did not work, only one attempt was made. For the setups where the stove guard worked, the test was repeated to verify the result. In the 68 different trials where a result was obtained, the stove guard performed as intended in 33 cases and failed in 35 cases.

Runefors and Frantzich have conducted a cost-benefit analysis of the installation of stove guards in Sweden [47]. The analysis is based on the system reducing the number of fatalities and injuries in fires and a reduced need for fire service rescue efforts. Additionally, reduced property damage in the dwelling because of a lower number of fires was accounted for. From a societal perspective, it was concluded that the installation of stove guards is not cost-effective. The savings do not compensate for the cost of installing stove guards in all homes, i.e. the benefit ratio is less than 1.0. However, there are indications that it may be socioeconomically profitable to install stove guards in homes for the elderly. But the uncertainty in estimating the prevention of personal injury is quite large which would require a more nuanced analysis to be performed.

6 Summary

Residential sprinkler systems were developed in the USA during the 1970s and 1980s and have proven an efficient means of improved protection against injury and life loss. Field experience from USA indicates that the death rate is in the order of 90% lower where sprinklers and hardwired smoke alarms are present. In addition, residential sprinklers do reduce the number of injuries in the event of a residential fire, medical costs, and total costs of injuries. Other benefits include a reduction of homeowner insurance premiums, uninsured direct property losses, and uninsured indirect costs. It is estimated that about 8% of homes in the USA are equipped with residential sprinklers. Although all U.S. model building codes include sprinkler requirements for all new, one- and two-family homes, each state can reject specific parts of the adopted code for their particular jurisdiction. This is the reason why residential fire sprinklers are not required in most areas, despite the model code requirements.

Residential sprinklers gradually started to be used outside of USA in the late 1990s, particularly in the Nordic countries and in the UK. Since July 2010, the Norwegian building code has required sprinklers in almost all new buildings, apart from single-family houses and some small buildings in which people do not sleep. In 2019, approximately 190,000 residential sprinklers were installed in Norway, which corresponded to almost 24% of all installed sprinklers. In 2007, England and Wales introduced requirements to fit sprinklers in new built apartment buildings higher than 30 m, along with several incentives to fit sprinklers in new three-storey and four-storey houses. In 2016, Wales became the first country to require sprinklers in all new housing. The British residential sprinkler market in 2020 is estimated to be over 500,000 sprinklers and expected to grow further with the new, upcoming requirements.

Water mist fire protection systems can provide similar protection to residential sprinklers, using lower discharge densities. There are recognized fire test procedures as well as design and installation standards that increase the market opportunities for the systems. In Norway, residential water mist nozzles had a market share of about 10% of the residential sprinkler market in 2019. Fixed-installed or mobile pre-engineered fire protection systems may also result in reduced water flow rates, as they typically are activated by a smoke and heat, or flame detector, which result in earlier activation. The systems are intended to be used as an alternative, or complement, to residential sprinklers for a particular part or parts of a dwelling. A mobile system may consist of a unit containing a smaller-sized water tank, a pump, a fire alarm panel, and an integrated water mist nozzle. The unit should be strategically positioned inside the room to be protected and is connected to an electric power supply. Additional nozzles, for example above specific fire hazard areas, the bed, or in adjacent rooms, can be connected to the unit if the pre-engineered design supports this functionality. Document field experience is limited, but experience indicates that life has been saved by these types of systems.

Many fires start in the kitchen in connection with cooking on the stove. A stove guard is a technical device that monitors the stove. When there is a risk of fire, it alarms and disconnects the power supply to the stove. The device can have detectors that respond to smoke, heat, movement, or a combination of these. All stove guards marketed in the EU and ESS must be designed and manufactured in accordance with EN 50615:2015, be type tested, and CE marked. There are currently no available studies showing to what extent the use of stove guard has reduced the number of kitchen fires.

References

1. America Burning (1973) The Report of The National Commission on Fire Prevention and Control
2. Woodruff ME (2016) The Residential Sprinkler is Born. April 1981: The Grinnell Model F954 receives UL listing. NFPA Journal® Special Issue Home Fire Sprinklers
3. Coleman R (1985) Alpha to Omega: the evolution in residential fire protection. Phenix Publications, San Clemente
4. Arvidson M (2001) En sammanställning av väldokumenterade brandförsök med bostadssprinkler ('A compilation of experiences from well-documented residential fire sprinkler tests'). SP Rapport 2001:03. ISBN 91–7848–844-3
5. Coleman R (1991) Residential sprinkler systems: protecting life and property. National Fire Protection Association, Quincy
6. Fleming R (1991) Fast response sprinklers: a technical analysis. In: Automatic sprinkler systems handbook, 5th edn. National Fire Protection Research Foundation, Quincy, pp 664–791
7. NFPA 13D (2019) Standard for the installation of sprinkler systems in one- and two-family dwellings and manufactured homes. National Fire Protection Association, Quincy
8. NFPA 13R (2019) Standard for the installation of sprinkler systems in low-rise residential occupancies. National Fire Protection Association, Quincy
9. Isman K (2001) NFPA 13 and NFPA 13R different levels of protection. Sprinkler Q 115:37–41
10. Sprinkler requirements https: //www.nfpa.org/Public-Education/Staying-safe/Safety-equipment/Home-fire-sprinklers/Fire-Sprinkler-Initiative/Legislation-and-adoptions/Sprinkler-requirements. Accessed 8 Dec 2020
11. Sprinklersystem i bostadshus med högst fyra våningar ('Sprinkler systems in apartments not exceeding four floors'). Svenska Brandförsvarsföreningen (1997), Stockholm
12. Östman B, Arvidson M, Nystedt F (2002) Boendesprinkler räddar liv: Erfarenheter och brandskyddsprojektering med nya möjligheter ('Residential sprinkler saves lives: experience and fire protection design with new possibilities'). Trätek, Stockholm. ISBN: 9188170292
13. Installation av boendesprinkler, utgåva 1 ('Installation of residential sprinklers, first edition'). Svenska Brandförsvarsföreningen (2002), Stockholm
14. Video Boendesprinkler räddar liv ('Video Residential sprinkler saves lives') (2001) SP Sveriges Provnings- och Forskningsinstitut, Borås
15. SS 883001:2009/INSTA 900-1 (2009) Brand och räddning – Boendesprinkler – Utförande, installation och underhåll ('Residential sprinkler systems – Design, installation and maintenance'). Svenska institutet för standarder, Stockholm
16. INSTA 900-2:2010 (2010) Residential sprinkler systems – part 2: requirements and test methods for sprinklers and their accompanying rosettes. Svenska institutet för standarder, Stockholm
17. UL 1626 (2008) Standard for residential sprinklers for fire-protection service. Underwriters Laboratories, Inc., Northbrook
18. INSTA 900-3:2014 (2014) Residential sprinkler systems – part 3: requirements and fire test methods for watermist nozzles. Svenska institutet för standarder, Stockholm
19. Sprinkler statistics from Sprinklerfrämjandet (2020) Sprinklerfrämjandet, Stockholm
20. Sprinkler statistics 2019 (2020) The Norwegian Fire Industry Association
21. BS 9251:2014 (2014) Fire sprinkler systems for domestic and residential occupancies, code of practice. British Standards Institution (BSI), London
22. BS 9991:2015 (2015) Fire safety in the design, management and use of residential buildings, code of practice. British Standards Institution (BSI), London
23. Barker N (2020) Government confirms 11m sprinkler threshold among raft of building safety reforms. https://www.insidehousing.co.uk/news/news/government-confirms-11m-sprinkler-threshold-among-raft-of-building-safety-reforms-65942. Accessed 2 Apr 2020

24. Brady D (2020) Sprinklers required in all new social homes in Scotland from next year. https://www.insidehousing.co.uk/news/news/sprinklers-required-in-all-new-social-homes-in-scotland-from-next-year-68909. Accessed 3 Dec 2020
25. EN 16925:2018 (2018) Fixed firefighting systems – automatic residential sprinkler systems – design, installation and maintenance. Comité Européen de Normalisation, Brussels
26. EN 12259-14:2020 (2020) Fixed firefighting systems – components for sprinkler and water spray systems – part 14: sprinklers for residential applications. Comité Européen de Normalisation, Brussels
27. Weatherby S (2009) Benefits of residential fire sprinklers: Prince George's County: 15-year history with its single-family residential dwelling fire sprinkler ordinance. Home Fire Sprinkler Coalition, Upper Marlboro
28. Ford J (1997) Automatic sprinklers a 10 year study, a detailed history of the effects of the automatic sprinkler code in Scottsdale, Arizona. Rural/Metro Fire Department, Scottsdale
29. Ford J (1997) One city's case for residential sprinkler systems. NFPA J 91:40–44
30. Ford J (2001) 15 years of built-in automatic fire sprinkler: the Scottsdale experience. Rural/Metro Fire Department, Scottsdale
31. Ahrens M (2017) U.S. experience with sprinklers. National Fire Protection Association, Quincy
32. No author given (2017) Efficiency and effectiveness of sprinkler systems in the United Kingdom: an analysis from fire service data. Optimal Economics Ltd, Edinburgh
33. Gritzo L, Bill R Jr, Wieczorek C, Ditch B (2011) Environmental impact of automatic fire sprinklers: part 1. Residential sprinklers revisited in the age of sustainability. Fire Technol 47:751–763
34. Wieczorek C, Ditch B, Bill R Jr (2011) Environmental impact of automatic fire sprinklers: part 2. Experimental study. Fire Technol 47:765–779
35. Hall J Jr, Ahrens M, Evarts B (2012) Sprinkler impact on fire injury. The Fire Protection Research Foundation, Quincy
36. Butry DT (2009) Economic performance of residential fire sprinkler systems. Fire Technol 45:117–143
37. Fraser-Mitchell J, Williams C (2012) Cost benefit analysis of residential sprinklers – Final report, BRE Global, Prepared for: The Chiefs Fire Officers Association (CFOA), Clients report number 264227 rev1.1, March 1, 2012
38. Final Report, Feasibility Study of Water Mist Applications for Residential Fires (1995), Contract No. EMW-93-4247, U.S. Fire Administration, Federal Emergency Management Agency, Emmitsburg
39. Bill RG Jr, Stavrianidis P, Hill EE Jr, Brown W (1995) Water mist fire protection in residential occupancies. Factory Mutual Research, Norwood
40. Bill RG Jr, Ferron R, Braga A (2000) Water mist (fine spray) fire protection in light hazard occupancies. J Fire Prot Eng 10(3):1–22
41. Automatic Sprinkler Performance Tables, 1970 Edition (1970). Fire Journal
42. Arvidson M (2017) An evaluation of residential sprinklers and water mist nozzles in a residential area fire scenario, RISE report 2017:40. RISE Research Institutes of Sweden, Borås
43. UL 2167 (2002) Standard for water mist nozzles for fire protection service, 1st edn. Underwriters Laboratories Inc., Northbrook
44. BS 8458:2015 (2015) Fixed fire protection systems. Residential and domestic watermist systems, code of practice for design and installation. British Standards Institution (BSI), London
45. Lätt monterbara automatiska släcksystem ('Easily mounted automatic extinguishing systems') (2007) Räddningsverket (Swedish Civil Contingencies Agency) and Direktoratet for samfunnssikkerhet og beredskap (The Norwegian Directorate for Civil Protection (DSB))
46. Individuellt brandskydd med mobila boendesprinklers räddar liv ('Individual fire protection with mobile residential sprinklers saves lives') (2015), Fokus samhällssäkerhet
47. Runefors M, Frantzich H (2017) Nyttoanalys av spisvakt och portabelt sprinkler system vid bostadsbränder ('Cost-benefit analysis of stove guards and portable re-engineered sprinkler systems in dwelling fires'). (LUTVDG/TVBB; Nr. 3210). Lund University, Department of Fire Safety Engineering, Lund

48. EN 50615:2015 (2015) Household and similar electrical appliances. Safety. Particular requirements for devices for fire prevention and suppression for electric hobs (cooktops). Comité Européen de Normalisation, Brussels
49. Stølen R, Steen-Hansen A, Stensaas J, Sesseng C (2011) Brann til middag? Undersøkelse av sikringstiltak mot branner på komfyr ('Fire for dinner? An investigation of measures against fires in cooktops'), NBL A11111, 2011-05-04
50. Komfyrvakt. https://brannvernforeningen.no/gode-rad/brannvern-i-hjemmet/komfyrvakt/. Accessed 8 Dec 2020
51. Hjohlman M (2011) Provning av spisvakter ('Testing of stove guards'), report PX14609, 2011-11-16, SP Sveriges Tekniska Forskningsinstitut, project for Södertörns Brandförsvarsförbund

Mr. Magnus Arvidson is a Fire Protection Engineer graduated from Lund University in 1989 and has been working at RISE Research Institutes of Sweden since 1991. He has served as a member in the NFPA 750 and CEN technical committees on the installation of water mist fire protection systems and has been active in the Sub-Committee on Fire Protection at the International Maritime Organization. He is currently a member of the Scientific Council of the International Water Mist Association. In 2020, he presented a licentiate thesis on water mist fire protection systems.

Chapter 12
Residential Fire Rescues: Building a Model of Rescue Types for Supporting the Fire Service

Margrethe Kobes and Ricardo Weewer

Abstract Firefighters take great risks when rescuing victims from residential fires. Therefore, insight from practice is essential for supporting the fire service in the choices that must be made during rescue operations. Despite the fact that generally little is known about the circumstances of rescue operations worldwide, tentative information is already known at the local level.

This chapter describes the development of a model of rescue types for supporting the fire service in the (preparation for) the organization of rescue operations and for the prevention of fires where rescue becomes necessary. The presented model is based on data from a multiyear survey by the Dutch fire service and is illustrated by descriptions from practice. Due to possible differences in the execution of fire rescue operations between countries, it may be necessary to adapt the presented model to local conditions.

Furthermore, insight is given in the preliminary indicators for an increased chance of survival. Survival appears to be mainly related to the location of the victim, degree of physical vulnerability to fire, and the physical capacity to escape. The speed of fire discovery and the response time of the fire service seem to have less influence on the survival of the fire.

Keywords Residential fires · Fire fatality · Urgent rescues · Emergency response · Model for rescue operations

---

M. Kobes (✉) · R. Weewer
Netherlands Institute for Public Safety (NIPV), Arnhem, Netherlands
e-mail: Margrethe.Kobes@nipv.nl

© The Author(s), under exclusive license to Springer Nature Switzerland AG 2023
M. Runefors et al. (eds.), *Residential Fire Safety*, The Society of Fire Protection Engineers Series, https://doi.org/10.1007/978-3-031-06325-1_12

1 Introduction

Saving lives, by fire rescue operations, is an important mission of the fire service. Fire rescue operations have a major social impact because they affect the direct lives of those involved and of those living around them. Besides, they also demand a lot from the fire service, both in the psychophysiological field for the firefighters involved and in terms of preparing and managing the rescue operation. Information is needed to support the fire service in this. Step-by-step knowledge is expanding about the possibilities and limitations of firefighter's capabilities under severe conditions: some recent studies focus on psychophysiological responses of firefighters to day and night rescue interventions [13], on heat stress, fatigue and recovery practices [5], or on crawling speeds of search and rescue operations during interior firefighting [12]. However, there is little data from practice available on rescue operations by the fire service. Even data on how many victims are rescued annually is difficult to find. However, in some countries, initial data collection has started, such as in Sweden [15], the Netherlands [11], and the United States (Firefighterrescuesurvey.com).

Rescue is needed when occupants in a building on fire cannot escape by themselves. Sometimes a rescue operation results in a fire fatality. Compared to fire rescue operations, more research has been conducted into fire fatalities worldwide for some time now [1, 6, 7, 9, 16]. The studies show, among other things, that most fatalities occur in residential fires. In addition, research has shown that modern residential fires develop faster and produce more smoke than before [2, 3, 10]. The smoke often spreads faster and further than the actual fire. The smoke contains poisonous gases and people can become intoxicated or disoriented as a result. Besides, a residential fire not only leads to unsafe situations for people in the direct vicinity of the fire but also for people in surrounding areas with smoke [3, 14]. In those circumstances, the occupants fail to evacuate by themselves (or cannot due to disability) and the need for rescue by the fire service will be inevitable. However, there are also limits to the fire service's ability to rescue people. For example, when there is heavy smoke development, a rapid fire spread, large numbers of people who need to be rescued, or a combination of these. These circumstances make it increasingly difficult for the fire service to rescue people from fires in the home and this raises the question to what extent this is still possible at all.

In this chapter, we present a model categorizing the various types of rescue operations. This model can be used to prepare for rescue operations, dimension the fire service capabilities and to prevent rescue operations to be necessary. The model is based on data from an extensive data collection on rescues of victims of residential fires by the Dutch fire brigade. We recognize that there will be differences in the execution of fire rescues between countries, because there may be a difference in the organization of the fire service and in building types. However, the model can be adapted to local differences by using local data on rescues. Based on the circumstances of victims who had to be rescued by the fire service, we distinguish several types of rescue operations. Furthermore, we give insight into differences in circumstances of victims who did or did not survive the fire. To demonstrate the applicability of the model, we conclude with an overview of critical findings from practice that are important for saving lives by rescue operations by the fire service.

2 Methodology

From literature, it appears that in general there is little data available on rescue operations by the fire brigade, especially on the circumstances of the victims who need to be rescued. To gain more insight into the circumstances during rescues by the fire brigade in residential fires and fatal residential fires, the Fire Service Academy of the Institute for Safety has started collecting data about these types of residential fires in the Netherlands. The data collection takes place in collaboration with qualified fire investigators of the Dutch fire service, using a digital questionnaire. The questions relate to four aspects that affect fire safety, namely, the fire characteristics, building characteristics, human characteristics, and intervention characteristics.

There are several views on what can be understood by "rescue from a residential fire." In this study, it was decided to use the following definition:

A rescue from a residential fire is an evacuation by the fire brigade of a civil person who cannot or does not want to escape independently and would have been in a worse situation without the intervention of the fire brigade. The fire took place in a building with a residential function or another "housing related" object, including fires that are caused intentionally.

The data about rescues from fire are compared to data about fatal residential fires:

A fatal residential fire is a fire involving civil fatalities due to fire, which took place in a building with a residential function or another "housing related" object and is not caused intentionally[1].

The study is therefore limited to rescues and fatalities from a building with a residential function or other "residential-related" object[2]. It is limited to rescues in the event of fire incident type, to rescues carried out by the fire brigade, and to rescues where the rescued person survived the fire. The study on fatalities is limited to unintended fires. First of all, it is because of the initial scope of the data collection and also because detailed data from a crime scene will not be available for the survey.

---

[1] These are the residential fires with fatal outcome where it is certain that there was no arson, murder, or suicide. Residential fires with a fatal outcome intentionally caused by accountable adults are excluded from the research. Other types of arson are included in the analysis, for example, fires caused by children playing or adults with mental health issues.

[2] The criterion for "residential function"/"residential-related" is that there must be more or less permanent residence and the rescued person's familiarity with the environment. Rescues of people from nursing homes were therefore included in the study, but rescues from (for example) hospitals were not. Rescues from mobile homes and sheds (if they belong to a home) were also included in the study.

The analysis of fatalities is based on data from the period 2008–2019 and the dataset contains information about 338 incidents and 366 victims. See for an annual review example [8]. The analysis of rescues is based on the data of incidents from 2016, 2017, and 2018 in The Netherlands. In total, approximately 750 people have been rescued by the fire brigade in about 245 incidents; these incidents are more or less evenly distributed over the years. In 90% of the incidents, a maximum of six persons had to be rescued, and generally (70%) there were one or two rescues per incident. Thus, there have been relatively few large-scale rescues. For efficiency reasons, the information regarding the rescued persons for most of the large-scale rescue operations was queried per group of victims that were rescued in comparable circumstances. In the other incidents, the information is registered per individual victim. In total, there is data available of about 400 victims on an individual level, rescued from 215 incidents (88%), and of about 350 victims on a group level.

The collected cases have been clustered into several common types of rescue. This characterization helps to gain a better understanding of the problems and possibilities for the fire service in terms of prevention, preparation, and operation of rescues. To distinguish different common types of rescue, we first divide between small-scale and large-scale rescue operations. In the former type, six or fewer victims per incident were rescued by the fire service, and in the latter type, more than six victims per incident. This is an approach from the point of view of the organization of the fire service. Another, complementary approach, is that from the point of view of the victims' circumstances. To distinguish between these circumstances, a model has been developed, based on the three stages of the escape process [4]. The basic principle for fire safety in buildings is that those present should escape from the home by themselves in the event of a fire. Rescues are necessary when those present cannot escape by themselves. The escape process consists of the following stages:

- Discovering the fire
- Decision making, based on an assessment of the situation by the resident
- Escape to a safe place

In these different phases, the ability to escape can be impeded, so that a rescue becomes necessary. The impediments can be caused by the physical and mental condition of the persons, by the fire situation, or by building characteristics. The combination of the three phases of the escape process and the three types of causes of impediments (impediment due to a physical disability, obstruction by fire or smoke, and obstruction by the building elements) has resulted in six potential rescue types. Since most of the incidents were small-scale rescues (6 victims or less), we only apply the aforementioned six rescue types for the small-scale rescues. To incorporate the large-scale rescues, two rescue types have been added to the model, namely the nonurgent rescues in large-scale rescue operations (type 7) and the urgent rescues in large-scale rescue operations (type 8).

Because there is a hierarchy in the reasons for the need for rescue, a rescue can, for example, fit in *rescue type 3*, while there is also serious injury from fire or a physical disability. In that case, the blocked escape route is considered more relevant for the allocation to a rescue type than the serious injury or the physical disability. In order to escape, it is first of all important that the escape route is available. Thereafter, an impediment due to serious injury is considered more relevant than an existing physical disability. In the event of serious injury there is a risk of loss of consciousness and there is usually no possibility to escape. With an existing physical disability, there is often still a possibility to escape, but this takes more time and effort, so that a rescue may still be necessary. Furthermore, *rescue type 3* is divided in the blocked escape route for the victims in the residential unit on fire (3a) and in the blocked escape route for the victims in the neighboring apartments (3b).

For the assignment of the rescues to the distinct rescue types, additional use has been made of the flow chart as shown below.

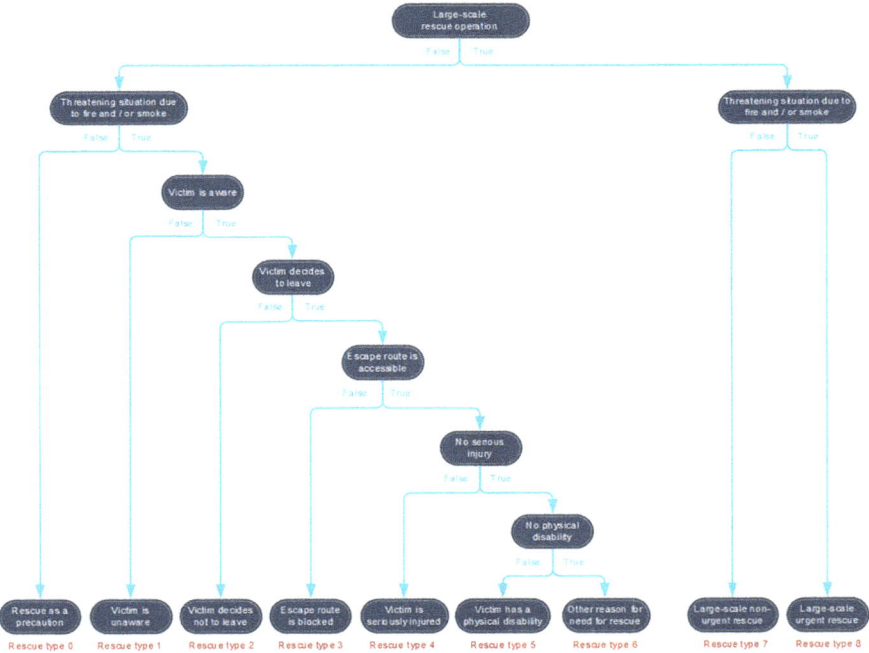

3 Survey Data as the Foundation of the Model

Developing a model for rescue operations requires a good understanding of the circumstances under which the rescue operations took place. This section describes the various rescue operations per clustered type of (similar) rescue operations. The first step of categorizing the types of rescues by the fire brigade is from the point of view of the organization of the rescue operation. The data of the Dutch survey is used to indicate the extent to which the various rescues in the major categories took place.

3.1 Characterization of the Rescues by Scale and Urgency of the Rescue Operation

First of all, a distinction is made in the scale of the operation. Nearly all incidents involved small-scale rescues, while only 60% of the victims were rescued in these fires with six or fewer victims per incident. The other 40% of the rescued victims were involved in large-scale incidents. Large-scale incidents have a social impact on society and it is challenging for the fire service to evacuate many victims in threatening circumstances. Therefore, the large-scale incidents are also included in the model, even though they are not decisive in the frequency of occurrence.

Second, a distinction can be made between urgent rescues and rescues as a precaution. In an urgent rescue, there is a direct threat to life, for example, because the victim is near the seat of the fire, there is heavy smoke development near the victim or it seems the victim is going to jump. In a rescue as a precaution, there is no immediate threat to the victim, but the fire situation is deteriorating. Most of the rescues involved small-scale urgent rescues (62 incidents and 117 victims annually).

Some of the victims who were rescued from a residential died at a later moment as a result of their injuries. A comparison of the circumstances of rescue operations with fatal residential fires can give insight into indicators of an increased chance of survival. The data on fatal residential fires are therefore included in the survey data. The fatal residential fires are almost exclusively small-scale operations.

Compared to fatal residential fires, there were about two times more small-scale rescue operations, and about three times more victims involved.

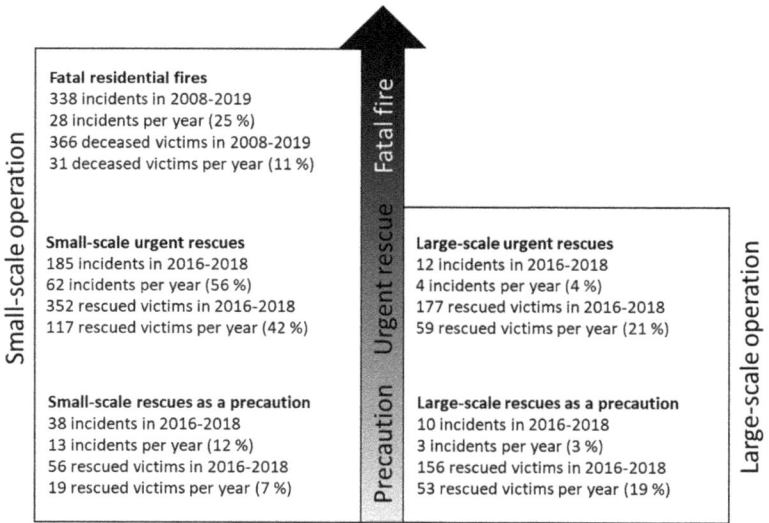

In the following sections, more detailed information is given on the circumstances of rescue operations and the fatal residential fires. Most of the rescues (measured by number of victims) in the Dutch survey concern small-scale urgent rescues, large-scale urgent rescues, and large-scale rescues as a precaution. Therefore, the focus of the detailed descriptions is on those three major categories. In addition, the small-scale urgent rescues will also be compared with fatal residential fires. In the comparison, the focus will be on the incidents where the victim was in the residential unit on fire.

3.2 General Features of Rescues by the Fire Brigade

First, the similarities between the small-scale, large-scale, urgent, and nonurgent rescues are discussed here. Where applicable, the similarities between rescues and fatal residential fires are also included.

Building and Human Characteristics The rescued victims were usually found outside the fire room. Both rescued and deceased victims were slightly more often male than female, although the percentages are around the average. Furthermore, the rescued or deceased victims were as often awake as they were asleep, only in the large-scale nonurgent rescues the victims were awake twice as often as they were asleep.

Fire Characteristics Incidents with a large fire size occur, but most of the incidents involve a fire that was limited to the room in which the fire started, including the fatal residential fires. In small-scale rescues, the fire was often even limited to the object of origin. However, these relatively small fires produce such an amount of smoke that shortly after the fire started the escape route gets blocked by smoke. In half of the cases, it concerned the hallway of the residential unit in which the fire started, and a victim who was found in a room other than the fire room. The other half of the cases concerned the common interior hallway or stairwell of an apartment building, probably because the resident had escaped from the apartment in which the fire started and left the front door open.

Intervention Characteristics Typically, incidents wherein rescue is needed occur in the evening or at night. In a fire in the evening or at night, the residents were often asleep and therefore less likely to discover the fire. However, despite the late time of the event, the fire was in general rapidly discovered and reported to the fire brigade, namely within 15 min after the start of the fire and even often within 5 min after the start of the fire. Fatal residential fires were also in general rapidly discovered and reported. The time between fire start and discovery was estimated by fire investigators, sometimes based on eyewitness statements. It should be noted, however, that it is not always possible to make a good estimate of the time between the moment of the start of fire and the moment when the fire was reported to the fire brigade. The response time of the fire brigade can be determined with more precision. Generally, also the fire brigade arrived rapidly on the scene, on average within 7 min for small-scale rescues and fatal residential fires and within 8 min for large-scale incidents. Thereafter, the victims are also quickly located: in almost all small-scale urgent rescues within 5 min after the arrival of the fire brigade, and in almost all the large-scale or fatal incidents within 15 min, and in 60% of the cases even within 5 min. Rarely, it took more than 15 min for the firefighters to locate and rescue the victim, and it occurred almost solely in large-scale rescues and fatal residential fires.

When the victims need to be rescued from the balcony, the use of a rescue vehicle turned out to be essential, as nearly 50% of the victims in the large-scale rescues were rescued via a turntable ladder or hydraulic platform, about as often as in the small-scale rescues. In the large-scale rescues, 25% of the victims were escorted outside without protective equipment, twice as often as in the small-scale rescues. In a rescue using a turntable ladder or hydraulic platform, the victims do not have to be exposed to the smoke in the blocked escape route.

3.3 Features of Large-Scale Rescue Operations by the Fire Service

Although it concerns a limited number of incidents yearly, in the Netherlands about seven per year, they are incidents that demand the utmost from the fire service as there are large numbers of people who need to be rescued, about 100 victims a year. In half of the large-scale incidents, between 7 and 10 people were rescued, in a quarter between 11 and 20 people, and in the other quarter more than 20 people were rescued, with about 55 people in the largest rescue operation. In all cases, but especially in the case of large-scale incidents, the challenges for the fire service are great when it comes to (many) victims who have to be rescued urgently. While many incidents concern rescues as a precaution, there is also an alarming number of incidents with many victims in a life-threatening situation.

Building Characteristics The incidents mostly took place in a porch flat, which is a multifamily apartment building, where the front doors of two adjoining apartments on each floor lead to a shared staircase. Furthermore, the incidents often occurred in an apartment building in which the front doors of the apartments are per floor connected to an interior common corridor. Large-scale rescue operations usually involve rescues from apartments adjacent to the apartment in which the fire started. Usually, it concerns apartments that share a common interior corridor or stairwell with the home in which the fire started. In these incidents, sometimes also a victim is rescued from the apartment in which the fire started.

In most cases, the victims were rescued from another apartment than where the fire started. Only 10% of the victims in the large-scale rescue operations had to be rescued from the apartment in which the fire started. In those rescue operations, also victims from the neighboring apartments were rescued. Although the victims were usually found outside the fire room, in the large-scale rescue operations also some victims (2%) were rescued from the fire room. In the nonurgent rescues, the victims who were rescued within half an hour after arrival of the fire brigade were mostly in their apartment, while the victims who were rescued after half an hour were often on the balcony.

Human Characteristics In large-scale rescues, the victims were frequently vulnerable elderly or children, though in the nonurgent situations (80%) more often than in the urgent situations (67%). In urgent situations, 50% of the victims were asleep, while 67% of the precautionary rescued victims were awake at the time of the fire. In 75% of the nonurgent rescues, limited mobility was the main reason for the need for rescue.

Fire Characteristics In the large-scale urgent operations, a rescue was mostly needed because the escape route was blocked by smoke. The victims to be rescued were frequently the neighbors of the apartment in which the fire started. They were often unable to escape because the common corridor of the stairwell, their only escape route, was full of smoke. In 20% of the cases, the neighbors were not only threatened by the smoke, but the fire spread to other apartments as well. These are the most difficult situations for the organization of the rescue operation: it concerns not only a large-scale rescue operation but also a large-scale firefighting operation.

Intervention Characteristics The large-scale rescue operations most often took place in the last three months of the year (50%), when it is getting colder outside and people are more often at home.

In the rescues as a precaution, the victims were mainly escorted outside by the firefighters without protective equipment (56%) or were rescued using a manual ladder (16%) or the revitox (12%), a device that is connected to the firefighter's breathing apparatus. In a few cases, the victim was dragged outside or rescued with the help of an evacuation chair.

3.4 Urgent Rescues: Small-Scale Compared to Large-Scale Operations

In an urgent situation, the firefighters may take more risks and endanger themselves, compared to situations where the victims are not in immediate threat or where there are no more victims inside. There are some differences between the small-scale and large-scale rescues, which have a consequence for the rescue operation. First of all, the number of victims that are involved in the rescue operation is relevant, as it has implications for the capabilities of the rescue operation. Second, a rescue operation in which several residential units are threatened by the fire (smoke) is more complex than a rescue operation that is limited to one residential unit. However, a rescue from one residential unit can already be qualified as complex.

To gain more insight into the main differences between small-scale and large-scale urgent rescues, the characteristics of both types of incidents are described below.

Building Characteristics The large-scale rescues almost exclusively took place in apartment buildings with shared interior hallways, mostly in porch flats. The small-scale rescues also often took place in such apartment buildings, although relatively less often compared to the large-scale rescues. In 25% of the small-scale rescue operations, the victims were rescued from a single-family home, while this type of housing was rarely involved in the large-scale rescues.

The large-scale operations usually involved rescues from several neighboring residential units, while more than 50% of the small-scale operations involved rescues from the residential unit in which the fire started.

In large-scale urgent rescues, the victims who were rescued within half an hour were mostly outside, on the balcony, or hanging from the window, while those who were rescued after half an hour were usually in their bedrooms. The victims in the small-scale urgent rescues were mostly located on the balcony or in a bedroom.

Human Characteristics In the large-scale urgent rescues, the victims were frequently vulnerable elderly or children, while the victims in the small-scale urgent rescues were generally mobile person between 21 and 60 years old. In both types of rescues, about 50% of the victims were not alert, for example as they were asleep. The victims in the small-scale rescues were often injured, namely in 80% of the cases, which is twice as often as in the large-scale rescues.

Fire Characteristics In most of the urgent rescues, the rescue was necessary because the escape route was blocked by smoke. Many small-scale urgent rescues were necessary due to rapid fire development or heavy smoke development, although the fire was often contained within the room where the fire started.

In large-scale urgent rescues, there was almost always smoke development in the vicinity of the victim, roughly as often heavy as light smoke development, sometimes also when the victim was standing on the balcony.

Intervention Characteristics In most of the small-scale rescues, the victim was injured to such an extent that the victim was dragged out by a firefighter, and some were escorted outside with the support of the fire crew. In large-scale urgent situations, the victims were most often rescued with the help of a turntable ladder or hydraulic platform (46%) or escorted outside by the firefighters without protective equipment (27%) or with the aid of an escape mask (15%). In large-scale incidents, the firefighters often had difficulty entering the residential unit as the front door had to be forced.

3.5 Small-Scale Urgent Rescue Operations Compared to Fatal Residential Fires

To gain insight into the aspects that make the difference between surviving and not surviving a residential fire, the small-scale urgent rescues were compared with fatal residential fires.

In the small-scale rescue operations, 60% of the victims were rescued from the residential unit in which the fire started, while this applies to almost all victims in the fatal residential fires. Therefore, we focus on the circumstances of the victims who were rescued from the residential unit on fire. For the other rescued victims, we assume that they survived the fire because they were not in the residential unit in which the fire started. Every year, in the Netherlands, it concerns about 48 incidents with 65 victims who were rescued from a residential unit on fire and about 28 incidents with 31 victims who deceased from a fire in their home. Some significant differences were found between the conditions in rescue operations and fatal residential fires.

Building Characteristics Both small-scale urgent rescues and fatal residential fires, wherein the victim was trapped by a fire in their residential unit, took place most often in a single-family house, namely in about 40% of the cases in both types. The first major difference between both incident types is that the deceased victims were mostly found in the fire room, while the rescued victims were usually rescued from another room than the fire room. About 30% of the rescued victims could escape to a certain extent as they stood on the balcony. And, more importantly, 10% of the victims were rescued from the fire room. This indicates that the efforts to rescue from the fire room are effective: To give an idea of the proportions, in the Netherlands, yearly about 17 victims deceased because they were in the room where the fire started, of whom six were initially rescued but they deceased later from the consequences of their injuries, and about 12 victims were rescued from the fire room.

Human Characteristics For the deceased victims as well as for the victims in small-scale urgent rescues, limited alertness played an important role in the fatality or the need for rescue. The victims who survived the fire were often mobile persons between 21 and 60 years old, while the deceased victims were more often frail elderly. Thus, regarding their physical conditions before the fire, the rescued victims were less vulnerable to fire than those who deceased from the fire. Nevertheless, in both the small-scale urgent rescues and the fatal residential fires, the victims were unable to escape without help. The rescued victims often needed help because of a blocked escape route and the deceased victims mainly because of a physical disability. About 30% of the deceased victims were still alive and initially rescued by the fire crew.

Fire Characteristics Rapid fire development or intense smoke development played an important role in the fatal residential fires, more often than in the rescues. Near the deceased victims, there was significantly more often heavy smoke than among the rescued victims. Nearly 50% of the rescued victims were slightly injured, 50% were seriously injured, and the rest was uninjured.

Intervention Characteristics Most fires were discovered and reported within fifteen minutes after their start; it applies to 67% of the rescued victims and to 50% of the deceased victims. There is, however, an important difference in the number of fires that are discovered and reported more than half an hour after they started. The late discovery applies to 10% of the rescue operations and to 25% of the fatal residential fires. It should be noted, however, that most of the victims had probably already deceased before the fire was discovered.

3.6 Summary of the Survey Data

The following figure summarizes the critical findings from practice that are important for the prevention, preparation, and execution of rescue operations.

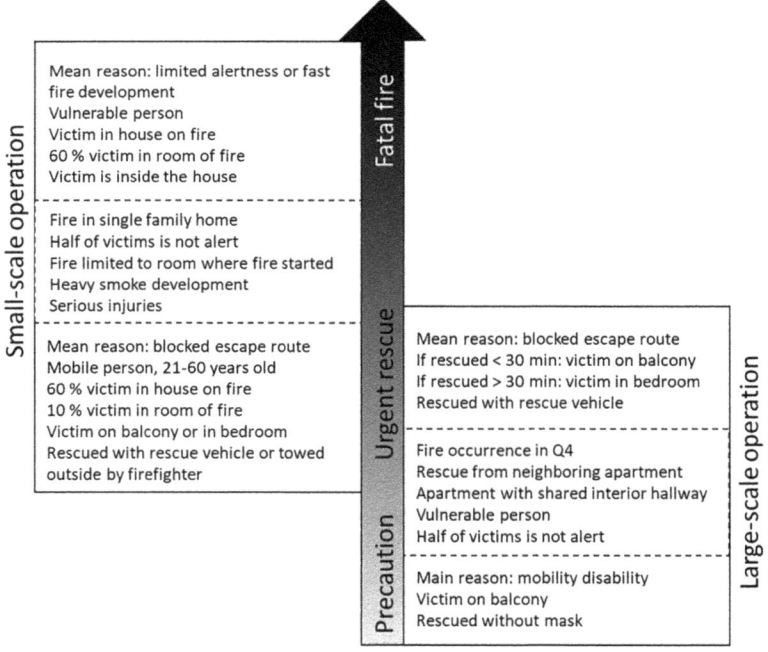

4 Building a Model for Common Types of Rescue

4.1 Introduction

The previous sections discussed the characteristics of large-scale and small-scale rescues and urgent and nonurgent rescues. In size, both in terms of the number of incidents and the number of victims rescued, the urgent small-scale ones are the most relevant. These types of rescues are subdivided into rescue types that are related to the escape process, from the victim's point of view. How the rescue operations can be assigned to different rescue types is described in detail in the methodology section.

In the table below, an overview is given of the various rescue types. First, there is a division into four major categories based on the scale and urgency of the rescue operation and the small-scale urgent rescues are subdivided into seven categories based on the escape process. To illustrate the expected distribution of incidents and victims over the rescue types, the distribution that emerged from the Dutch study is also shown.

Rescue types	Incidents	Rescued victims
Small-scale rescues as a precaution		
Rescue type 0: The victim is rescued as a precaution	15%	8%
Small-scale urgent rescues		
Rescue type 1: The victim is unaware of the fire	14%	6%
Rescue type 2: The victim decides not to escape	14%	6%
Rescue type 3a: The escape route of the residential unit on fire is blocked by smoke	19%	12%
Rescue type 3b: Smoke blocks the escape route for the neighboring apartments	15%	14%
Rescue type 4: The victim is seriously injured by the fire	7%	3%
Rescue type 5: The victim has a physical disability	4%	1%
Rescue type 6: Other reasons for the need for rescue	3%	1%
Large-scale rescues as a precaution		
Rescue type 7: Large-scale rescue operation, rescues as a precaution	4%	22%
Large-scale urgent rescues		
Rescue type 8: Large-scale rescue operation, urgent rescues	5%	25%

A description of an incident example has been made based on the information obtained from the analysis per rescue type. This includes the most common circumstances for the incident. In practice, the actual circumstances per incident may differ in parts from the example.

4.2 Rescue Type 0: The Victim Is Rescued as a Precaution

There is no life threat and impediment. The person is in an environment with no fire and in which no or hardly any smoke is present.

Example
 A fire breaks out in a porch apartment or apartment connected to a shared interior corridor. A few occupants need to be rescued from both the apartment on fire and the apartments on the floor above. The occupants are young adults, or mobile elderly people, twice more men than women. They were awake when the fire started. The fire was discovered within 5 minutes after it started and reported to the fire brigade. The fire remains small, within the room in which it originated. But because of the smoke in the common stairwell, the occupants cannot leave their apartments and they escape to the balcony. There is no smoke there. The fire crew arrives 9 minutes after the call and first rescues the occupant of the burning apartment by dragging him outside. The other residents are then removed from the balcony with the aid of a turntable ladder or escorted outside via the ventilated staircase without protective means. The victims suffered no or minor injuries from the fire.

4.3 Rescue Type 1: The Victim Is Unaware of the Fire

There is an impediment during the discovery phase, for example, because the person is asleep at that moment.

Example
 During the night, a fire breaks out in the living room of an apartment occupied by a 30-year-old man. The occupant is sleeping in the bedroom. Ten minutes later, a passer-by, walking the dog, sees that there is a fire and calls immediately the fire brigade. The smoke has now spread to the bedroom. Only the sofa in the living room is on fire, but the hallway is now full of smoke. The fire brigade arrives 6 minutes after the call. They force the front door and wake the occupant. The occupant suffers from slight smoke inhalation and is escorted outside with an escape mask. The neighbors have also awakened and encountered the smoke that has entered the stairwell as a result of the rescue operation. Without an escape mask, they are escorted outside by the fire crew.

4.4 Rescue Type 2: The Victim Decides Not to Escape

Impediment during the decision-making phase, for example, because the person has mental health issues or does not want to leave the home for some other reason.

Example
 A fire breaks out in an apartment. A single male 50-year-old occupant with mental health issues is in the fire room. He is under the influence of alcohol and is suicidal. The man starts a fire and observes that the things he has collected in recent years catch fire. He does not want to leave the residential unit. The room soon becomes full of heavy smoke. The neighbors hear some noises, smell fire, and call the fire brigade. The fire crew arrives after 7 minutes and discovers the occupant inside. He has serious burns and is taken outside without a mask by the fire crew.

4.5 Rescue Type 3a: The Escape Route of the Residential Unit on Fire Is Blocked by Smoke

During the escape phase, there is an obstruction due to building characteristics, for example, when the person is locked in a room because of smoke in the landing.

> *Example*
> In a semidetached single-family house, a fire breaks out at night. A young couple is sleeping in the bedroom on the first floor when the fire starts. Suddenly, they wake up and discover that there is a fire on the ground floor. The staircase is full of smoke, but they try to escape. One person manages to escape, but the other does not dare to use the stairs and goes back to the bedroom. The smoke develops rapidly and the occupant can no longer escape. The fire brigade crew after 7 minutes. There is then heavy smoke development in the bedroom. The firefighters rescue the occupant by using a manual ladder. The occupant is suffering from severe smoke inhalation.

4.6 Rescue Type 3b: Smoke Blocks the Escape Route for the Neighboring Apartments

During the escape phase, there is an obstruction due to building characteristics, for example, when the only, shared escape route (stairwell) is completely filled with smoke.

> *Example*
> A fire breaks out in an apartment of a porch flat. The fire is discovered within 15 minutes after it started and reported to the fire brigade. The fire and smoke develop quickly and the young adult occupants of the apartments above are alerted by the neighbors. They escape to the balcony, as it is impossible to leave the porch flat via the stairwell due to the smoke development. The fire spreads to a neighboring apartment and light smoke is now hanging on the balconies. The fire crew arrives after 7 minutes and rescues the occupants from the balconies with a turntable ladder. As a result of the fire, the occupants are suffering from light smoke inhalation.

4.7 Rescue Type 4: The Victim Is Seriously Injured by the Fire

During the escape phase, an impediment occurs due to the fire situation, for example, a loss of consciousness due to smoke inhalation.

> *Example*
> In one of the last months of the year, a fire breaks out in the apartment of a healthy 50-year-old occupant. The occupant is smoking in the living room and his clothing suddenly catches fire. The occupant discovers that the sofa has also caught fire and he is just able to call the fire brigade. The fire rapidly spreads to other items in the living room and soon the living room fills with heavy smoke. The fire crew arrives after 6 minutes and discovers the occupant unconscious in the living room. The occupant is dragged out by the firefighters. The victim suffered minor burns and severe inhalation trauma.

4.8 Rescue Type 5: The Victim Has a Physical Disability

During the escape phase, an impediment occurs due to mobile limitations, for example, because a wheelchair user cannot descend the stairs.

> *Example*
> At night the sofa in the living room catches fire in the apartment of an 85-year-old occupant. He is using a wheelchair and cannot leave the apartment without help. The fire crew arrives after 7 minutes and discovers the occupant in the living room which is filled with heavy smoke, even though only the sofa is on fire. The occupant suffers from severe smoke inhalation and is dragged outside by the firefighters.

4.9 Rescue Type 6: Other Reasons for the Need for Rescue

During the escape phase, an impediment occurs that is not covered by the other rescue types.

> *No example description because of a limited number of cases*

4.10 Rescue Type 7: Large-Scale Rescue Operation, Rescues as a Precaution

There is no life threat and impediment. Several persons need to be rescued from multiple locations. They are located in an environment with no fire and where little or no smoke is present.

> *Example*
> In the evening in one of the last months of the year, a fire breaks out in an apartment in a residential complex for seniors. Most of the apartments' occupants have a physical disability. Rapidly, the hallway and stairwell are full of black smoke. The occupants escape to the balcony. The smoke has not yet spread to the balconies and the apartments, but the people on the balcony do not feel safe. The fire crew arrives after 8 minutes. The firefighters ventilate the stairwell and escort the occupants outside without an escape mask. The occupants were not injured as a result of the fire.

4.11 Rescue Type 8: Large-Scale Rescue Operation, Urgent Rescues

Several persons need to be rescued from multiple locations. They are located in an environment that is threatened by the fire or by the effects of fire (smoke).

Example
　Late in the evening in one of the last months of the year, a fire breaks out in an apartment complex for seniors. The fire started because the occupant had put a frying pan on the stove, but fell asleep on the sofa. The occupant has a physical disability and escapes to the stairwell. The front door remains open, and quickly the stairwell fills with smoke. Some occupants of the other apartments notice the fire and escape to the balcony. Others are sleeping in their bedroom and do not notice the fire. The smoke is now also spreading to the balconies and apartments. When the fire crew arrives, they hear several occupants calling for help from the balconies. In the stairwell, they discover the unconscious occupant of the burning apartment. Meanwhile, the rescue vehicle has also arrived and the other occupants can be rescued from the balconies and their bedrooms. The occupant of the apartment in which the fire started deceased on the way to the hospital. The occupants of the other apartments were not injured.

5　Application of the Model

To demonstrate the applicability of the model, we give an overview of critical findings from the practice that are important for saving lives by rescue operations by the fire service. In this section, we described the circumstances of victims who had to be rescued by the fire service and discussed the differences between the death or survival of fire.

　It is found that fires in apartments that are accessed from a shared interior hallway cause the greatest difficulties for a safe escape, both for the persons in the apartment on fire and for the persons in the neighboring apartments. Occupants of this type of apartment often became trapped because the corridor, their only escape route, was full of smoke, see for example *rescue types 3a and 3b: the escape route is blocked by smoke*. Building regulations, in the Netherlands but conceivably also in other countries, include measures to ensure that fire in one home will not cause a problem for other homes. In practice, residents do appear to face a life-threatening situation if a fire breaks out in a neighboring apartment. Often it was a porch-flat, where the front doors of two adjoining apartments on each floor lead to a common staircase. Furthermore, it often occurred in an apartment building in which the front doors of the apartments are per floor connected to an interior corridor.

　In some incidents, it is known that the smoke has spread because the resident of the burning apartment left the front door open during the escape. From other incident descriptions, it is known that heavy smoke entered the corridor or stairwell after the fire brigade forced the front door of the apartment in which the fire started; even when the fire extent was limited to the first ignited object. Some fire investigators (respondents) indicated that there was "a disproportionate amount of smoke," a degree of smoke spread that did not meet the expectations of the firefighters. This picture needs to be adjusted, supported by results from recently conducted field experiments on smoke dispersion in residential buildings [3]. From this, it appears that in the event of a fire in a sofa, an open front door quickly leads to life-threatening concentrations of gases in the adjacent corridor and surrounding apartments, especially for vulnerable people. The experiments also showed that, even though no smoke was visually discovered, there were still high concentrations of toxic gases. The neighbors are consequently threatened by the fire or do not have a safe escape route, even if the hallway or stairwell appears to be almost smoke-free. Therefore, a quick and safe rescue of neighbors is vital in the event of a fire in an apartment that is connected to a shared corridor. Preferably, the rescue should take place through the smoke-free outdoor air, or indoors using a mask.

In addition to rescuing many neighbors, a large number of residents were also rescued from the residential unit in which the fire started, even from the room on fire, see for example *rescue type 4: the victim is seriously injured by the fire* and *rescue type 5: the victim has a physical disability*. Moreover, in numbers, as many people in the room on fire were saved as deceased. Entering a burning residential unit for a rescue operation involves major risks for the firefighters, but it appears to be worthwhile. The comparison between urgent rescues from the apartment in which the fire started indicates that the difference between survival and death in the event of a residential fire is mainly related to the victims' physical vulnerability and the degree of smoke development in the direct vicinity of the victim. From this, it is assumed that survival is most likely when the victim is between 21 and 60 years old, or if the victim has escaped to a relatively safe place due to a good mobility ability.

In all types of rescues, as well as fatal residential fires, the fire is mostly rapidly discovered and reported, and the fire brigade arrives quickly on the scene after reporting. However, a considerable number of fatal fires were discovered after more than half an hour from the start of the fire. Where there is a late discovery, the victims are often not alert, for example, because they are asleep, see the example under *rescue type 1: the victim is unaware of the fire*. A preventive measure to discover the fire more quickly, such as a smoke detector, can be effective in reducing the number of victims in a fire, provided that the residents are not vulnerable and have a normal mobility ability. For the frail elderly victims, a faster discovery has less effect, as it is found in the fatal fires that in about 25% of the incidents a smoke detector was activated, mostly when an older, physically impaired victim was involved. Measures for rapid firefighting and limiting smoke production or preventing fire ignition are more suitable. The home furnishings, particularly sofas and matrasses, have a major influence on smoke production.

The *rescue type 2: the victim decides not to escape* often involves a person with mental health issues or suicidal person. In some incidents, it is known that the victim set fire. When someone sets fire in an apartment that is connected to a common interior corridor or stairwell, the victim endangers not only himself but also the neighbors. To prevent such fires, measures that can influence the behavior of potential arsonists are most appropriate. The solutions therefore mainly lie in the field of social support. An apartment with a shared entrance is the most dangerous and therefore least suitable type of housing for people with mental health issues. Another type of housing would be more suitable to prevent neighbors from becoming fire victims.

About 20% of the victims become trapped in their residential unit by smoke that has spread to the corridor after the fire breaks out in a room elsewhere in the residential unit (*rescue type 3a*). In these situations, most victims were often not alert or at least not aware of the fire. A smoke detector in the potential fire room, such as the living room, kitchen, and bedrooms, ensures a faster discovery. This increases the probability that the fire will be discovered before the escape route is already full of smoke. Closing all interior doors when the residents go to sleep will also keep the escape route smoke-free for a longer time.

In some of the small-scale urgent rescues, neighbors have become trapped because the shared interior hallway is full of smoke (*rescue type 3b*). This is also the case in all large-scale urgent rescues (*rescue type 8*). In some cases, the rescue operation involved both rescued and deceased victims. Such incidents have a major impact, both on the residents of the apartment building and the fire crew. Although the victims in the neighboring residential units are often not injured, after the incident they may no longer feel safe in the apartment building. For the rescue operation, the focus is not only on the residential unit on fire, but the working area is larger. The operation requires several fire crews that are not immediately present at the scene of the incident. This makes the rescue operation extra complex. Furthermore, the use of a rescue vehicle appears to be essential for these types of rescues. Most residents are on the balcony and as the escape route is full of smoke, rescue via the turntable ladder or hydraulic platform is the safest way to rescue.

The fatal residential fires often occur in single-family homes as well as in apartments. This also applies to urgent rescues in which the victims need to be rescued from the residential unit on fire; proportionally this housing type is involved about as often as in the fatal residential fires. This indicates that a fire in a single-family home more often leads to a very urgent situation than a fire in another housing type. Probably, this is affected by a relatively late discovery of the fire in single-family homes compared to other housing types, as the data reveals. An explanation for the faster discovery of apartment fires can be that one of the neighbors in an apartment building will quickly discover the fire because the smoke spreads to the shared corridor of stairwell, while it takes more time for single-family home neighbors to discover a fire next door.

Finally, in the case of rescues, it is noticeable that while driving to the incident location, the fire crew often receives little information from the fire dispatch center about the situation on site. It is often not known in which apartment the fire is, but only that the stairwell is full of smoke or even only that smoke has been discovered. It is also regularly not known whether people are inside. This limits the possibilities of the fire crew because upscaling is often necessary, while the information for this decision is not available until the fire crew arrives on site. This wastes valuable time for upscaling. To have this information available earlier, the fire dispatch center should, where possible, inquire about specific characteristics that are related to rescues or should have more specific information in their database. This includes the housing type, whether it concerns a fire in an apartment with a shared interior hallway or not, and the details of the residents, whether it concerns residents who are vulnerable to fire.

6 Conclusions

6.1 A First Step Toward a Model of Rescue Types for Supporting the Fire Service

Although the understanding of fire rescue operations by the fire service is still limited, certain insight is gained from a Dutch survey in which qualified fire investigators provided data on rescues by the fire service. The survey data are used as the basis to build a model on residential fire rescues in order to support the fire service. This model is applicable in (preparation for) the organization of rescue operations by the fire service and for the prevention of fires where rescue becomes necessary. Due to possible differences in the execution of fire rescue operations between countries, it may be necessary to adapt the presented model to local conditions. Therefore, the methodology for building the model is described and can be applied in the same way to categorize a local dataset on fire rescues.

6.2 Main Findings from the Dutch Survey

The following findings can be drawn from the Dutch dataset on residential fire rescues and fatalities:

- Fire rescue operations occur typically in the evening or at night.
- Generally, the fires are rapidly discovered and reported to the fire brigade, and after reporting, the fire brigade arrives on average within 8 min on the scene.
- Most of the rescue operations are small-scale urgent rescues, i.e., a maximum of 6 victims need to be rescued from a life-threatening situation.
    - The main reason for the need for rescue is a blocked escape route.
    - The rescued victims are usually mobile persons between 21 and 60 years old.
    - A fast majority of the victims are trapped in single-family house on fire. Ten percent of the victims is rescued from a room on fire.
    - Most victims are rescued from the balcony or the bedroom.
    - Most victims are rescued by using a rescue vehicle or are towed outside by a firefighter.
- Fatal fires can be expected in single-family houses with vulnerable occupants.
    - The main reason for fatality is a limited alertness or a fast fire development.
    - A fast majority of the victims are in a room on fire.
- In both fatal fires and small-scale urgent rescues, the fire size is usually small, mostly limited to the room where the fire started, but heavy smoke development can be expected.

- Half of the victims are not alert (sleeping).
- Most of the victims have serious injuries.

- Large-scale rescue operations are rare and can be expected in fires in apartment buildings with a shared interior corridor or stairwell.
  - Most rescued victims are neighbors from the apartment on fire.
  - Most victims are vulnerable persons and half of the victims are not alert (sleeping).
  - The main reason for urgent rescues is a blocked escape route and victims are mostly on the balcony or in the bedroom.
  - The main reason for a rescue as a precaution is the victims' physical disability and most victims are rescued from the balcony.

6.3 Indicators for an Increased Chance of Survival

Despite the rapid discovery and the relatively small fire size, some victims deceased from the fire. Based on the comparison of the circumstances of residential fires wherein the victims were trapped in a residential unit on fire, some indicators for an increased chance of survival are found.

Given the few differences between the residential fires where victims were rescued or deceased, the assumption is that survival is mainly related to the location of the victim, degree of physical vulnerability to fire, and the physical capacity to escape. A victim in the fire room, an elderly victim, and a victim with a physical disability are less likely to survive than a mobile victim between 21 and 60 years old, who can bring themself to safety to a certain extent (escape to the balcony). The person's physical vulnerability, in combination with the life-threatening environmental conditions, probably resulted in a fatality, while the less vulnerable persons were able to await their rescue by the firefighter in a relatively less harmful environmental condition.

There were no significant differences found in the speed of fire discovery and in the response time of the fire service. These factors therefore seem to have less influence on the survival of the fire. However, it should be noted that in both types of incidents the fire was already rapidly reported and the fire crew arrived shortly after the fire call.

References

1. Büyük Y, Koçak U (2009) Fire-related fatalities in Istanbul, Turkey: analysis of 320 forensic autopsy cases. J Forensic Legal Med 16(8):449–454. https://doi.org/10.1016/j.jflm.2009.05.005
2. Fire Service Academy (2015) It depends – Descriptive research into fire growth and survivability. IFV, Arnhem

3. Fire Service Academy (2020a) Smoke propagation in residential buildings. The main report on the field experiments conducted in a residential building with internal corridors. IFV, Arnhem
4. Fire Service Academy (2020b) Fire rescues 2016–2018. IFV, Arnhem. (in Dutch: Reddingen bij brand 2016–2018)
5. Fullagar HHK, Schwarz E, Richardson A, Notley SR, Lu D, Duffield R (2021) Australian firefighters perceptions of heat stress, fatigue and recovery practices during fire-fighting tasks in extreme environments. Appl Ergon 95. https://doi.org/10.1016/j.apergo.2021.103449
6. Hasofer AM, Thomas I (2006) Analysis of fatalities and injuries in building fire statistics. Fire Saf J 41(1):2–14. https://doi.org/10.1016/j.firesaf.2005.07.006
7. Holborn PG, Nolan PF, Golt J (2003) An analysis of fatal unintentional dwelling fires investigated by London Fire Brigade between 1996 and 2000. Fire Saf J 38(1):1–42. https://doi.org/10.1016/S0379-7112(02)00049-8
8. IFV (2017) Fatal residential fires in The Netherlands. Annual review 2016. Institute for Safety (IFV), Arnhem
9. Jonsson A, Bonander C, Nilson F, Huss F (2017) The state of the residential fire fatality problem in Sweden: epidemiology, risk factors, and event typologies. J Saf Res 62:89–100. https://doi.org/10.1016/j.jsr.2017.06.008
10. Kerber S (2012) Analysis of changing residential fire dynamics and its implications on firefighter operational timeframes. *Fire Technol* 48(4):865–891. https://doi.org/10.1007/s10694-011-0249-2
11. Kobes M, Van Den Dikkenberg R (2016) An analysis of residential building fire rescues: the difference between fatal and nonfatal casualties. In: Interflam 2016: 14th International fire science and engineering conference, pp 353–364
12. Lambert K, Merci B, Gryspeert C, Jekovec N (2021) Search & rescue operations during interior firefighting: a study into crawling speeds. Fire Saf J 121. https://doi.org/10.1016/j.firesaf.2020.103269
13. Marcel-Millet P, Groslambert A, Gimenez P, Grosprêtre S, Ravier G (2021) Psychophysiological responses of firefighters to day and night rescue interventions. Appl Ergon 95. https://doi.org/10.1016/j.apergo.2021.103457
14. Purser & McAllister (2016) Assessment of hazards to occupants from smoke, toxic gases, and heat. In: Hurley MJ et al (eds) SFPE handbook of fire protection engineering, pp 2308–2428. https://doi.org/10.1007/978-1-4939-2565-0
15. Runefors M (2020) Measuring the capabilities of the Swedish fire service to save lives in residential fires. Fire Technol 56:583–603. https://doi.org/10.1007/s10694-019-00892-y
16. Runyan CW, Bangdiwala SI, Linzer MA, Sacks JJ, Butts J (1992) Risk factors for fatal residential fires. N Engl J Med 327:859–863. https://www.nejm.org/doi/full/10.1056/NEJM199209173271207

Dr. Margrethe Kobes received the Ph.D. degree in Social Sciences in 2010 from VU Amsterdam and holds a M.Sc. degree in Science and Innovation Management from Utrecht University and a B.B.E. in Building Engineering and Architecture from Hanze University of Applied Sciences. She started her working career as a fire prevention assessor at several Dutch fire brigades. Since 2002 she has been working as a researcher and project leader at the Netherlands Institute for Public Safety (NIPV). Margrethe has experience in a range of subjects, from statistics on fires, fire fatalities and rescue operations, field lab research into human behavior in fire, fire protection and firefighting techniques, to developing research methodologies, and evaluating policy instruments for fire service organization.

Prof. Ricardo Weewer is professor of fire service science at the Netherlands Institute for Public Safety (NIPV). He holds a MSc in materials science and electrochemistry and and a Ph.D. in technical sciences. His main objective is to connect practice and science, and to connect prevention and suppression. Before he started working at the Fire Service Academy he went through the ranks and was Deptuy Chief Officer from 2004–2015 in the Amsterdam Fire Service. He was or is in charge of a number of studies into fire fighting tactics and techniques as well as command and control.

Chapter 13
Cost-Benefit Analysis of Fire Safety Measures

Henrik Jaldell

Abstract Ignoring costs when evaluating different measures is not a very rational way to deal with fire safety. Finding efficient measures to increase fire safety is a necessary, but not sufficient condition for choosing the relevant measure. The measure in question must also be economically efficient, that is, the benefits must outweigh the costs, both measured in monetary values. Cost-benefit analysis, CBA, is a method used to find out if that is true or not. This chapter describes what CBA is and how to use it for evaluating fire safety measures. The problem of choosing values for lives and injuries is discussed. The chapter also includes a short list of CBA results for residential fire safety measures. The main conclusion of the chapter is that more CBA studies evaluating fire safety measures should be done.

Keywords Economic evaluation · Benefits and costs · Monetarise · Economically efficient · Value of statistical life

1 Introduction

Having efficient fire prevention and suppression in terms of organization, staff, and equipment is important. We want smoke detectors and sprinklers to be able to save people from injuries and fatalities efficiently. We want fire and rescue services to prevent and suppress fires efficiently. However, other public activities in sectors such as health and traffic safety could also save injuries and fatalities, since resources are limited. From a social point of view, the question then is where a given amount

H. Jaldell (✉)
Economics, Karlstad Business School, Karlstad University, Karlstad, Sweden
e-mail: henrik.jaldell@kau.se

of money will prevent most injuries and fatalities and save most property values. To be able to answer that question, information about the effectiveness of the measures is not sufficient; we also need to consider the costs for them. Given that we can save the same number of people through two different activities, that is they are equally efficient, we should, from an economic point of view, choose the least costly activity. However, in many cases the outcomes are not directly comparable. Fires lead to a range of consequences such as fatalities, property losses, and personal injuries. To be able to compare different measures in terms of effectiveness, we then need to weigh them together using some sort of an index.

The economic way of constructing such an index is to use money as weights. The economic cost-benefit analysis, CBA, uses money to weigh benefits and costs, respectively, together. From an economic standpoint, the relation between benefits and costs shows economic efficiency. The more benefits outweigh costs, the better it is from a social point of view and the higher economic efficiency the activity in question have. Since both the benefits and the costs are measured using the same values, it is also possible to compare fire-related activities to activities in all other sectors, not only fire safety or safety in general.

Cost-benefit analyses are relatively straightforward when it comes to devices such as smoke detectors. If the benefits of the smoke detector outweigh its costs, it is economically efficient. The costs are the purchase price plus the installation cost. The benefits are the people warned and rescued and thus the prevented injuries and fatalities and the saved property. The costs are, mostly, quite easy to calculate using monetary values, for instance using the purchase price. The benefits are harder to quantify, both when it comes to the effect and what values to use. Given a known effect, monetary values must be set, not only on property saved, but also on reduced personal injuries and fatalities.

A more complex cost-benefit analysis could also analyze the effects of a relocation of the fire and rescue service. Is it economically efficient to move the fire station to another place in order to decrease the response times? Yes it is, if the benefits outweigh the costs. Here, the costs are associated with the construction of the new fire station. The benefits are the effects of the decreased response time calculated, in a cost-benefit analysis, as the aggregated monetary benefits of all reduced injuries, fatalities, and properties due to responses of the fire and rescue services to all different missions: fires, traffic accidents, drownings, and so on, in the future.

This chapter will discuss how cost-benefit analyses can be performed for fire safety measures. The next section will present the purpose and the method of cost-benefit analyses in a somewhat more detailed fashion. The section after that will give some examples of results from cost-benefit analyses for residential fires. After that, some complications associated with cost-benefit analyses will be discussed, especially regarding how to value lives in monetary values and how to generalize the results.

2 The Ten Major Steps in Performing an CBA

1. Explain the purpose of the CBA
2. Specify the set of alternative projects
3. Decide whose benefits and costs count (specify standing)
4. Identify the impact categories, catalogue them, and select metrics
5. Predict the impacts quantitatively over the life of the project.
6. Monetize all impacts
7. Discount benefits and costs to obtain present values
8. Compute the net present value of each alternative.
9. Perform sensitivity analysis
10. Make a recommendation

According to Boardman et al. [3]

The ten steps in performing a cost-benefit analysis, CBA, will be described in short using the two examples of smoke detectors and relocation of the fire station.

2.1 Explain the Purpose of the CBA

The main purpose of a CBA is to evaluate whether a public project leads to improved welfare in a society. The difference of economic cost-benefit analyses compared to other evaluations of fire safety is that the cost-benefit analyses compare costs to benefits. That is the same as comparing resources (measured in monetary units) to the welfare outcome for society (measured in monetary units). It is important that resources for prevention lead to fewer fires and greater knowledge about how to deal with fires when they occur. It is also important that fire and rescue services can efficiently suppress fires when they do happen. However, from an economic point of view, the interesting thing is the relation between the resources put into the system and the welfare that people get from it. The resources can be measured as monetary costs. The welfare, due to saved lives, fewer injuries, less property damaged, and an increased feeling of safety, can, according to economists, also be measured in monetary units.

The purpose of the CBA is to evaluate whether or not a public project leads to increased welfare.[1] Therefore, the interesting question is whether the government could "help" the market in some way, for example by more information, different taxation, subsidizing, or even nationalization.[2]

---

[1] A policy or market that leads to highest possible welfare is called (Pareto) efficient in economic theory. The purpose of a cost-benefit analysis can be said to evaluate so-called "market failures." A "market failure" exists, according to economic theory, when the free market itself does not lead to highest possible welfare in society.

[2] The very fact that the fire and rescue services are run by national, regional, or local governments is due to market failures (according to economists): once a fire and rescue service exists, it is hard

The problem with smoke detectors is that people do not buy and install them. The reason could be that it is too expensive, too complicated, or the problem may be that people are not aware of the positive effects regarding risk reduction when it comes to smoke detectors. Another effect people may not think about is the positive side effect (externalities) of having a smoke detector which also reduces the risk for neighbors. However, if the benefits to society outweigh the costs, there may be reason to either inform people more about installing smoke detectors, to give out detectors for free, or to make them mandatory using legislation. The economic problem of a new relocated fire station is whether the benefits of reduced response times leading to saved lives, fewer injuries, and less property damaged outweigh the costs of construction.

2.2 Specify the Set of Alternative Projects

Considering the smoke detector problem, alternative projects could be a smoke detector in a block of flats or a detached house. It could also be considered in a specific neighborhood or nationwide. Should legislation be used or just information? Considering the location problem of a fire station, there are many alternative geographical locations. The new alternative must be compared to something and usually the easiest and most interesting base alternative is the current state, that is, the present location of the fire station.

2.3 Decide Whose Benefits and Costs Count (Specify Standing)

Considering smoke detectors, those who have standing are those living in the area of interest, which could be a block of flats, a neighborhood, a city, a region, or a country. Considering the location problem of the fire station, those who have standing are those served by the local fire and rescue service. That means mainly the local residents (and who will have to pay it through their taxes have to pay for it), but not only them. It would be strange not to include visiting people in a CBA such as hotel guests and those in cars passing by.

---

to collect fees for it since many, not paying fees, can free-ride on the outcome of the service (this is called the public good problem).

2.4 Identify the Impact Categories, Catalogue them, and Select Metrics

Questions that must be answered before performing a CBA for smoke detectors are: Who will benefit from more smoke detectors? (That is, people who have already installed smoke detectors.) What is the risk of fires in their specific homes? How can these people and their risks be measured? How can the risk reduction, when it comes to injuries, fatalities, and property be measured, that is, what is the potential effect of a smoke detector for different risk groups? To perform a CBA, all these questions must be answered in numbers. This means that data either from official statistics or from a survey performed for the specific CBA must be available.

Questions that must be answered before doing a CBA for relocation of the fire station are: How much will the response times be changed for different rescue categories? How many rescues are there for each category? How can the risk reduction when it comes to injuries, fatalities, and property be measured, that is, what is the effect of a changed response time for different rescue categories? To perform a CBA, all these questions must be answered in numbers. Here, data from official statistics for the fire and rescue services are needed.

2.5 Predict the Impacts Quantitatively Over the Life of the Project

Both smoke detectors and the relocation of the fire station have impacts that extend over a long time. Changes in the future should be taken into account. If the population covered by the local fire and rescue service increases over time, the benefits of it will also increase over time. What is the lifespan of the smoke detector? Is it five or ten years? That affects the cost per year, since it is only the depreciation that should be included in a CBA. And what happens when the battery stops working after a year? Will the owner change the battery immediately or forget about it? The latter would mean that, over time, fewer and fewer smoke detectors will be working. Such predictions for the future are of course hard to make. Often these numbers must be established in specific studies, and therefore the task of the CBA researcher will be to collect data from previous research on the effectiveness of specific fire prevention measures. Examples of such effectiveness numbers are presented in Runefors et al. ([35, 36] [and Chapter 14 in this anthology]).

The important thing about effectiveness numbers is that they represent the difference between the changed condition with the action taken and the expected condition without the action taken, and not only the changed condition with the action taken (see Fig. 13.1). The expected condition without the action taken will depend on other factors and is especially relevant when there are multiple fire safety prevention measures taken at the same time or if risks will change over time, for example, due to a more elderly population or more immigrants who may be expected to lack fire safety knowledge.

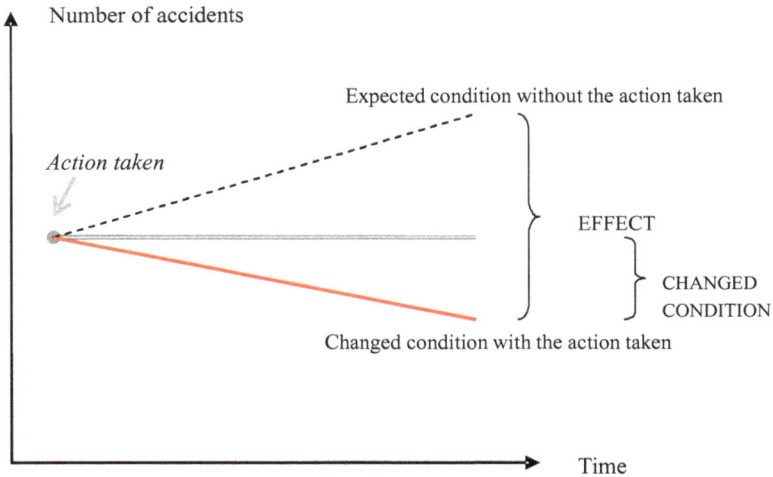

Fig. 13.1 Difference between effect and changed condition. (Reference: [10]).

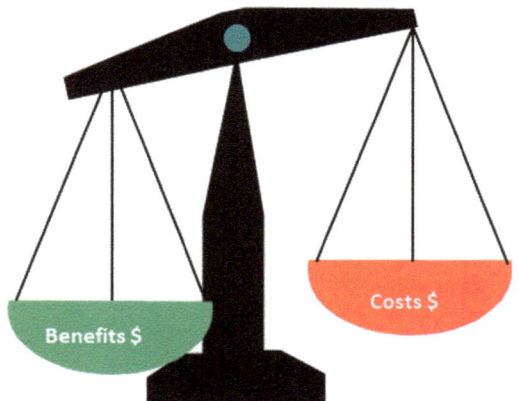

Fig. 13.2 The cost-benefit scale

2.6 Monetize All Impacts

Once all effects have been measured in physical units, they have to be monetized to be put on the same scale (Fig. 13.2). For things that have market prices, this is quite easy. The cost of smoke detectors can, for example, easily be found by comparing prices on the internet. A value for the installation time should also be added. If the smoke detectors are given out or offered using a local campaign, the labor and other costs of the campaign should also be included. Costs of labor include not only direct wages, but also payroll taxes, pension, and health fees.[3]

The main benefits of smoke detectors are reduced personal injuries, fatalities, and property. Values of property losses could be found from insurance companies. For monetary values of fatalities and personal injuries, the analyst must rely on estimates made by other researchers and most countries have set official so-called values of statistical lives, VSL, and statistical injuries. The VSL is a specific value for a life in dollars or euros. Most of these official values are used and developed for the traffic sector where CBAs have been used widely. One question therefore is whether the same values could be used for fire safety. The simple answer is yes (a life is a life), but it is not obvious since there are different base risks and people have been found to have different preferences for different risk contexts.[4]

For the relocation problem, the time factor must be monetized to be able to compare the benefits of reduced response time to the construction cost.[5]

By monetizing all impacts, explicit weights are put on each impact. If the value of a statistical life is six times the value of a severe injury, then the weight in the CBA on each saved life will be six times higher than for each saved injury.

2.7 & 2.8 Discount Benefits and Costs to Obtain Present Values, and Compute the Net Present Value of Each Alternative

A project taking place today normally results in benefits for many years in the future. Since we have positive interest rates in the world, people in general think that the future is worth less and less, and thus should be discounted. The present value of the installation of smoke detectors is the discounted value for all social benefits, B, and all social costs, C, during the life span of the project. If the life span is 10 years and the social discount rate to be used is s, then the net present value, NPV, could be calculated as

$$\text{NPV} = \sum_{t=0}^{10} \frac{B_t - C_t}{(1+s)^t}$$

---

[3] The monetary values are measured by studying how the input market and output market affect consumer surplus, producer surplus, effect on environment, effect for government, and other changes. For sizable government projects, this is not straightforward to calculate. Thus, just multiplying price with quantity often does not give the correct social opportunity cost (see an introductory textbook on CBA, e.g. [3]).

[4] Both Sanderson et al. [38] and Carlsson et al. [6] found that the value of statistical life for fires was about 2/3 of the used value for traffic accidents.

[5] Mattsson and Juås [27] describe how to value the time factor from an economic perspective for all responses by fire and rescue services, while Jaldell [21] concentrates on the relation between the time factor and saving lives.

The problem here is to choose the social discount rate, s. The social discount rate deviates from the market interest rate because we are dealing with government projects. The government may diversify risks easier than the private sector, thus the risk is lower and therefore the discount rate should be lower. Most countries have officially set social discount rates which makes choosing the rate more easily.

If the NPV is positive, the project is said to increase economic efficiency (relative to the base status quo alternative). Therefore, the decision rule is to choose projects with positive net social benefits. If there are more projects, or if we like to compare projects between different sectors, the ratio of benefits and costs could be compared.

$$\text{Benefit-to-cost ratio} = \sum_{t=0}^{10} \frac{B_t}{(1+s)^t} / \sum_{t=0}^{10} \frac{C_t}{(1+s)^t}$$

The benefit-to-cost ratio describes how much each extra invested monetary unit gives back in return.[6] The greater ratio, the better from an economic point of view.

2.9 Perform Sensitivity Analysis

Most numbers used in a CBA are uncertain in larger or smaller amounts. We cannot know the exact effect smoke detectors will have on reduced injuries, fatalities, and property losses, neither for a country as a whole nor, especially, for a specific studied neighborhood. Even if there are official numbers for values of statistical lives, statistical injuries, and the social discount rate, our results may be sensitive to the choice of these numbers.

A simple sensitivity analysis for smoke detectors could be to check how the results change if prices increase by, for example, 25%. Another could be to see what size of the percentage impact of the smoke detector on injuries, fatalities, and property losses leads to the net benefit being zero. Even if the effect is uncertain, this calculated percentage may be so low that it is reasonable to assume that the net benefit is mostly positive.

---

[6] Yet another way is to present the results as net benefit ratios. If the net benefit ratio is positive, the policy is economically efficient, if negative the policy is not economically efficient.

2.10 Make a Recommendation

If there is only one alternative policy, the recommendation will be to adopt the policy if the net benefit is positive, and not to adopt the policy if the net benefit is negative. If there are many policies, the recommendation is to adopt the policy with the highest positive net benefit or highest benefit-to-cost ratio.

However, the decision-maker takes the decision, not the CBA analyst. Not all effects can be measured and made quantitative, which means that there are things left out from the CBA that the decision-maker may regard as important.

3 Some CBA Results: Residential Fires

Some results from CBAs for fire safety measures for residential fires are presented here (Table 13.1). The results presented should be seen as examples, so this is not a literature review, a systematic review, or a meta-analysis.

In the table, the benefit-to-cost ratios are presented for different alternatives, together with the country and the year of the publication of the study. To indicate the effect on saving lives, effectiveness figures from Runefors et al. [35] are also shown.[7] However, remember that a CBA should include all benefits, not just saved lives. Areas where no CBA has been found have also been noted.

The table shows that there are not many CBA studies done on fire safety measures, which makes it hard to draw general conclusions about the economic efficiency. (See also Sect. 4.2 about how to think about generalizations from results). Smoke detectors seem to be economically efficient, but even such programmes might fail from an economic point of view. However, even if the benefit-to-cost ratio is below 1, there may be lessons learned from such a study regarding why the specific programme was not economically efficient. For other measures, the economic efficiency seems to depend on the circumstances of the specific programmes. Also, note that the studies on portable fire extinguishers show economic efficiency, even if it is doubtful that they save lives. The results are thus driven by prevented injuries and property damage.

---

[7] Numbers are from Runefors et al., i.e. not the numbers used in the actual CBA study. Only those with numbers greater than 10%, or with CBAs found, are listed.

Table 13.1 List of cost-benefit analyses for residential fire safety measures

Category	Safety measure	Subarea	Effect on saving lives [35]	B/C-ratio	Country	Year (published)	Reference
Building, etc.	Well-maintained electrical systems		14%				None found
	Chimney sweeping		4%				
		Wood – five times a year		0.3	Sweden	2004	a
		Wood – once a year		1.7	Sweden	2004	a
		Oil – three times a year		0.3	Sweden	2004	a
		Oil – once every second year		1.7	Sweden	2004	a
	Emergency exits		–				None found
Products	Flame-resistant clothes		11–24%				None found
	Flame-resistant furniture		15%				None found
	Ignition-proof cigarettes		40%				None found
	Quit smoking		–				None found
	Stove guards		5%	0.1–0.2	Sweden	2017	b
Fire alarms	Smoke detectors		37%				
	General	Average home		3.0–7.5	USA	1997	c
		Detached houses: network – batteries short life – long life		2.3–9.2-10.0	Sweden	2011	d

(continued)

Table 13.1 (continued)

Category	Safety measure	Subarea	Effect on saving lives [35]	B/C-- ratio	Country	Year (published)	Reference
		Apartment buildings: network – batteries short life – long life		3.1–12.5-13.3	Sweden	2011	d
	Give-away programmes	Give-away programme		29	Oklahoma, USA	2001	e
		Give-away programme		0.15	Inner London, UK	2005	f
		Give-away and installation programme		2.1–2.3	Hypothetic representative community, USA	2012	g
		Give-away programme		18–177	Baltimore, USA	2014	h
		Installation programme		3.2	Dallas, USA	2018	i
Fire extin-guishers	Portable fire extinguisher		~0%				
		Residential houses		2	Norway	1998	j
		Households		2.5	Australia	1999	k
		Detached houses		4.8	Sweden	2011	c
		Apartment houses		1.4	Sweden	2011	c
Sprinklers	Installed		68%				
		Detached houses		0.4	Sweden	2004	a
		Apartment buildings					
		Colonial-style, townhouse, ranch-style		2.5–2.6-6.0	USA	2009	l
		Care homes		1.2	Wales	2013	m

(continued)

Table 13.1 (continued)

Category	Safety measure	Subarea	Effect on saving lives [35]	B/C-- ratio	Country	Year (published)	Reference
		Nursing homes for elderly – existing and new buildings (saved lives)		0.7–1.7	Sweden	2012	n
		Nursing homes for elderly – existing and new buildings (saved life years)		0.3–1.1	Sweden	2012	n
	Portable		30% (all)				
		For elderly people (all >65 years and only smokers >65 years)		0.3–2.5	Sweden	2017	b
FRS organization and complementary missions							
	Help from private security companies		–	3.3	Sweden	2018	o
	Home visits		–	7–10	Sweden	2019	p

References
a. Mattsson [26] updated results from Juås and Mattsson [22]
b. Runefors and Frantzich [37]
c. Miller and Levy [28]
d. Jaldell [19]
e. Haddix et al. [15]
f. Ginnelly et al. [14]
g. Liu et al. [24]
h. Diamond-Smith et al. [9]
i. Yellman et al. [46]
j. Mostue [29]
k. Beever and Britton [2]
l. Butry [5]
m. Fraser-Mitchell and Williams [13]
n. Jaldell [20]
o. Sund and Jaldell [40]
p. Sund et al. [39]

4 Some Complications in Doing and Using CBAs

4.1 Valuing Non-market Units

The monetary valuations in CBAs should be done using market values, but some things do not have a market value.[8] Loss of life, health effects, and loss of ecological goods are examples of so-called intangible effects that do not have market values. How should these values be chosen and is it ethical to set monetary values on lives and injuries?

Monetary values on life are used to be calculated using production losses due to fatalities. If you were expected to work for 25 additional years, how much would you have produced during those years and what is the value of that lost production? A simple way to calculate this is your lost wages. Life is however much more than just work, so this estimate (called production loss or human capital approach) is a very conservative valuation. This value is also zero for people who have retired.

Today, there are two main methods used to establish the values of non-market goods and services. One is called revealed preferences and the other is called stated preferences. Stated preferences are about asking people directly, while revealed preferences are about finding values from observing people's behavior (indirect measure). An example of revealed preferences is how much people pay for smoke detectors. Given the risk reduction associated with smoke detectors, it is possible to calculate the monetary value for a given reduced risk of fatality.[9] Another example of revealed preferences valuation is to compare how much higher salaries have to be in more risky jobs to attract workers. Stated preference questions are about trying to let people value small risk changes (not their lives as a whole). If you think your willingness to pay for reducing your risk by 1/100000 is €90, then we can estimate your valuation of a statistical life, VSL, to be 100,000*90 = 9,000,000.[10] Finding the values of injuries could be done in the same way, but it could also be found by weighting the VSL with medical weights for different injuries.

Estimates of VSL vary. Recent meta-analyses point toward an average of about $10,000,000 in the US [45]. The official values from US agencies are similar [23]. The official values of other countries lie lower. For example, the OECD recommendation is $3.6 million ($2012), the UK £1 million (£1997), and Sweden SEK 40.5 million (SEK2020).[11] Viscusi and Masterman argue for the values in other countries

---

[8] To be used in a cost-benefit analysis, the market value should reflect the social marginal cost. There may be discrepancies between the market price and the social marginal cost due to non-competitive markets, external effects, or asymmetric information between buyers and sellers. However, this problem will not be discussed further here.

[9] Dardis [8] used the revealed preferences methods and purchases of smoke detectors for estimating the willingness to pay for risk reductions.

[10] This value is called the value of a statistical life, VSL, in the economic literature, but in other literature, it is called the value of a prevented fatality, VPF.

[11] OECD [30]; UK: HM Department of Transport [16]; Sweden: Trafikverket [44].

to be calculated using the ratio of the gross domestic product (GDP) of each country compared to the GDP of the United States, which would lead to higher estimates for VSL in other countries.

The word "statistical" in VSL emphasizes that this is a statistical concept and not a number trying to value real persons. We do not, in a planning situation, know who will be saved from fires. It can be you, me, or someone else. So setting values on lives does not mean that we value specific individuals. That would be impossible. We instead value the statistical risk of fatalities. Another objection to setting a monetary value on life is that some say that the value of life is unlimited or infinite. However, that is not the way people in general behave. We take risks by driving cars, crossing streets with heavy traffic, travelling, or using candlelight, which means that people in general do not behave as if the value of life is infinite.

One advantage of setting an explicit monetary value on life is that the number can be criticized and discussed. Another thing to remember is that there is always an implicit value set in public safety projects. Say that the local government thinks it is too expensive to spend €5,000,000 on sprinkler systems in nursing homes, which they believe would save two persons from dying. This means that the local government has, implicitly, assumed that the monetary value of life is lower than €2,500,000.

Some argue that monetary value of life years, VSLY, should be used instead of VSL. A related question is whether different values should be used for different ages, for example children versus elderly, since using VSLY instead of VSL implies that children are weighted higher than the old people. Using different values hinges on the fact that the safety measure in question can be limited to one group or another.

For example, when evaluating sprinklers in nursing homes in Sweden, the benefit-to-cost ratio for installation in new buildings was reduced from 1.7 to 1.1 using VSLYs instead of VSLs [19]. People's valuation of a risk reduction can also depend on other factors such as the baseline risk, income, controllability, and psychological factors such as fear or dreadfulness.

The difficulties in monetarizing values of lives and other problems in defining, measuring, and monetarizing relevant aspects of welfare (see e.g [41]) have led some researchers to leave the standardized methods of CBA (e.g [17]). The problem with doing that is that the results become hard to understand and are incomparable to other CBA studies.

4.2 Generalizations and Benefit-Transfers

Could the result from one CBA study be generalized outside the object of the study? I would say that it depends on several things. The study is done taking specific baseline risks into account, assuming specific effects and using specific values. This means that it seems reasonable to generalize to similar risk-specific areas, where the effect of the fire safety device would be similar and where people's valuation of safety is similar. To be able to generalize to other areas, it might be a good idea to present the results in units such as per flat or per detached house.

If the study is done on a general country level, it could be used within this country. On the other hand, if the study is done on a specific area, it is not certain that the results could be generalized if this specific area diverges when it comes to risk and risk behavior from the area where you want to use the results. Considering monetary values, benefits are valued the same and things cost about the same within a country, but the prices could be different when crossing borders. The monetary value of a statistical life differs, sometimes considerably, between countries.

A similar problem arises if you would like to perform your own CBA study of fire safety. Normally, you cannot find all the required values on your own, so you need to use already estimated values. Using already estimated values for impacts is called benefit-transfer. Could, for example, values based on US research be used in European studies? Boardman et al. [3] point out four specific sets of factors to take into account: (1) differences in income and other socioeconomic factors, (2) differences in physical surroundings (e.g. different risk contexts), (3) differences in the projects themselves, and (4) the fact that things change over time. Results from a CBA study on smoke detectors in general in a country are perhaps not relevant to use for a specific risk group (e.g. elderly people or smokers), neither in that country nor in other countries. A study done for detached houses is perhaps not relevant for a block of flats. A study on giving smoke detectors away for free is not relevant for an information campaign. If people buy the smoke detectors themselves, the incentive may be higher for also installing them (correctly) and buying new batteries (and changing them) after a year or two. The effect of smoke detectors 10–20 years ago may be different from today, due both to better technology and to changed awareness of how to behave when the alarm sounds.

To be specific, could the benefit-to-cost ratio for smoke detectors in Sweden of 10.0 be generalized to all detached houses in Sweden, in Scandinavia, in Europe, in the western world, in the world? For Sweden I would say yes, because the purpose of the study was to receive a general ratio for Sweden. Of course, there may be very large or small houses, or houses in very risky or non-risky regions, or houses using different heating systems that may lead to different conclusions. However, the ratio 10 is well above the limit of 1 and therefore the result that smoke detectors are economically efficient will generally hold. The prices and costs are about the same all over Sweden and the same value of statistical life is used within a country. Comparing the Scandinavian countries, I would say that the risk levels and the sizes of the detached houses are quite similar. The problem may be that prices and costs are quite different between the countries. Another problem is that the value of statistical life also varies between the countries, and as discussed above, there seems to be a correlation between the VSL and the income level, but again, since the ratio is 10 to 1 I would say that the result of the study indicates that smoke detectors are economically efficient all over Scandinavia. However, I would hesitate to generalize further to other countries, since houses, risk levels and behaviors, prices, costs, and the value (and thus preferences) of statistical lives may differ too much. An additional problem is whether the results from a 10-year-old study can still be used. Both effects and costs change over time.

4.3 CBAs Are Non-budget Calculations

The numbers and values used in a cost-benefit analysis are calculated for the society as a whole including the welfare of everyone in that society. They are not for a specific agency or a local or national government. A CBA that results in benefits outweighing costs does not mean that managing such a public project will lead to more revenues or a better economic result for the agencies involved. This is true even if there are positive net benefits that are directly connected to a specific agency. The budget effects for the agency could even be the other way around. If smoke detectors are shown to have positive net benefits in a CBA, this may allow the fire and rescue service to save resources and money since there will be fewer and less damaging fires to suppress. However, the major benefits are for people involved and for the health sector having to take care of fewer injuries. It may even be the case that the decision-makers think it is a good idea that the fire and rescue service put more (expensive) emphasis on fire prevention by informing about smoke detectors and perhaps even installing them for free. A relocation of the fire station is most surely more expensive and thus leads to negative budget effects for many years. The positive effect of saving more people will not directly affect the local government's budget. It will instead directly affect the people living in the community, the insurance companies, the health sector, and so on, which all make up a local society.

4.4 CBAs Evaluate Marginal Increases in Fire Safety, Not Perfect Fire Safety

Economic theory mostly deals with marginal – that is, small – changes and tries to evaluate whether or not marginal benefits outweigh marginal costs. Installing one additional smoke detector is an example of a small additional change. In Fig 13.3, we have a theoretical marginal cost curve of reducing fire fatalities to zero starting from today's numbers (that is going from right to left). The marginal benefit curve is horizontal implying that each saved life has the same value. According to economic theory, we should continue saving lives from fires as long as marginal benefits are greater than marginal costs, that is to the point where they are equal. Moving further to the left from this point is not economically efficient. In other words, then we could do better things with our resources. For example, we could

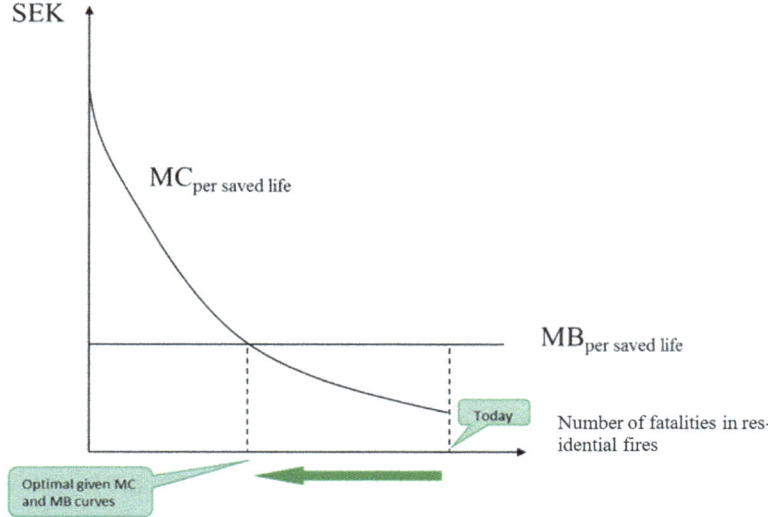

Fig. 13.3 Marginal cost, MC, and marginal benefit, MB, of safety measures

use them to save lives in cheaper ways from other safety projects.[12] When doing a CBA, only marginal changes along short stretches of the curves are evaluated, not all points on the curves.

It is reasonable to assume that the marginal cost curve gets steeper and steeper the further we move to the left. The additional cost for saving each life becomes greater and greater. Some argue that eventually, if you invest too much in fire safety the effect will even be negative, since money invested in fire safety leads to less money left for people, which may in turn lead to people investing even less in fire safety [1, 4].

"Vision Zero" is the long-term goal that no one should die or become seriously injured in fires discussed by Andersson (Chapter 15 this anthology). How does the cost-benefit analysis compare to "Vision Zero"? The simple answer is that the economic policy of only performing public projects where the benefits outweigh the costs is a completely different view compared to "Vision Zero." In "Vision Zero" no costs are mentioned and only personal benefits are interesting. In contrast, in a CBA, all benefits, not only reduced fatalities and injuries, should be included. The monetary valuation puts weights on the different benefits and makes it possible to compare the benefit-to-cost ratios across all sectors, not only fires and not only safety (see e.g [11]).

---

[12] Another problem with not using marginal valuation is that there may be economies of scale, which means that average costs are decreasing. This has for example been considered by Parmer et al. [31] when it comes to giving out smoke detectors.

4.5 Difference from Other Economic Evaluation Methods

There are other economic evaluation methods. The one closest to the cost-benefit analysis is the cost-effectiveness analysis, CEA.[13] In a CEA only one benefit is considered at a time. For residential fires, this is normally saved lives or saved life years. The costs are calculated in the same way as in a CBA. The implication is that different fire safety devices could be compared in terms of their cost efficiency. The cheaper a life year could be saved, the better the fire safety measure. The advantage of CEA is that monetary values of lives or life years do not have to be set and used. The drawback is that the result of the study does not imply economic efficiency. Since only one benefit is used, most often saved lives, and other benefits are disregarded (reduced injuries and property losses), the result of a CEA does not show whether benefits outweigh costs, and thus we cannot from the result establish whether the welfare of society increases or decreases by implementing the fire safety measure in question.[14] Examples of surveys including these values are given by Tengs et al. ([42]; fourteen fire-related studies out of 587) and Ramsberg and Sjöberg ([33]; seven fire-related studies out of 165).[15]

4.6 For the Sceptical Reader

When two things are compared, one sometimes hears the expression "But you cannot compare apples and oranges!" The saying means that two things are so different that they cannot be compared. Cost-benefit analysis is a method taking this problem into account. Since all benefits and all costs are measured in the same units, money, everything can be compared.[16]

However, CBA is no panacea for decisions to increase fire safety. The results do not show the absolute truth, but rather possible directions. However, when performing a CBA, a structural listing of all resources used in the project and the consequences from it must be completed. Moreover, using results from CBAs also makes

---

[13] Cost-of-illness, COI, is another method trying to estimate the size of a problem using monetary values. However, a COI does not give information about what to do about the problem, just about the total cost of the problem. This means that numbers from COI cannot be used in economic evaluations since economic evaluations rely on marginal changes. It is seldom relevant to totally eliminate a problem. Currie et al. [7] and Rice [34] debate the pros and cons of COI.

[14] A variant of the CEA is the cost-utility analysis, CUA, that measures the benefits using quality adjusted life years, QALYs. QALY weigh life years with health quality. The health quality index goes from 0 to 1, where 0 is death and 1 is a perfect healthy functional life.

[15] I have chosen to include only the CEAs in Table 13.1 that have weighted saved lives with the value of statistical life. Again, also notice that portable fire extinguishers were found to be economically efficient even if the effect on saving lives is about zero.

[16] Miller and Levy [28] evaluate smoke detectors from an economic efficiency perspective, but it is also a good short and pedagogical example of how to perform an economic analysis.

it natural not to forget about costs. If you are sceptical of the CBA study in question, try to ask the following questions about the analysis (from Ref. [43]):

(i) Is the project clearly specified?
(ii) Does the design of the project used in the calculations correspond to the project that is actually planned?
(iii) Are the assumptions based on realistic forecasts and do they seem reasonable?
(iv) Have all important conditions and risks been taken into account?
(v) Have the effects been evaluated according to an accepted method?
(vi) Have all effects been treated – even those that could not be valued?
(vii) Have sensitivity analyses been performed?
(viii) What other decision basis does the decision-maker have access to?

5 Conclusions

Finding effective measures to increase fire safety is a necessity, but not a sufficient condition. The measure in question must also be economically efficient, which means that the benefits must outweigh the costs. Cost-benefit analysis is a method which makes it possible to evaluate if that is true or not. Not taking costs into account when evaluating different fire safety measures may lead to not making rational decisions on which measures to use.

The CBA analyst should follow the standardized way as for example formulated in textbooks in general (e.g [3]) and by Farrow and Viscusi [12], for safety projects. If the analyst openly shows the values used and calculations done, the results will be easy to comprehend and possible to criticize and correct if needed.

Considering two surveys of CBAs for accident-related measures, there were only very few fire safety-related studies included, four [32] and three [25], respectively. The results from CBAs presented in this chapter also do not make up a particularly long list. So there is room for more CBA studies evaluating fire safety measures to be undertaken.

References

1. Ashe B, de Oliveira FD, McAneney J (2012) Investments in fire management: does saving lives cost lives? Agenda J Policy Anal Reform 19(2):89–103
2. Beever P, Britton M (1998) Research into cost effective fire safety measures for residential buildings. Victoria University of Technology, Melbourne
3. Boardman AE, Greenberg DH, Vining AR, Weimar DL (2018) Cost-benefit analysis: concepts and practice. Cambridge University Press
4. Broughel J, Viscusi WK (2021) The mortality cost of expenditures. Contemp Econ Policy 39(1):156–167
5. Butry DT (2009) Economic performance of residential fire sprinkler systems. Fire Technol 45(1):117–143

6. Carlsson F, Daruvala D, Jaldell H (2010) Value of statistical life and cause of accident: a choice experiment. Risk Anal 30(6):975–986
7. Currie G, Kerfoot KD, Donaldson C et al (2000) Are cost of injury studies useful? Inj Prev 6:175–176
8. Dardis R (1980) The value of a life: new evidence from the marketplace. Am Econ Rev 70(5):1077–1082
9. Diamond-Smith N, Bishai D, Perry E, Shields W, Gielen A (2014) Economic evaluation of smoke alarm distribution methods in Baltimore, Maryland. Inj Prev 20(4):251–257
10. Ekonomistyrningsverket (2006) Effektutvärdering Att välja upplägg. Rapportnummer 2006:8
11. Elvik R (1999) Can injury prevention efforts go too far? Reflections on some possible implications of Vision Zero for road accident fatalities. Accid Anal Prev 31:265–286
12. Farrow S, Viscusi WK (2011) Towards principles and standards for the benefit-cost analysis of safety. J Benefit-Cost Anal 2(3):5
13. Fraser-Mitchell J, Williams C (2013) Cost-benefit analysis of residential sprinklers for Wales. BRE Fire and Security Client report number 276803v3
14. Ginnelly L, Sculpher M, Bojke C, Roberts I, Wade A, Diguiseppi C (2005) Determining the cost effectiveness of a smoke alarm give-away program using data from a randomized controlled trial. Eur J Public Health 15(5):448–453
15. Haddix AC, Mallonee S, Waxweiler R, Douglas MR (2001) Cost effectiveness analysis of a smoke alarm giveaway program in Oklahoma City, Oklahoma. Inj Prev 7(4):276–281
16. HM Department of Transport (2020) TAG UNIT A4.1 Social Impact Appraisal
17. Hopkin D, Spearpoint M, Arnott M, van Coile R (2019) Cost-benefit analysis of residential sprinklers–application of a judgement value method. Fire Saf J 106:61–71
18. Jaldell H (2002) Essays on the performance of fire and rescue services. PhD dissertation, memorandum 116, Göteborg University
19. Jaldell H (2011) Kostnadsnyttoanalyser och evidens av brandskydd i hemmet. Myndigheten för samhällsskydd och beredskap, MSB:309–311
20. Jaldell H (2013) Cost-benefit analysis of sprinklers in nursing homes for elderly. J Benefit-Cost Anal 4(2):209–235
21. Jaldell H (2017) How important is the time factor? Saving lives using fire and rescue services. Fire Technol 53(2):695–708
22. Juås B, Mattsson B (1994) Economics of fire technology. Fire Technol 30(4):468–477
23. Kniesner TJ, Viscusi WK (2019) The value of a statistical life. Vanderbilt University Law School,Legal Studies Research Paper Series, Working Paper Number 19–15
24. Liu Y, Mack KA, Diekman ST (2012) Smoke alarm giveaway and installation programs: an economic evaluation. Am J Prev Med 43(4):385–391
25. Mahalingam M, Peterson C, Bergen G (2020) Systematic review of unintentional injury prevention economic evaluations 2010–2019 and comparison to 1998–2009. Accid Anal Prev 146:105688
26. Mattsson B (2004) Vad är lagom säkerhet nu? P21–448/04. Räddningsverket
27. Mattsson B, Juås B (1997) The importance of the time factor in fire and rescue service operations in Sweden. Accid Anal Prev 29(6):849–857
28. Miller TR, Levy DT (1997) Cost outcome analysis in injury prevention and control: a primer on methods. Inj Prev 3(4):288
29. Mostue BA (2000) Evaluering av tiltak mot brann, Har røykvarsler, håndslokningsapparater og sprinkleranlegg hatt effekt på brannsikkerheten i Norge?, SINTEF Rapport, SF22A00853
30. OECD (2012) Mortality risk valuation in environment. Health and Transport Policies, Paris
31. Parmer JE, Corso PS, Ballesteros MF (2006) A cost analysis of a smoke alarm installation and fire safety education program. J Saf Res 37(4):367–373
32. Polinder S, Segui-Gomez M, Toet H, Belt E, Sethi D, Racioppi F, van Beeck EF (2012) Systematic review and quality assessment of economic evaluation studies of injury prevention. Accid Anal Prev 45:211–221

33. Ramsberg JA, Sjöberg L (1997) The cost-effectiveness of lifesaving interventions in Sweden. Risk Anal 17(4):467–478
34. Rice DP (2000) Cost of illness studies: what is good about them? Inj Prev 6:177–179
35. Runefors M, Johansson N, van Hees P (2016) How could the fire fatalities have been prevented? An analysis of 144 cases during 2011-2014 in Sweden. J Fire Sci 34(6):515–527
36. Runefors M, Johansson N, van Hees P (2017) The effectiveness of specific fire prevention measures for different population groups. Fire Saf J 91:1044–1050
37. Runefors M, Frantzich H (2017) Nyttoanalys av spisvakt och portabelt sprinklersystem vid bostadsbränder. LUTVDG/TVBB; Nr. 3210. Lund University, Department of Fire Safety Engineering
38. Sanderson K, Goodchild M, Nana G, Slack A (2007) The value of statistical life for fire regulatory impact statements. New Zealand fire service commission research report 79. Business and Economic Research Limited, Wellington
39. Sund B, Jaldell H, Jakobsson N, Bonander C (2019) Do home fire and safety checks by on-duty firefighters decrease the number of fires? Quasi-experimental evidence from southern Sweden. J Saf Res 70:39–47
40. Sund B, Jaldell H (2018) Security officers responding to residential fire alarms: modelling the effect on survival and property damages. Fire Saf J 97:1–11
41. Sunstein CR (2018) The cost-benefit revolution. MIT Press
42. Tengs TO, Adams ME, Pliskin JS, Safran DG, Siegel JE, Weinstein MC, Graham JD (1995) Five-hundred life-saving interventions and their cost-effectiveness. Risk Anal 15(3):369–390
43. Trafikverket (2012) Introduktion till samhällsekonomisk analys. 2012:220
44. Trafikverket (2020) Analysmetod och samhällsekonomiska kalkylvärden för transportsektorn. ASEK 7.0
45. Viscusi WK, Masterman CJ (2017) Income elasticities and global values of a statistical life. J Benefit-Cost Anal 8(2):226–250
46. Yellman MA, Peterson C, McCoy MA, Stephens-Stidham S, Caton E, Barnard JJ et al (2018) Preventing deaths and injuries from house fires: a cost–benefit analysis of a community-based smoke alarm installation programme. Inj Prev 24(1):12–18

Dr. Henrik Jaldell is an associate professor (docent) and senior lecturer in economics at Karlstad University. He has a bachelor's degree in economics from Karlstad University and a Ph.D. in economics from the University of Gothenburg. He mainly teaches courses in microeconomics and public economics. His Ph.D. thesis was called "Essays on the Performance of Fire and Rescue Services". Research is about risks, accidents, injuries, and cost-benefit analyses. He has regularly since 1994 worked on projects in collaboration with the Swedish Civil Contingencies Agency (MSB).

Chapter 14
Sociodemographic Patterns in the Effectiveness and Prevalence of Preventive Measures

Marcus Runefors

Abstract The sociodemographic gradients in the exposure to fatal fires are well known in the literature. However, less is known about the gradients for preventive measures, including their respective prevalence and effectiveness. This chapter partly fills this gap with an analysis based on data from both 1856 fire fatalities in Sweden between 1999 and 2018 and a national survey performed in Sweden in 2018. This implies that the results are specific for Sweden, but there is reason to believe that the situation is similar in most other western countries.

The results indicate, for example, that the effectiveness of smoke alarms decreases with age, especially for smokers, and therefore, additional measures are needed for these groups. Examples of effective additional measures are detector-activated sprinkler systems, fire-resistant clothing and safe cigarettes (e.g. e-cigarettes).

Concerning the prevalence of preventive measures, the result shows that non-Europeans living in Sweden have a much lower level of fire protection. Also, for example, low income, being divorced and living in a rented apartment are all linked to a lower protection level. Younger individuals tend to own smoke alarms to the same extent as older individuals, but they tend not to test them, which give room for improvement. Younger people, however, own extinguishers and fire blankets to a larger extent than older people, but homeownership was the strongest determinant for ownership of extinguishers.

Keywords Sociodemographic · Smoke alarm · Effectiveness · Cost-Benefit Analysis · Risk groups · Residential sprinklers

---

M. Runefors (✉)
Division of Fire Safety Engineering, Lund University, Lund, Sweden
e-mail: marcus.runefors@brand.lth.se

1 Introduction

In Sect. 1 of this anthology, the strong sociodemographic gradients in the exposure to the risk of fatal fires were presented and this serves as a fundamental basis for the design and implementation of a fire safety strategy. However, to link the exposure to a strategy, information about the tools available and their respective effectiveness is needed. This information can be used both to determine how the risk-level of specific individuals and groups can be reduced and to assess who would benefit most from a specific measure. Those concepts are fundamentally different since a slight reduction in the risk of high-risk groups can decrease the societal risk more than a large reduction for low-risk groups. As such, this information can be used both for targeted interventions (see Chap. 17) and cost-benefit analysis (see Chap. 13) for the entire population as well as for different population groups.

Another important aspect to acknowledge when interventions are not targeting specific individuals, but rather broad population groups in, for example, the form of campaigns or legislation are the patterns where specific preventive measures are already implemented. For example, a smoke alarm campaign targeting high-income families owning their home is likely to have limited impact since the coverage, as is presented later in this chapter, in this group is almost 100%, at least in Sweden. A smoke alarm campaign targeting low-income divorced non-European immigrants in rental homes in Sweden has a much larger potential since fewer in this group have a smoke alarm. This is further reinforced by that most of those factors are also linked to higher exposure to the risk of fatal fires.

This chapter aims to answer three questions:

1. What measures are effective for different population groups?
2. Where will the installation of a specific measure provide the largest benefit?
3. Who currently owns different fire preventive measures?

All results are based on Swedish data, but there is reason to believe that the results would be similar also for most other western countries (see Sect. 4).

2 Effectiveness of Different Measures

In a previous study [1], a dataset with 1856 fire fatalities in Sweden in the period from 1999 to 2018 has been analysed to derive factors (e.g. cause of the fire, type of building, alcohol, etc.) that influence the effectiveness of different preventive measures. The data in the analysis is a combination of data from the fatal fires database maintained by the Swedish Civil Contingencies Agency and the database "*Rättsbase*" maintained by the National Board of Forensic medicine. The former is based on reports from the fire service and police, while the latter is based on autopsy data. For details about the data, see the cited paper. The methodology to derive if a specific measure would have been effective in preventing a specific fatal fire was developed and validated in a previous paper [2].

In this chapter, the same data is presented, but instead of presenting factors that influence the effectiveness, the absolute effectiveness for different groups is presented. It should be acknowledged that the effectiveness can be expected to vary within each group, but it is still judged to be useful to have group average values rather than population average, which is the alternative when designing prevention strategies.

First, the effectiveness for different age groups is presented in Table 14.1. The division into age groups is based primarily on the widely adopted MeSH age groups [3], but age groups from newborn to adolescent (i.e. from 0–19 years) are merged due to few fatalities among children in Sweden [4] and therefore a lack of data. The MeSH division has been found to be a good proxy for changes in health and disease over the life span [5] and can therefore be expected to also be a reasonable division for the effectiveness of different measures.

The effectiveness is defined as the fraction of current fatalities that could have been prevented if everyone would have had that specific measure installed and functional. The fractions in Table 14.1 are the fraction of cases where it would have been effective among the cases where the effectiveness is known. This assumes that cases where it has not been possible to analyse the effectiveness of a measure (for example, due to missing data) are similar to cases where it has been possible. This is not necessarily true since cases with missing data have been found to differ on a number of variables compared to cases without missing data [6], but correcting for this has not been possible in the current study.

Table 14.1 Effectiveness of preventive measures for different age groups and relative risk (RR)

	Age					
	All	0–19 years	20–44 years	45–64 years	65–79 years	80+ years
	n = 1856	n = 70	n = 240	n = 573	n = 534	n = 439
RR	1 (ref)	0.16	0.40	1.19	2.31	4.44
Measure						
Safe electrical system	10%	31%	9%	8%	8%	12%
Safe cigarettes	42%	0%	19%	49%	55%	39%
Fire-resistant bedding	17%	3%	10%	21%	21%	16%
Fire-resistant sofas	11%	7%	11%	15%	14%	5%
Fire-resistant clothes	10%	7%	2%	3%	11%	24%
Stove guards	7%	5%	11%	8%	7%	4%
Sprinklers	82%	95%	89%	79%	77%	86%
Detector sprinklers	59%	59%	56%	58%	59%	63%
Smoke alarm	42%	42%	44%	52%	42%	31%

Interestingly, while a previous study found that the effectiveness of a sprinkler system continuously decreases with age [2], this study indicates a slight increase for the oldest age group. The difference between the publications is probably due to a small data set in the previous study, resulting in few cases in the oldest group (85+ years in that study). This slight increase in the effectiveness for the oldest group in this study is coherent with the decrease in effectiveness for safe cigarettes[1] for this group since smoking-related fires tend to ignite objects in the direct proximity to the victim for which the sprinkler system has been found to be non-effective [7].

The relative decrease in the number of smoking-related fires for this group might be due to an increase in exposure to other types of fires due to functional limitations (see Chap. 5). This is coherent with the increase in the effectiveness of a safe electrical system which also previously has been found to be a major risk factor for this group [2], but where the victim is further away from the fire, and therefore the sprinkler system generally has the potential to prevent the fatality.

It has previously been shown [2] that the effectiveness of different measures is very different between smokers and non-smokers. Therefore, the effectiveness for smokers and non-smokers for the three oldest age groups (where the number of smoking-related fires is substantial) is presented in the table below, both separate for each age group and for the three age groups combined. The Relative Risk (RR), which is the risk for one group compared to the population average, is also presented.

In line with the previous discussion, sprinkler systems are very effective for non-smokers, but have lower effectiveness for smokers. It can also be found that fire-resistant clothes are very effective for smokers in the oldest group, while fire-resistant sofas (and to some extent bedding) are more effective for younger smokers. Stove guards are less effective for the oldest group, even among non-smokers, compared to the second oldest group.

For smokers, safe cigarettes are very effective, indicating that fires related to smoking dominate other potential sources of fire. It can also be found that the presence of smoking is a stronger determinant of risk level than is age, but it is when those factors combine, the risk level can become very large (up to 22.1 times the general public for smokers who are 80 years or older).

This chapter has provided information in relation to a limited set of variables (i.e. age and smoking) which are judged sufficient for most practical situations. For more information about the influence of other sociodemographic factors (e.g. living conditions, type and size of municipality and alcohol consumption), the reader is referred to [1].

---

[1] Note that safe cigarette is not the same as RIP-cigarette which has been found to be not effective (see Chap. 10), but rather, for example, e-cigarette, changing to safer smoking habits or even stop smoking entirely.

Table 14.2 Effectiveness of preventive measures for smokers and non-smokers and relative risk (RR)

Age	All (45+ years)		45–64 years		65–79 years		80+ years	
Smoker	Yes	No	Yes	No	Yes	No	Yes	No
RR	4.03	0.69	2.73	0.83	7.95	1.43	22.1	3.3
Measure								
Safe electrical system	2%	16%	3%	13%	2%	15%	2%	19%
Safe cigarettes	87%	0%	84%	0%	88%	0%	92%	0%
Fire-resistant bedding	32%	7%	36%	5%	33%	6%	25%	10%
Fire-resistant sofas	19%	5%	24%	5%	20%	6%	9%	3%
Fire-resistant clothes	17%	6%	5%	0%	17%	4%	39%	14%
Stove guards	2%	10%	3%	12%	2%	12%	1%	6%
Sprinklers	65%	94%	67%	91%	62%	94%	65%	97%
Detector sprinklers	76%	46%	78%	40%	75%	42%	74%	57%
Smoke alarm	46%	40%	63%	43%	43%	40%	21%	37%

3 Benefit from the Installation of Different Measures

While Tables 14.1 and 14.2 provide information about which measure has the highest potential to reduce the risk of a fire fatality for a specific group, this is not necessarily the same as where a specific preventive measure would provide the greatest absolute risk reduction in society. This is because it might result in more lives saved to reduce the risk of a high-risk group by a small percentage, compared to reduce the risk of a low-risk group with a higher percentage. Therefore, a complementary measure is needed, which also account for the risk level, and that has been labelled the *"Benefit Proxy"* [2]. The benefit proxy is a measure of the number of lives saved every year per million people protected by the specific measure under the assumption that it is perfectly reliable. For a cost-benefit analysis (see Chap. 13), the actual level of reliability should be taken into account, but when comparing the benefit between groups, this factor is cancelled. In mathematical terms, the benefit proxy is the effectiveness of the measure, presented in the tables above, multiplied by the individual risk. The measure can be used in a cost-benefit analysis using the equation below.

$$BC_{A,B} = \frac{BP_{A,B} \cdot R_B \cdot V}{C_B} \sum_{t=0}^{T} \frac{1}{(1+i)^t}$$

In the equation, $BC_{A,B}$ is the benefit-cost quota which should be above one for the measure to be cost-effective. The variable $BP_{A,B}$ is the benefit proxy for group A and measure B, presented in the tables below. R_B is the reliability of measure B, and V is the value of statistical life (see for example [8]). C_B is the cost of installation per individual protected, i is the interest rate, and T is the expected lifetime of the installed measure.

Table 14.3 Benefit for installation of preventive measures for different age groups. The unit of the benefit is lives per year saved per 1 M protected by the measure

	Age					
	All	0–19 years	20–44 years	45–64 years	65–79 years	80+ years
	n = 1856	n = 70	n = 240	n = 573	n = 534	n = 439
RR	1 (ref)	0.16	0.40	1.19	2.31	4.44
Measure						
Safe electrical system	1.1	0.5	0.4	1.0	2.0	6.1
Safe cigarettes	4.7	0.0	0.8	6.5	14.2	19.2
Fire-resistant bedding	1.9	0.1	0.4	2.7	5.4	7.7
Fire-resistant sofas	1.2	0.1	0.5	2.0	3.6	2.6
Fire-resistant clothes	1.1	0.1	0.1	0.4	2.9	11.8
Stove guards	0.8	0.1	0.5	1.0	1.7	1.8
Sprinklers	9.1	1.7	3.9	10.5	19.8	42.4
Detector sprinklers	6.6	1.1	2.4	7.7	15.3	31.2
Smoke alarm	4.7	0.7	1.9	7.0	10.8	15.2

Table 14.4 Benefit for installation of preventive measures for smokers and non-smokers. The unit of the benefit is lives per year saved per 1 M protected by the measure

Age	All (45+ years)		45–64 years		65–79 years		80+ years	
Smoker	Yes	No	Yes	No	Yes	No	Yes	No
RR	4.03	0.69	2.73	0.83	7.95	1.43	22.1	3.3
Measure								
Safe cigarettes	47.9	0.0	25.6	0.0	77.9	0.0	227.3	0.0
Fire-resistant bedding	17.8	1.0	11.1	0.4	28.9	0.9	61.2	3.6
Fire-resistant sofas	10.5	0.7	7.4	0.5	17.5	1.0	22.3	1.0
Fire-resistant clothes	9.1	0.9	1.5	0.0	14.7	0.6	95.8	5.2
Sprinklers	35.4	14.1	20.5	8.5	54.8	15.0	160.2	35.8
Detector sprinklers	41.6	6.9	23.7	3.7	66.6	6.7	183.0	20.9
Smoke alarm	25.3	6.0	19.2	4.0	38.4	6.3	50.7	13.7

The result per age groups is presented in the table below (Table 14.3).

It can be seen that most measures have a steadily growing benefit with increasing age. The only two exceptions are stove guards and fire-resistant sofas, which have a decreasing benefit between the second oldest groups and the oldest group. Interestingly, even if the effectiveness of smoke alarms decreases for the oldest group compared to the second oldest, the benefit per installation increases, which illustrates the need for those complementary measures.

As for the effectiveness, the benefit proxy is divided for smokers and non-smokers below. Only measures that are, to some extent, are related to smoking are presented. For other measures (electrical system and stove guards), the benefit per installation can be expected to be the same for both smokers and non-smokers since they are equally exposed to that risk (Table 14.4).

For smoking individuals, some very large benefits per installation can be found, which illustrates the importance of targeted interventions towards this group (see Chap. 17). Cigarettes, sprinklers and detector-activated sprinklers give the highest benefit, but the benefit of safe clothes is also very high – especially accounting for the much smaller investment.

4 Sociodemographic Patterns in Current Level of Residential Fire Protection

As previously described, the sociodemographic patterns of fatal fires are well known in the literature. The most widely cited is probably age, where high age is related to increased risk exposure, but also low income, rented apartments and low education have been found to be correlated with an increased risk of fire fatality [9]. However, to design interventions, it is also relevant to identify factors linked to a lower level of fire protection since this indicates where there is room for improvement.

There are some studies on the sociodemographic patterns of smoke alarm prevalence, which show that, for example, the factors below are linked to increased ownership.

- High income [10–12].
- Homeownership [10, 11].
- Single-family homes [12].
- Employment [12].
- Central heating [10].
- Speaking the national language [11].
- Having children at home [11, 12].

No studies investigating the ownership of other fire prevention measures (e.g. fire extinguisher, stove guard) have been identified in the literature.

In this chapter, the results of a Swedish national survey performed by Statistics Sweden (SCB) on behalf of the Swedish Civil Contingencies Agency (MSB) in 2018 have been investigated. The survey was distributed to 43,600 individuals between 18 and 79 years, among which 18,466 responded (42%). The survey included a few sociodemographic variables such as marital status and type of house. Also, more variables of this type (income, age, gender and education level) were further matched from other databases based on the survey identification number.

The survey included a range of different questions relating to safety, and among those questions, there were questions about smoke alarm (ownership, functionality and testing) as well as ownership of fire blankets and fire extinguishers. In the tables below, the sociodemographic patterns in fire safety measure prevalence are presented as odds ratios (ORs) based on logistic regression. An odds ratio below unity implies that the presence of that factor decreases the prevalence of that safety measure (keeping all other included factors constant).

As presented in Table 14.5, country of origin is a strong predictor of smoke alarm ownership in Sweden. Individuals from non-European countries, despite

Table 14.5 The influence of sociodemographic patterns on smoke alarm ownership, functionality and testing presented as odds-ratio (OR) with 95% confidence interval. Bold factors are statistically significant ($p < 0.05$)

Variable	Value	Smoke alarm ownership	Smoke alarm functionality	Smoke alarm testing
Gender	Female	1 (reference)	1 (reference)	1 (reference)
	Male	**0.77 (0.65–0.92)**	**0.81 (0.7–0.94)**	**1.18 (1.07–1.31)**
Age group	18–29 years	1.07 (0.78–1.46)	0.91 (0.69–1.21)	**0.46 (0.38–0.55)**
	20–49 years	1.00 (0.77–1.3)	0.96 (0.75–1.21)	**0.73 (0.63–0.85)**
	50–64 years	1 (reference)	1 (reference)	1 (reference)
	65–79 years	1.03 (0.82–1.3)	0.99 (0.81–1.21)	1.13 (0.99–1.3)
Marital status	Unmarried	**0.71 (0.55–0.90)**	0.83 (0.67–1.04)	**0.86 (0.75–0.99)**
	Married	1 (reference)	1 (reference)	1 (reference)
	Divorced	**0.64 (0.5–0.84)**	**0.71 (0.56–0.9)**	**0.84 (0.71–0.99)**
	Widowed	0.85 (0.56–1.27)	0.97 (0.67–1.4)	**0.72 (0.56–0.93)**
Income group (quintiles)	0–19%	**0.74 (0.58–0.94)**	**0.75 (0.6–0.94)**	**0.81 (0.7–0.95)**
	20–39%	0.99 (0.77–1.28)	0.94 (0.75–1.18)	0.9 (0.77–1.05)
	40–59%	1 (reference)	1 (reference)	1 (reference)
	60–79%	**1.52 (1.13–2.04)**	**1.44 (1.11–1.87)**	0.88 (0.75–1.03)
	80–100%	**1.56 (1.15–2.13)**	**1.33 (1.02–1.73)**	0.89 (0.76–1.05)
Education	Compulsory	0.84 (0.68–1.04)	0.84 (0.69–1.02)	1.09 (0.94–1.27)
	High-school	1 (reference)	1 (reference)	1 (reference)
	University	1.15 (0.95–1.4)	1.09 (0.92–1.29)	**0.83 (0.75–0.92)**
Household type	With children	1.01 (0.78–1.32)	1.07 (0.84–1.37)	1.02 (0.88–1.17)
	With only adults	1 (reference)	1 (reference)	1 (reference)
	Living alone	**0.48 (0.38–0.59)**	**0.48 (0.39–0.58)**	**0.79 (0.69–0.91)**
Country of origin	Sweden	1 (reference)	1 (reference)	1 (reference)
	Other Nordic	0.78 (0.5–1.23)	0.92 (0.6–1.41)	1.08 (0.79–1.47)
	Other European	**0.41 (0.3–0.57)**	**0.48 (0.35–0.65)**	**0.67 (0.53–0.83)**
	Non-European	**0.16 (0.13–0.21)**	**0.19 (0.15–0.24)**	**0.48 (0.39–0.6)**

(continued)

Table 14.5 (continued)

Variable	Value	Smoke alarm ownership	Smoke alarm functionality	Smoke alarm testing
House type	Single-family house	**2.06 (1.63–2.6)**	**2.1 (1.71–2.57)**	**1.58 (1.37–1.81)**
	Owned apartment	1 (reference)	1 (reference)	1 (reference)
	Rented apartment	0.98 (0.78–1.23)	0.97 (0.79–1.19)	**0.8 (0.69–0.94)**
	Other	1.08 (0.67–1.75)	1.2 (0.78–1.85)	**1.9 (1.33–2.72)**
		n = 17,596	*n = 16,881*	*n = 16,569*

constituting only 4% of the respondents, account for 22% of the individuals without smoke alarm. This is particularly interesting given that people from non-European countries living in Sweden have a significantly lower risk of dying in fires [9].

Smoke alarm ownership and reported functionality are similar for all age groups, but the youngest group, to a large extent, reports that they never test their alarm. Therefore, it is important to continue to stress the importance of smoke alarm testing for this group.

Further, the results appear to be concurrent with previous research in that high income and living in single-family houses increase the prevalence of smoke alarms. However, no influence of having children at home was found, but living alone (which is also a risk factor for fire fatality [13]) was found to be associated with a lower prevalence of smoke alarms and the same was found for divorced and unmarried individuals.

In the table below, the influence of the same factors on the ownership of suppression equipment (i.e. fire blanket and fire extinguisher) is presented (Table 14.6).

The results revealed similar patterns as for smoke alarms with low income, living alone and originating in a non-European country as important factors. However, living in a single-family house has a much larger influence on extinguisher ownership than on smoke alarms. Also, there seems to be an age-based gradient where younger people seem to have more of both fire extinguishers and fire blankets.

5 Limitations

As stated above, all the results in this chapter are based exclusively on Swedish data, and therefore, the applicability of the results to other countries needs to be discussed. Even if this is difficult to prove, there is reason to believe that the situation is similar in most western countries. One reason is that the same risk factors appear to be found across countries (see Chap. 2), but also that the studies on the effectiveness of different measures in the literature appear to give similar results regardless of the country [14].

Table 14.6 The influence of sociodemographic patterns on ownership of fire extinguishers and fire blankets presented as odds ratio (OR) with 95% confidence interval. Bold factors are statistically significant ($p < 0.05$)

Variable	Value	Extinguisher	Fire blanket
Gender	Female	1 (reference)	1 (reference)
	Male	1.05 (0.97–1.15)	**0.86 (0.81–0.92)**
Age group	18–29 yrs	1.17 (1–1.38)	**1.22 (1.06–1.4)**
	20–49 yrs	**1.19 (1.04–1.36)**	**1.26 (1.14–1.4)**
	50–64 yrs	1 (reference)	1 (reference)
	65–79 yrs	**0.85 (0.77–0.95)**	0.98 (0.9–1.07)
Marital status	Unmarried	**0.74 (0.66–0.83)**	**0.76 (0.7–0.84)**
	Married	1 (reference)	1 (reference)
	Divorced	**0.78 (0.68–0.89)**	**0.81 (0.73–0.9)**
	Widowed	0.83 (0.68–1.02)	0.94 (0.79–1.12)
Income group (quintiles)	0–19%	**0.78 (0.68–0.88)**	**0.81 (0.73–0.9)**
	20–39%	0.91 (0.8–1.03)	**0.84 (0.76–0.92)**
	40–59%	1 (reference)	1 (reference)
	60–79%	1.04 (0.91–1.18)	1.02 (0.93–1.12)
	80–100%	**1.18 (1.03–1.35)**	**1.18 (1.06–1.3)**
Education	Compulsory	1.02 (0.91–1.15)	**0.9 (0.82–0.99)**
	High-school	1 (reference)	1 (reference)
	University	0.98 (0.9–1.07)	**1.14 (1.06–1.22)**
Household type	With children	0.95 (0.84–1.08)	**1.3 (1.18–1.43)**
	With only adults	1 (reference)	1 (reference)
	Living alone	**0.67 (0.6–0.75)**	**0.77 (0.69–0.85)**
Country of origin	Sweden	1 (reference)	1 (reference)
	Other Nordic	**0.76 (0.61–0.95)**	**0.76 (0.63–0.92)**
	Other European	**0.53 (0.44–0.64)**	**0.48 (0.4–0.57)**
	Non-European	**0.35 (0.29–0.42)**	**0.33 (0.27–0.4)**
House type	Single-family house	**5.03 (4.52–5.59)**	**1.57 (1.43–1.74)**
	Owned apartment	1 (reference)	1 (reference)
	Rented apartment	**0.61 (0.54–0.68)**	**0.87 (0.78–0.99)**
	Other	**6.23 (4.57–8.48)**	**1.49 (1.21–1.83)**
		$n = 17{,}560$	$n = 17{,}560$

This implies that a reasonable hypothesis is that the results in this chapter can be applied also to other western countries, but it is strongly recommended to challenge this hypothesis by performing a similar analysis also in other countries. Awaiting such studies, however, it is recommended to base strategies on the results presented in this chapter in the absence of indications that they should not be applicable.

A second important discussion is the difference between a causal and non-causal risk factor which has been thoroughly discussed in Chap. 2. There is no reason to believe that there is a causal relationship between most of the factors mentioned in this chapter and the effectiveness or ownership of preventive measures. Instead, the factors are *indicators* of effectiveness and ownership. However, the purpose of the results presented is not to modify the factors but rather to use them to identify where specific preventive measures can be expected to be effective and/or present.

Finally, the large variations between individuals within each group should also be acknowledged. There are, of course, many older adults in good health and many divorced individuals without the specific causal risk factors present. However, on average, some measures are more effective in some groups compared to within other groups. Therefore, the results in this chapter should not be seen as a universal blueprint of prevention for a specific individual, but as a good starting point for individualized prevention. It is also judged to be very useful for designing strategies on a more generic level, for example, selecting communication channels for smoke alarm campaigns.

6 Conclusions

This chapter has been based on three questions for which an answer is attempted below, based on the data presented in this chapter. It should, however, be noted that the numbers are based on Swedish data.

6.1 What Measures Are Effective for Different Population Groups?

For most groups, smoke alarms are very effective in reducing the risk of a fatal fire – especially given the limited investment. However, for high-risk groups such as older people in general and specifically older smokers, a smoke alarm will generally not be enough. This conclusion is based on both the reduction of smoke alarm effectiveness, from 42% for the general public to 31% for people at 80 years or above and 21% for smokers in that group, and the steep increase in the risk level for those groups. The risk level for a smoker of age 80 or above is more than 22 times that of the general public.

A range of different options exists for additional interventions towards this group. For smokers, an intervention to reduce the hazard of the smoking material is very appealing, which makes the limited performance of the recently introduced RIP-cigarettes [15] problematic, but other options exist in the form of, for example, e-cigarettes. Also, interventions to prevent the ignition are quite effective, and especially the substitution of clothing materials for synthetic or animal fibres (see Chap. 10), which do not typically ignite by a cigarette, is favourable. The effect on flaming ignition sources is not as pronounced for these fabrics, but the risk of deep burns is generally lower since the melted material insulates the skin from the flame temperature [16]. There are also options in relation to suppression and, given that sprinkler systems generally are too slow to activate, a detector-activated suppression system is often a better choice (see Chap. 11).

6.2 Where Will the Installation of a Specific Measure Provide the Largest Benefit?

As previously described, the distribution of fire risk is very uneven in society. Hence, even a limited reduction in the risk of high-risk individuals can provide substantial risk reduction on the societal scale. This information is important to investigate where a specific measure is most motivated (in contrast to the previous question, which had the individual as a point of departure).

The increase in risk with age typically outweighs the reduction in effectiveness for most measures (for example, for smoke alarms), making the installation more beneficial on a societal scale for older individuals. The only two exceptions are stove guards and fire-resistant sofas, for which the benefit per installation decreases between the second oldest (65–79 years) and the oldest group (80+ years).

It should also be noted that some very large benefits per installation can be found among smokers and especially older smokers where safe cigarettes, sprinklers and detector-activated sprinklers give the highest benefit, but also fire-resistant clothing.

6.3 Who Currently Owns Different Fire Preventive Measures?

Country of origin and especially being born outside Europe seem to be strongly correlated with a low prevalence of smoke alarms, extinguishers and fire blankets in Sweden. Interestingly, however, the same group has been found to have a reduced risk of dying in fires [9], but this can probably be reduced even further with wider adoption of, particularly, smoke alarms. Also, smoke alarm testing seems to be lower for the youngest age groups, but they seem to have more extinguishing equipment available.

Apart from this, it is clear that men living alone in apartments with a low income have a substantially lower level of protection and, at the same time, a higher risk and should therefore probably be a focus of future campaigns.

The results are rather coherent with previous studies from other countries looking at similar factors, which indicate that the results are likely to be similar in other countries. The predictor "country of origin" should, however, be interpreted with caution in an international context even if factors relating to immigration (e.g. spoken language [11]) have previously been found as a strong predictor also in other countries.

References

1. Runefors M, Nilson F (2021) The influence of sociodemographic factors on the theoretical effectiveness of fire prevention interventions on fatal residential fires. Fire Technol. https://doi.org/10.1007/s10694-021-01125-x
2. Runefors M, Johansson N, van Hees P (2017) The effectiveness of specific fire prevention measures for different population groups. Fire Saf J 91:1044–1050
3. NLM (2020) Introduction to MeSH. Natl Libr Med. https://www.nlm.nih.gov/mesh/introduction.html. Accessed 30 Dec 2020
4. Jonsson A, Runefors M, Särdqvist S, Nilson F (2016) Fire-related mortality in Sweden: temporal trends 1952 to 2013. Fire Technol 52:1697–1707. https://doi.org/10.1007/s10694-015-0551-5
5. Geifman N, Cohen R, Rubin E (2013) Redefining meaningful age groups in the context of disease. Age (Omaha) 35:2357–2366. https://doi.org/10.1007/s11357-013-9510-6
6. Jonsson A, Runefors M, Gustavsson J, Nilson F. Residential fire fatality typologies in Sweden: results after 20 years of high-quality data. Unpubl Manuscr
7. DCLG (2007) Sprinkler effectiveness in care homes – final research report: BD 2546. Department of Communities and Local Government, London
8. Hultkrantz L, Svensson M (2012) The value of a statistical life in Sweden: a review of the empirical literature. Health Policy (New York) 108:302–310. https://doi.org/10.1016/j.healthpol.2012.09.007
9. Jonsson A, Jaldell H (2019) Identifying sociodemographic risk factors associated with residential fire fatalities: a matched case control study. Inj Prev:1–6. https://doi.org/10.1136/injuryprev-2018-043062
10. Jones AR, Thompson CJ, Davis MK (2001) Smoke alarm ownership and installation: a comparison of a rural and a suburban community in Georgia. J Community Health 26:307–329. https://doi.org/10.1023/a:1010478116532
11. Harvey LA, Poulos RG, Sherker S (2013) The impact of recent changes in smoke alarm legislation on residential fire injuries and smoke alarm ownership in New South Wales, Australia. J Burn Care Res 34:168–175. https://doi.org/10.1097/BCR.0b013e318257d827
12. EHS (2014) English housing survey 2012 to 2013: fire and fire safety report. Department for Communities and Local Government, UK Government
13. Nilson F, Lundgren L, Bonander C (2020) Living arrangements and fire-related mortality amongst older people in Europe. Int J Inj Contr Saf Promoto:1–7. https://doi.org/10.1080/17457300.2020.1780454
14. Runefors M (2020) Fatal residential fires – prevention and response. Lund University
15. Bonander CM, Jonsson AP, Nilson FT (2016) Investigating the effect of banning non-reduced ignition propensity cigarettes on fatal residential fires in Sweden. Eur J Pub Health 26:334–338. https://doi.org/10.1093/eurpub/ckv180
16. Kadolph SJ (1987) A flammability hazard rating and index for women's apparel. J Consum Stud Home Econ 40(2):59903–59181. https://doi.org/10.1111/j.1470-6431.1987.tb00070.x

Dr. Marcus Runefors is a Lecturer at the Division of Fire Safety Engineering at Lund University in Sweden, where he also finished his PhD in the beginning of 2020. The topic of his PhD was fatal residential fires from both a prevention and response perspective, focusing on the effectiveness of different measures to prevent fatal fires for different groups in the population.

Part III
Implementing Evidence-Based Fire Safety Promotion

Chapter 15
Vision Zero for Fire Safety

Ragnar Andersson and Thomas Gell

Abstract The so-called Vision Zero policy has become an inspiration and model for systematic safety work in many fields. In short, Vision Zero combines an ethical approach – that it is never acceptable to let people die or become seriously injured in environments where the risks are clearly preventable – with a scientific approach to the principles of prevention. The Vision Zero was introduced in Sweden applied to road safety and has since spread to other countries and other problem domains. In this chapter, we wish to illustrate Vision Zero as it was originally formulated, and what a Vision Zero model, according to the same principles, would imply if transferred to fire safety. Finally, it is discussed what challenges it entails to introduce a Vision Zero on fire, based on Swedish experience where a Vision Zero for fire safety was launched already in 2010.

Keywords Fire safety · Vision Zero · Policy · Implementation · Systems approach · Management by objectives

---

R. Andersson (✉)
Centre for Societal Risk Research, Karlstad University, Karlstad, Sweden
e-mail: ragnar.andersson@kau.se

T. Gell
The Swedish Fire Research Foundation (Brandforsk), Brandforsk, Sweden

© The Author(s), under exclusive license to Springer Nature Switzerland AG 2023
M. Runefors et al. (eds.), *Residential Fire Safety*, The Society of Fire Protection Engineers Series, https://doi.org/10.1007/978-3-031-06325-1_15

1 Introduction

"Good solutions" to societal problems are not proven good until they have been put into practice and shown to fulfill expected results under realistic circumstances. For this, just promising innovations are not enough. A societal implementation process is also needed to ensure that the solutions come into place. Policies need to be developed and implemented, employing steering instruments available to society. These can be laws and regulations, information, financial stimuli, and the like. Organizational structures and practices may also need to be strengthened to make the governance more efficient. Finally, the measures taken need to be evaluated to ascertain that they really lead to the expected effects.

An upcoming model for societal development in the field of safety is the so-called Vision Zero, initially developed for road safety [7]. The model was first introduced in Sweden in the 1990s and has since spread widely to other countries, as well as to other problem domains. There is yet no unambiguous and standardized definition of a Vision Zero. But in road safety, the model is described as a paradigm shift that has revolutionized perceptions of safety work [2]. The most apparent element is what has become known as the "ethical approach." Fatalities and serious injuries can never be seen as acceptable. The only acceptable alternative, therefore, is a continuous strive toward zero. Fundamental to the new philosophy is also a radical shift in perceptions of responsibility. According to Vision Zero, the responsibility for road safety should be seen as shared between road users and those designing the road transport system. Besides the individual performance of the road users, it is evident that the frequency and severity of accidents largely depend on road and vehicle design, regulations, etc. The Swedish Vision Zero on traffic places, the ultimate responsibility on the "system designers" since the system's design, ultimately determines its inherent risks. Previously, the primary responsibility was placed on the individual road user, regardless of the technical, environmental, and regulatory conditions set by others. The Vision Zero model, as initially applied to traffic safety, is described in more detail below.

The purpose of this chapter is to illustrate what a Vision Zero on fire safety could mean in the light of its role model on traffic safety. We wish to pinpoint conditions that appear particularly challenging when applied to fire safety, as compared to traffic, and how these challenges can be tackled in future fire safety work. The Vision Zero policy on fire safety adopted in Sweden in 2010 is analyzed and discussed as an example.

2 The Role Model: Vision Zero on Road Traffic

In addition to the ethically based ultimate goal – that no one should die or sustain serious injury in road traffic – Vision Zero rests on a profound scientific basis. One of the essential components is the adoption of a systems approach where the previously dominating individual-oriented perception of traffic accident causation, the "human factor," is replaced by a more multifactorial view. This view is based on a conception of how road users, vehicles, and the traffic environment interact and where weaknesses in one part of the system can be compensated by improvements directed at other parts [11]. Human error is considered particularly difficult to eliminate; why technology, roads, and regulations should be designed to reduce negative consequences of human shortcomings (so-called forgiving systems). Another central component is the biomedical understanding of the injury mechanisms. Vision Zero aims at reducing the severity of traffic injuries (killed and seriously injured), which is not the same as reducing the number of accidents. What causes deaths and injuries in traffic accidents is exposure to energies, usually mechanical, in quantity and intensity exceeding the human body's tolerance thresholds. Therefore, the core issue is to control the release of these energies and their further transmission to human tissues. One way of doing this is still to prevent the occurrence of accidents, e.g., through various types of technical driver support. However, since accidents most likely will continue to occur frequently due to inherent and long-lasting system imperfections, powerful complementary strategies are needed to limit postaccident consequences. This broadens the scope of traffic safety work and raises the responsibilities of a multitude of societal actors, especially those who in some respect can be regarded as system designers.

In the spirit of Vision Zero, a number of innovative safety systems have been developed regarding driver performance as well as vehicles and the traffic environment [17]. Although this development cannot be explained solely by the Vision Zero adoption, it bears the Vision Zero philosophy's apparent features. In Sweden's case, the implementation of several innovative measures is judged to have been accelerated by Vision Zero, including the introduction of so-called 2 + 1 roads with a center barrier, plus a massive replacement of four-way intersections with roundabouts [7].

The Vision Zero has, as pointed out, diffused to several countries and now inspires road safety work internationally [18]. Vision Zero has also influenced other domains outside road safety. In Sweden, national Vision Zero policies are adopted in areas such as fire safety, occupational safety, patient safety, and suicide prevention, plus in several areas other than injuries, such as social and environmental problems [9]. In both cases (other countries and problem domains other than traffic safety), it has turned out that the content of the Vision Zero philosophy has been interpreted quite differently depending on the context in which the model has been introduced. The same applies to the possibilities of practically implementing systematic safety management in the spirit of Vision Zero. Hence, there is a need to clarify Vision Zero's essential characteristics to prevent the term from being distorted and reduced to just an empty political slogan. Among other things, there is an obvious risk of confusion with the concept of Zero Tolerance, which usually refers to strict intolerance of certain behaviors, i.e., the exact opposite of the "forgiving" and harm-reducing philosophy of Vision Zero [1, 10]. A recent comparative content analysis points out the importance of scientific grounding, a holistic view, a long-term commitment, and functional governance in order for the Vision Zero approach to be considered fully applied [9].

3 A Vision Zero on Fire Safety: Rationale and Challenges

Fire safety is a field developed mainly within a relatively narrow professional framework, initially the fire brigades and the insurance industry, and later on, with scientific contributions from construction and fire protection engineering. Now when (as a result of fire preventative and fire delimiting measures mainly) a situation has arisen where a growing majority of those who die in residential fires do so due to their individual vulnerability, there are strong reasons to broaden the perspective and view the problem as a wider societal problem requiring new approaches. We believe that such a change in perspective and management is necessary to pave the way for the next step in further reducing the death toll due to fire, especially in light of the fact that the proportion of single and vulnerable elderly people will continue to increase in the coming decades (see Chaps. 2 and 3). Here, a Vision Zero-based safety philosophy offers an ethically defensible, scientifically anchored, and socially inspiring approach for risk management with promising potential.

Elsewhere, we have pointed out five factors as essential for systematic risk management at the societal level [1].

1. The system intended to control, including its components, how they interact, and the nature of the system's inherent risks, needs to be understood. The system's main actors and their incentives need to be identified as well.
2. The variables intended to control must be possible to monitor. This applies to both the undesirable outcomes (in this case, deaths and serious injuries) and their modifiable underlying determinants generating these outcomes.
3. The variables intended to control must also be possible to influence by means of well-known measures ("tools") considered effective.
4. There must exist a sustained political commitment to the necessity of control, and an organization and a set of governing instruments ensuring that the intentions are carried out.
5. The work needs to be targeted, not only in the form of long-term visions but also by timed operational subgoals for outcomes and determinants, to facilitate ongoing accomplishment and evaluation.

In the following, points 1–4 are commented on in more detail concerning a possible application of a Vision Zero approach to fire safety.

4 The Systems Approach

Deaths and serious injuries from fire occur in several environments and situations. Usually, they relate to residential settings, including nursing homes, but life-threatening fires also occur in traffic and public environments. Fire is thus a risk that affects several subsystems in society. The incidents are usually unintentional, but intentional fires resulting in death or serious injury happen as well. In common, fire-related injuries and deaths result from exposure to the emissions from fire – heat, and/or toxic gases – in amounts that exceed the human organism's tolerance thresholds. Indirectly, and more rarely, injuries may also occur in connection with rescue efforts or evacuation, such as falls, falling debris, jumps from balconies, etc.

Considering housing as a system, fire is one risk alongside many others, such as falls, poor indoor air quality, etc. The housing system components consist roughly of the residents themselves and their visitors, the building with its installations, furniture, products, etc. The systems' risks are determined by the hazards inherent in the living environment in combination with the residents' personal vulnerabilities and abilities to manage the hazards, whether manageable at all by the individual. Some ignition sources may appear beyond the control of the individual, such as fixed electrical installations. Upholstered furniture, common in most homes, poses a large potential fire load and generates gases with imminent lethal toxicity in the event of a fire, a danger of which many residents might be unaware. There is usually no consumer information on fire properties for furniture. Such dangers, beyond the control of the individual, must be managed by others; construction companies, property owners, manufacturers, suppliers, installers, etc., as well as the society's regulators and licensors. Therefore, all these actors belong to the system and should be attributed responsibility for the living environment's inherent risks. Concerning other risks, the moral responsibility can be seen as shared between the system's users and its designers in proportions to the degree users can be expected to cope with the dangers themselves in a safe manner. Among residents, there is one large group of minors who are unable to care for their own safety. Instead, parents or other caregivers are expected to step in and compensate. There is also a large group of elderly, disabled, and chronically ill, with impaired abilities in various respects. In terms of risk, these people constitute a very vulnerable group in a housing environment in practice designed for high-performing users in midlife. Particularly vulnerable are those who, in addition, live alone and thus lack someone in their vicinity who in critical situations can intervene and assist.

Housing is an arena traditionally characterized by the individual's right to privacy and self-determination. From this also stem a traditional view of individual responsibility in terms of home safety. As the population ages and more and more people are cared for at home, even for serious illnesses, the conflict between this traditional view and the requirement for safe housing has sharpened. Like in traffic, the system designers need to step forward and take more direct responsibility for the growing share of residents who cannot reasonably be expected to care for themselves in critical situations. Concerning fire, there is convincing evidence indicating that the elderly, the disabled, and the socially disadvantaged constitute an increasingly dominant group among those killed and seriously injured, especially in high-income countries. That these groups stand out in terms of risk does not seem to be primarily due to them having more fires than the general population, but to the fact that they face more difficulties in surviving if a fire occurs [13]. This fact, in turn, is due to a combination of increased medical vulnerability and a decreased ability to act adequately in the event of fire (see Chaps. 4 and 5). Rather, the occurrence of residential fires seems to be more common in well-off households with, on average, younger residents. However, these households are also better prepared to extinguish, evacuate, and call for help to avoid loss of life and health. Fires in which people die are often limited in magnitude, but become fatal because the involved individuals are extra vulnerable and lack the ability to handle the situation. This is a structural problem beyond the individual's control, indicating that the traditional view of the division of responsibilities in fire safety needs to be fundamentally revised. Housing, like road transportation, is a system where the system designers largely determine the risks and where, therefore, the ultimate responsibility needs to be attributed to them.

5 Measurability

Setting goals for something that cannot be measured is hardly rational. That is like acting in blindness. If the focus is on fatalities and serious injuries, these outcome variables need to be measured with adequate accuracy over time. This task is more challenging than one might think at first glance due to the common coexistence of different registration systems with different purposes, and thus, normally, different coverages. The accessibility and quality of the data captured vary as well. For example, the fire sector usually relies on the rescue service's reporting. However, this can lead to a considerable underestimation of the true number of people killed in fires, partly because the rescue services are not attending all fatal events and that some victims rescued alive die later from their injuries [8]. Also, rescue personnel are seldom well trained to assess the degree of injury severity among fire victims (see Chap. 6, Fire safety surveillance). The obvious solution is to match data from several sources (call-out reports, cause of death registers, in-patient registers, forensic registers) to obtain an adequate coverage of the outcomes in question and a richer and more valid set of information [8].

In addition to the outcomes subjected to reduction, it is also desirable to measure and follow underlying determining factors behind the outcomes. Of particular importance are factors subjected to intervention, such as the presence of smoke alarms, for example. All variables of interest to modify to reduce the number of fatalities and seriously injured should entail goals to enable program performance evaluation. The performance should be traced by an active management by objectives (MBO) system.

6 Controllability

Lacking instruments to influence what is intended to be controlled is as bad as not being able to measure. In that case, there is awareness of the problem but unawareness of what to do. This prompts continuous investments in what is often referred to as evidence and grounded experience. Research and experience gradually enhance the accumulated knowledge on the most effective measures. A toolbox with several credible countermeasures is needed to achieve the greatest possible effect of preventative efforts.

Historically, fire safety interventions have primarily focused on limiting large-scale fires in urban areas by preventing the spread from building to building [6]. Through urban planning with spacious streets and avenues, this type of fire has been replaced by more limited fires in individual buildings or building compartments (fire cells) designed to contain a fire [15]. Another line of development is the establishment of rescue services with the ambition of being able to carry out firefighting and rescue those in need within a reasonable time [14]. These efforts have undoubtedly had an effect, but there is still a problem with limited fires where people die and are injured without the rescue service arriving swiftly enough, if even alerted. The toolbox includes, e.g., smoke alarms, sprinklers, self-extinguishing cigarettes, information campaigns, and home visits. The scientific evidence for these measures is partly weak, but strengthens gradually. Among other things, we know today that self-extinguishing cigarettes are proven to be less effective than expected [3, 4]. Smoke alarms do not help those who, for various reasons, lack the ability to evacuate themselves [16]. Campaigns and home visits also have their obvious limitations. The incentives of innovation and the commercial driving forces regarding fire safety in living environments leave room for considerable improvements. While car manufacturers are competing to introduce new safety-enhancing technology in our cars, and vehicle safety has become a powerful commercial argument where consumers have access to qualified safety evaluations [5], the housing sector still seems characterized by the attitude that fire safety at home is the resident's own problem. Much research and innovation remain for the toolbox to be considered sufficiently complete, especially in terms of protecting the most vulnerable in the event of fire. Also, a shift to another mindset regarding fire safety as a commercial driving force is much needed.

7 Determination, Mandate, and Organization

To create real change, it is not enough to have access to a toolbox; it must also be ensured that the measures are implemented. Conflicts of objectives surround almost every political action, and the competition for limited resources is fierce. If an effort is to have priority, a strong political mandate is needed. As responsibilities are shared among many actors and affect several societal sectors, the mandate must be broad and supported by sufficient powers. The societal governance of fire safety needs to be conducted systematically and decisively by means of a balanced mix of effective measures at disposal. Society has different faces; parliament, government, authorities, regions, and municipalities. It also has various roles; policymaker, infrastructure developer, owner, and user. Finally, society has various instruments, such as regulation, education, information, and finances. Through effective governance, at appropriate levels and with broad community involvement, these various faces, roles, and means can all be utilized for the intended result.

8 Challenges and Opportunities in Adopting a Vision Zero for Fire Safety

Inspired by the Vision Zero on traffic safety, a Vision Zero was adopted on fire safety in Sweden in 2010. The wording of this vision is similar to the traffic area's Vision Zero – *"No one should die or be seriously injured because of fire."* A recent comparative analysis of five Swedish national Vision Zero policies, all with an injury prevention focus (traffic, fire, suicide, patient safety, and occupational fatalities), found significant problems associated with most of them, such as insufficient tools, lack of governance, difficulties in measuring and evaluation, and lack of a holistic/systems view [9]. To finalize, we here wish to comment on these challenges with reference to the Swedish Vision Zero on fire, and from there, point at the possibilities of refining effective Vision Zero work in this field.

The Vision Zero on traffic meant a clear break with an outdated perception of human error as the primary cause and individual responsibility as the main solution. Instead, it introduced a perspective of societal responsibility and a systems approach where the responsibility ultimately rests with the system designers, not its users. We cannot see that this view has yet permeated Swedish fire safety work, despite the adoption of Vision Zero. A Vision Zero is a societal commitment, i.e., a mission that society directs toward itself and which cannot be passed on to the citizens to realize. The systems view is, therefore, an indispensable part of a Vision Zero policy's theoretical basis. In our opinion, effective Vision Zero work in the fire area cannot be established without the "housing system" being modeled in the same way as the transport system. The housing risks, in analogy with the transport system risks, should be understood as inherent system properties for which the system designers bear an overall responsibility. Fire risks in settings other than housing, for example, in traffic, should be covered by the safety work within these.

The Vision Zero in the traffic area also meant a shift from the traditional view that safety work primarily aims to prevent "accidents," such as crashes or fires. Instead, the new focus is to limit the consequences of these events in the form of killed and seriously injured. The consequences always represent the burden of an accident. Therefore, it is ultimately the consequences that need to be reduced over time. It is also usually the consequences that are measured, evaluated, and compared in so-called accident statistics, as well as in research and analysis, and thus form the basis for prioritization and follow-ups. Preventing accidents is, of course, a way of preventing consequences. But, as discussed in Chap. 3, many accidents result in minor or insignificant consequences. This means two things; that accidents in many contexts are common and often trivial events, and, secondly, that there are usually several modifiable factors in addition to the accident event that contribute to the severity of the consequences. Some of these factors might be more meaningful to address in systematic safety work than spending resources on preventing accidents in general. The Swedish Vision Zero on fire safety, like the one on traffic, sends a clear message back to society to ensure that the consequences for life and health from fires are systematically reduced. However, the Swedish front organization to shoulder this mission, the rescue services, still perceives that their main task is to fight fires, i.e., to combat the accident as such. A new, consequence-focused goal-setting needs to permeate key actors and become expressed in new approaches and strategies, meaning that a deep-rooted professional culture needs to be challenged.

When establishing long-term work toward fewer killed and seriously injured by fire, it is necessary to create valid and comprehensive data collection systems for outcomes and determinants (indicators), something that still appears challenging, not least in Sweden. When Vision Zero was adopted for Swedish fire safety work, regular statistics on fatalities existed, but not on seriously injured. An extensive quality review of the Swedish fatal fire database, from which the data on fire fatalities is obtained, revealed that the national statistics on fatalities systematically underestimated the numbers by about 20% [8]. Some categories were more underestimated than others, including fire setting to commit suicide and fire in clothing. Underreporting and skewness have been gradually remedied through improved data collection routines, but there is still no accepted definition of serious injury, a category also encompassed by the vision. In the absence of this, attempts are made to estimate the extent and development over time by using various proxy variables, such as the number of in-patients treated for injuries caused by fire. Work is now underway to agree on definitions and inclusion criteria to allow that even this variable can be monitored and compared adequately over time; see Chap. 6.

An indicator-based management by objectives (MBO) system also presupposes the identification of relevant determinants on a scientific basis, which is a significant challenge in itself, as well as the establishment of valid and sustainable data collection systems for the corresponding variables [12]. The measures that can be implemented must be prioritized based on current knowledge of the expected effects in relation to their related costs, while continued research and development need to be directed toward better future solutions.

The biggest challenge is probably the establishment of a national cross-sectoral governance system. Such a system presupposes that the Vision Zero strategy is supported from the highest political level with a clear obligation for all sectors concerned to cooperate and that the issue is given the necessary priority. The Swedish Vision Zero on fire safety is so far only adopted by a single governmental agency, nationally responsible for fire safety, the Swedish Civil Contingencies Agency, MSB. Consequently, the overall political leadership, the parliament and the government, is thus not yet committed to the vision, which in turn means that other relevant sectors with major impact on fire safety, such as the construction sector, social services, and healthcare, are not obliged to contribute. What exists is a voluntary collaboration group including a number of national actors participating in the work. MSB's role is mainly informative, advisory, and educational vis-à-vis the public and the (formally independent) municipal-based rescue services. Hence, in reality, MSB has limited opportunities to influence the development that Vision Zero sets out.

9 Conclusions

That the Vision Zero model can serve as a powerful instrument for societal governance is shown in traffic safety. However, research discloses that misinterpretations and misunderstandings about the model can lead to theoretical distortion and undermined trustworthiness when applied to new problems. We believe that the Swedish Vision Zero on fire safety is an example of this. In order for a Vision Zero on fire to be perceived as a serious and credible approach, systematic efforts are required to address the weaknesses we have pointed out above, such as weak governance, inaccurate and insufficient monitoring systems, and ineffective preventative strategies and tools to protect life and health. Based on the above analysis and discussion, we here finally want to summarize what we perceive should constitute the key elements of a Vision Zero-based approach to residential fire safety. A Vision Zero:

- Expresses an ethical approach, that it is not ethically acceptable for people to die or become seriously injured in their homes due to fire.
- Shifts focus from the "accident" phenomenon (in this case, a residential fire) to the consequences thereof (fatally or seriously injured). The consequences from fire do not appear randomly but result from contributory and often modifiable factors. Therefore, harm reduction is a core element in every Vision Zero strategy.
- Applies a systems view. Housing is a system where several actors – system designers – have created the conditions for the home's inherent fire safety standard and where the residents can be regarded as "users" of the system.
- Takes into account that people cannot always be expected to behave correctly or have the ability to handle a fire incident themselves. It is the system designers' responsibility to design the system (the home) in such a (forgiving) way that a human lapse or inability does not result in death or serious injury.
- Is based on scientific knowledge about the human body's tolerance thresholds to fire-related hazards (mainly toxic gases and heat), the residents´ possibilities to handle a fire incident or to place themselves in safety, and for external rescue resources to intervene and assist.

References

1. Andersson R, Gell T (2021) The vision zero handbook - Theory, technology and management for a zero casualty policy. Springer International Publishing, 2019. ISBN 3030231763, 9783030231767
2. Belin MÅ, Tillgren P, Vedung E (2012) Vision Zero – a road safety policy innovation. Int J Inj Contr Saf Promot 19(2):171–179
3. Bonander C, Jonsson A, Nilson F (2016) Investigating the effect of banning non-reduced ignition propensity cigarettes on fatal residential fires in Sweden. Eur J Pub Health 26(2):334–338
4. Bonander C, Jakobsson N, Nilson F (2018) Inj Prevention 24:193–198
5. Euro NCAP, The European New Car Assessment Programme (2021). https://www.euroncap.com/en. Accessed 2021

6. Garrioch D (2019) Towards a fire history of European cities (late middle ages to late nineteenth century). Urban History 46(2):202–224. https://doi.org/10.1017/S0963926818000275
7. Johansson R (2009) Vision zero – implementing a policy for traffic safety. Saf Sci 47(2009):826–831
8. Jonsson A, Bergqvist A, Andersson R (2015) Assessing the number of fire fatalities in a defined population. J Saf Res 55:99–103
9. Kristianssen AC, Andersson R, Belin MÅ, Nilsen P (2018) Swedish vision zero policies for safety – a comparative policy content analysis. Saf Sci 103(March 2018):260–269
10. Kristanssen AC, Andersson R (2021) The vision zero handbook - Theory, technology and management for a zero casualty policy. Springer International Publishing, 2019. ISBN 3030231763, 9783030231767
11. Larsson P, Dekker SWA, Tingvall C (2010) The need for a systems theory approach to road safety. Saf Sci 48(2010):1167–1174
12. MSB (2019) Analys av utvecklingen inom bostadsbrand 2018 Målstyrning av brandsäkerhetsarbetet mot etappmålen 2020
13. Nilson F, Bonander C, Jonsson A (2015) Differences in determinants amongst individuals reporting residential fires in Sweden: results from a cross-sectional study. Fire Technol 51:615–626
14. Nyström L (1992) Lagar och ansvarsförhållanden i det svenska brandväsendets historia. Räddningsverket 1992
15. Rasbash DJ et al (2004) Evaluation of fire safety. Wiley 2004
16. Runefors M (2020) Fatal residential fires – prevention and response. Doctoral Thesis, Lund University
17. Volvo Cars (2021). https://group.volvocars.com/company/safety-vision. Accessed January 2021
18. WHO, World Health Organization (2009) European status report on road safety: towards safer roads and healthier transport choices. WHO Regional Office for Europe, Copenhagen, p 2009

Prof. Ragnar Andersson is a Senior Professor of Risk Management affiliated to Karlstad University in Sweden where he served as full professor from 2001 until retirement in 2015. His educational background is in engineering and public health. After serving for the Swedish National Board of Occupational Safety and Health in the 1970s and 1980s, he took his PhD in Social Medicine at Karolinska Institutet, Sweden, in 1991 on occupational injury prevention. Dr. Andersson's research is focused on accident and injury analysis and prevention, injury surveillance, and macro-level determinants of risk in broad fields such as occupational, traffic, product, child, senior, and fire safety.

Mr. Thomas Gell holds a Licentiate of engineering degree in Marine structural engineering from Chalmers University of Technology. For more than 25 years, he worked in various managerial positions with risk-related issues at the Swedish Rescue Services Agency and the Swedish Civil Contingencies Agency. In 2016-19, he was Head of Research and Innovation at the Swedish Fire Protection Association and director of Brandforsk, the Swedish Fire Research Foundation. He has been particularly focused on research-related development, especially learning from events and systematic safety work. He currently works as an independent consultant. He is chairman of Karlstad University's Center for Research on Societal Risks and a US Fire Protection Research Foundation board member.

Chapter 16
Fire Safety Education Campaigns

Charles R. Jennings

Abstract Public fire education, when properly designed, can be an effective means to reduce the toll of fires and related problems on the community. Public fire education must be carefully designed and based upon analysis of local incident data to include affected populations in order to properly target messages. In spite of a long history, success in implementing programs varies widely. In some cases, cultural factors and managerial challenges limit program development. The fire service must define the problem, and outside partnerships from academics and advertising and marketing specialists can improve the rigor of program designs, which must be planned to support systematic evaluation through data collection to measure results. Sustaining programs so they can produce measurable results are necessary. The ongoing evolution of marketing technologies associated with social media and widespread use of electronic devices creates both opportunities and challenges.

Keywords Fire prevention · Public education · Program evaluation · Community risk reduction · Fire risk

1 Introduction

Fire safety education campaigns are a critical component of residential fire safety. They offer the possibility of reducing fires or their severity by providing the public with information in an organized fashion. In spite of the importance of such campaigns and their existence going back many years, there remains a shortage of literature documenting effective campaigns, providing guidance to the fire services, and others attempting to design and implement such programs.

C. R. Jennings (✉)
Faculty of Security, Fire, and Emergency Management, John Jay College of Criminal Justice (CUNY), New York, NY, USA
e-mail: cjennings@jjay.cuny.edu

This chapter attempts to summarize the current state of knowledge, identify best practices, and provide approaches and commentary on designing programs using fire incident and other data. While an attempt is made to be representative, this chapter focuses primarily on English-language sources from the setting of developed nations. Considerable public education efforts in other contexts are well-established in places such as Japan, which inspired efforts in the United States and other countries [53, p. 77].

While there is no consensus on defining fire safety education campaigns, the functional definition we will use is that they involve an intentional effort to convey safety-related information to the lay public for purposes of awareness, use, or informing or protecting others. While campaigns may indeed exist to promote a particular policy, such as mandating automatic sprinklers in the building code, we will define such campaigns as influence operations, and they won't be considered here.

Fire and emergency services, particularly those that also provide emergency medical services, have often embraced a broader range of educational subjects. These have included injury prevention and lifestyle behavioral changes not strictly fire-related. This chapter will confine its examples to strict fire-related hazards, but the information is applicable to these broader efforts as well. Smoke detectors remain the dominant intervention to reduce the toll of fires [20]. Other hazards may be addressed based on local agency responsibilities, such as provision of emergency medical services, and may include initiatives such as water safety, poisoning prevention, seat belt usage, or traffic safety.

Lastly, this chapter is not intended as a treatise on the evolving fields of marketing and advertising, but rather will present general concepts. The reader planning to undertake such a program is referred to the references within the chapter for guidance.

2 History of Fire Safety Campaigns

2.1 Insurance Industry

Early fire safety campaigns were driven in large measure by the insurance industry. With the rapid development of urban centers, sometimes constructed with timber, the threat of conflagration was common in many national contexts. In the US, early efforts were concerned with avoidance of large-scale fires, as well as the promotion of fire-safe conditions in industrial and commercial properties. While its greatest emphasis was on the development of codes and standards for construction, maintenance and use of buildings, and hazardous processes, organizations such as the National Board of Fire Underwriters in the USA had very active propaganda campaigns, often centered around generalized public awareness of fire and its toll on life and the economy [23, p. 113]. The 1913 First American National Fire Prevention

Conference noted that there were 25 state-level fire prevention associations "comprised almost entirely of insurance personnel" [17, p. 26].

Many of these educational materials were crude by today's standards (see Fig. 16.1), but they are the antecedents of modern fire safety education campaigns.

2.2 Nonprofits and Community Groups

Perhaps most sustained efforts to promote fire safety education have come from nonprofit and community groups. Groups such as the National Fire Protection Association's Fire Marshals Association of North America endorsed fire prevention day on the 40th anniversary of the Great Chicago Fire of 1871. The fire prevention day would eventually grow into a nationally recognized day (and later week) by proclamation [36].

The National Fire Protection Association uses its statistical capabilities to develop a nationally themed fire prevention week campaign with materials designed to be used by local fire departments. These high-quality materials are widely adopted and are effectively a "turn-key" option for local agencies.

While many civil society groups have championed fire safety education campaigns, one of the most recent large-scale efforts in the USA is headed by the American Red Cross. Stimulated by their experience responding to assist people displaced by fires, they began a comprehensive campaign dedicated to the installation and maintenance of working smoke detectors in dwellings. That program which began in 2014 is credited with installing over two million smoke detectors and saving 864 lives [38].

Other groups are devoted to specific dimensions of the fire problem, such as burn prevention or juvenile firesetting. Countless community partnerships between local fire services, businesses, civil society groups, and neighborhood groups have been effective in spreading fire prevention messaging and having local impact.

2.3 Fire Service

The fire service plays a central role in design, delivery, and evaluation of public fire education campaigns across the world. The context varies globally according to long-standing cultural norms, occupational cultures, and societal resources.

2.3.1 United States/North American Context

The fire service can be considered the origin of much fire safety education. Fire prevention education within the fire service has gone hand-in-hand with fire prevention efforts such as code enforcement. Fire prevention education activity varies

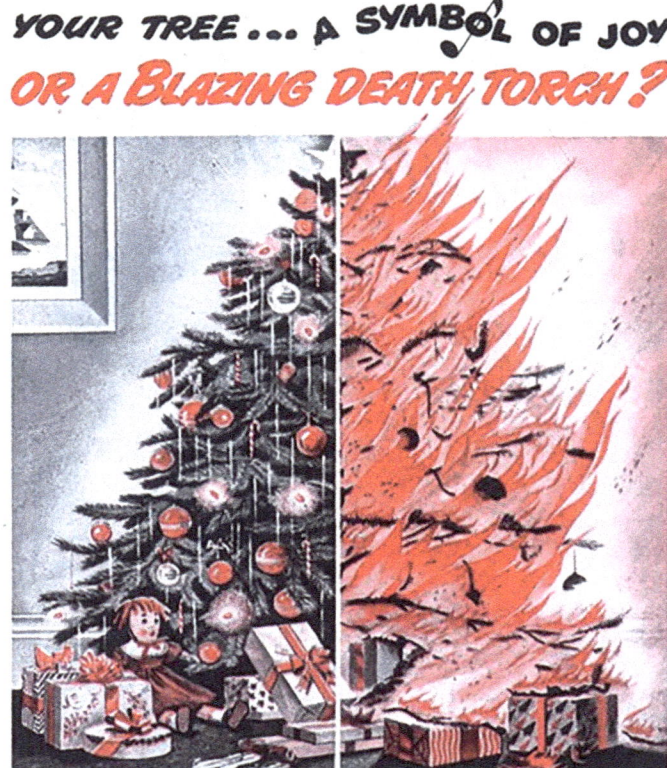

Fig. 16.1 National Board of Fire Underwriters Christmas Tree Safety advertisement c1960

greatly between fire departments, as there is little regulatory requirement to deliver public fire education. Professional qualifications for fire safety educators date back to 1977 with the NFPA's addition of these requirements to its standard on fire inspector, fire investigator, and fire prevention education officer [32].

Gaining buy-in and sustained interest in fire safety campaigns has been a long-term challenge in the USA [9], perhaps in part due to the fire service's highly decentralized and localized nature. A cultural bias toward the excitement and recognition of manual firefighting has undoubtedly played a role in North America [56]. The US National Fire Academy's model of community risk reduction explicitly mentions organizational culture as a component of implementing such programs [57, p. 6].

These challenges are also a reflection of lack of resources and expertise in many (especially smaller) fire departments. Too great an emphasis on fire prevention can be viewed by members of the fire service as a threat to firefighting jobs [21, p. 285]. Although some recent research suggests this attitude is changing [41], we have seen remarkable results in fire prevention among nations where the fire service is more regional or national in nature.

The persistence of this challenge is evident as "integrate … public fire education into the regular operations of the fire department" and was among the first items listed among strategies in a 2019 national conference on the fire problem [31]. Such pronouncements date back at least to 1913s First American National Fire Prevention Convention and were echoed later in the US's 1947 Presidential Conference on Fire Prevention (Fig. 16.2).

2.3.2 Rest of World Fire Service Public Fire Education Exemplars

The US context is by no means reflective of global practices. As indicated previously, larger or more regionalized fire services often have more resources and the capability to provide specialized staff and resources. Many international fire services require technical degrees for management and often employ specialist staff. While there has been considerable exchange of information between nations, a non-exhaustive sample of exemplary practices can be found among the following nations and major cities.

The European Union also identified the need for fire safety education as a component of national fire safety efforts. A recent report found "community fire safety programmes, at both the national and local level, are adopted around Europe" [49].

The United Kingdom has greatly increased its emphasis on fire prevention education, focusing on risk-based inspection and installation and testing of smoke alarms. Most Brigades maintained data analytic capability to target preventive efforts [52, p. 14].

Japan has a long-standing commitment to public fire education, with major cities devoting considerable resources to large, far-reaching programs that emphasize fire safety along with disaster preparedness. As an example, the Tokyo Fire Department reached over two million people with various combinations of evacuation drills,

N 73.60.2.1

OFFICIAL RECORD

of the

First American

National Fire Prevention Convention

Held at

PHILADELPHIA, PA., U. S. A.

October 13-18 (inclusive) 1913

Including all Papers, Discussions and Appendices

FIRE LOSSES IN THE UNITED STATES AND CANADA
1883-1913 (INCLUSIVE)

Year	Amount	Year	Amount
1913	$224,723,350	1898	$119,650,500
1912	225,320,900	1897	110,319,650
1911	234,337,250	1896	115,655,500
1910	234,470,650	1895	129,835,700
1909	203,649,200	1894	128,246,400
1908	238,562,250	1893	156,445,875
1907	215,671,250	1892	151,516,000
1906	459,710,000	1891	143,764,000
1905	175,193,800	1890	108,993,700
1904	252,554,050	1889	123,046,800
1903	156,195,700	1888	110,885,600
1902	149,260,850	1887	120,283,000
1901	164,347,450	1886	104,924,700
1900	163,362,250	1885	102,818,700
1899	136,773,200	1884	110,008,600

Total for 30 years $5,070,526,875
Average ....$ 169,017,562

Fig. 16.2 Philadelphia (PA, USA) Fire Prevention Conference, 1913

initial firefighting, and first aid training. In addition, they reported reaching over one million students through school-based life safety education [51, p. 27].

Similar efforts took place in many other countries, building on a renewed international interest in enhancing public fire education efforts. Notably, English-language efforts in Australia and New Zealand, among others, received emphasis in the 1990s [3, 11].

2.3.3 Summary

Some formal efforts impacting access to information on design of fire safety education campaigns came about recently, with the National Fire Protection Association Standard 1730 *Standard on Organization and Deployment of Fire Prevention Inspection and Code Enforcement, Plan Review, Investigation, and Public Education Operations* to address the conduct of such campaigns.

One of the greatest challenges facing public fire education within the fire service is the ability to sustain well-designed campaigns. Changes in leadership, inattention, and diversion to other priorities undermine success. This will be discussed more in the section of the chapter on "Implementation."

3 Major References and Milestones

The transition from broad awareness and publicity campaigns to a proper campaign was facilitated by a number of efforts initiated in the 1970s. While academic studies continued to trickle out beginning in the late 1970s, largely under US government sponsorship under the US fire Administration and its predecessor, these efforts had limited impact on fire service adoption of these practices, not being widely read among the fire service.

The US Federal Emergency Management Agency's US Fire Administration first published the guidebook *Public Fire Education Planning: A Five Step Process* [47] in 1980. This document was the first complete guide for the development of fire safety education program specifically targeted to the fire service.[1] This was most recently followed by a multiagency collaboration with the Centers for Disease Control to produce a significant expansion as a comprehensive toolkit [55].

Philip Schaenman and collaborators at TriData, a US-based consultancy and research firm, completed a series of extremely influential reports examining many aspects of fire prevention, including collecting international best practices. Under funding from the tobacco industry, and later US Centers for Disease Control and Prevention and other sources, these reports were widely disseminated and had

---

[1] The guide was most recently updated by the US Fire Administration in 2008 http://www.usfa.fema.gov/downloads/pdf/publications/fa-219.pdf

far-reaching impact to stimulate both more attention to fire prevention in the US fire service and also international collaboration and interest in adopting best practices [52, p. 11]. Unfortunately, these reports are not in print, and digital copies of the various reports are not in a single online repository.

Perhaps their most relevant report to this effort was the 1990 report *Proving Public Fire Education Works*, which was a seminal publication that identified and promoted the need for evaluation of fire safety education programs.

Overcoming an implicit bias toward suburban, nuclear families in much of the prevention literature, recognition of the need to engage meaningfully with diverse elements of the community, urban populations, immigrants, and even apartment dwellers was highlighted. One of the earliest recognitions of the need to focus on those members of the community most at risk was creation of a comprehensive toolkit titled *The Community-Based Fire Safety Education Handbook* [39]. This handbook included artwork and other aids to developing customized educational materials.

More recently, *Vision 20/20* (strategicfire.org) is a multiyear grant-funded effort to "provide a forum for sustained, collaborative planning to reduce fire loss in the United States" [24]. Beginning in 2008, this program has developed numerous tools and facilitated knowledge sharing and adoption of high-quality education campaigns in the context of community risk reduction, which in a broader term describing the process of community-wide risk assessment and development of interventions which may include public education. Vision 20/20 has guides for both Community Risk Assessment and development of a Community Risk Reduction Plan. The UK government published an evaluation guide for fire services programs in 2010 [10].

The National Fire Protection Association published its standard 1300, *Standard on Community Risk Assessment and Community Risk Reduction Plan (2020)* for the first time in 2019. This standard contains high-level guidance. The NFPA also has a standard for training fire service personnel to conduct community risk reduction.

4 How to Define a Campaign

As already noted, a public fire education campaign can be defined, for our purposes, as an intentional effort to convey safety-related information to the lay public for purposes of awareness, use, or informing or protecting others. These campaigns are almost exclusively targeted at people in their dwellings, although they can be directed at workplaces as well. However, reaching people in their homes is the most challenging dimension of public fire education.

Before we begin detailing the components of a public education campaign, we should briefly address what it is *not*. Much activity of the fire service that falls colloquially under the banner of public education does not meet this rigorous definition. Merely distributing literature, if not targeted to real-world fire problems of its audience, is little more than public relations. Indeed, some fire departments spend hours on activities that impart little or no actionable information or are so broad in their focus that they have limited use. Climbing on apparatus, spraying hoses, donning helmets, and such activities may captivate children, but can't substitute for a focused message delivered effectively. A last fallacy of public education programs is basing presentations on public requests. Such requests seldom come from the groups at highest risk, and waiting for the public to ask for information is often not likely to address a community's most serious risks or at-risk populations.

A campaign can be guided by the 5-step process. Figure 16.3 shows the 5-step process. The five steps begin with conduct of a community risk analysis. Risk analysis remains a challenge for many organizations, although there are several methods purporting to offer formulas or approaches. An important concept is that of fire frequency versus fire loss. Interventions often act on only one of these two dimensions of fire risk. For example, preparing a family escape plan does not necessarily reduce the frequency of fires, but reduces the risk of injury by enabling a household's members to evacuate and avoid reentering a structure [25, pp. 82–83].

A clear-eyed and incisive identification of the problems in your community must be undertaken. Developing a risk analysis also requires carefully identifying issues that are amenable to public education, as opposed to other approaches such as passing regulation, greater enforcement, or general advocacy.

The next step is to identify community partnerships. Almost any effort to undertake outreach to segments of a community based on location, demographic characteristics, or other risk profiles will require interaction with representatives of that community. Ideally, this relationship will be easy to establish, but it is important to understand norms, values, and local culture before crafting an intervention strategy. Community partnership may involve a community planning team, but this need not necessarily be rigid and formal. These relationships will assist in adoption of the program and add legitimacy to the fire department's efforts. Some effort may need to be made to identify members of the targeted community, perhaps even working through trusted intermediaries.

Once the problem is identified and knowledgeable and/or influential community representatives are identified, then an intervention strategy is developed. This strategy must again refine the target population and identify places for intervention and the specific interventions to be used. These may include combinations of in-person engagement, door-to-door visits, advertising, and outreach via popular and trusted locales such as faith or community groups, or popular businesses. Once these options are identified, necessary resources must be secured for costs such as design of program materials, printing, and hard costs for services such as data analysis or computer hardware such as tablet computers or phone-based apps to document activity. Do not neglect to account for availability of personnel to perform the outreach. This is where community partnership can add value by extending the reach or availability of personnel and resources. There will always be adjustment to account for limited resources, and this is where a good risk analysis will identify the most critical areas for intervention. Any strategy must incorporate identifying a measurable change in the problem being targeted.

Once a strategy is designed, the next step is implementation. A pilot administration of the program, or testing of materials should always be undertaken before it is

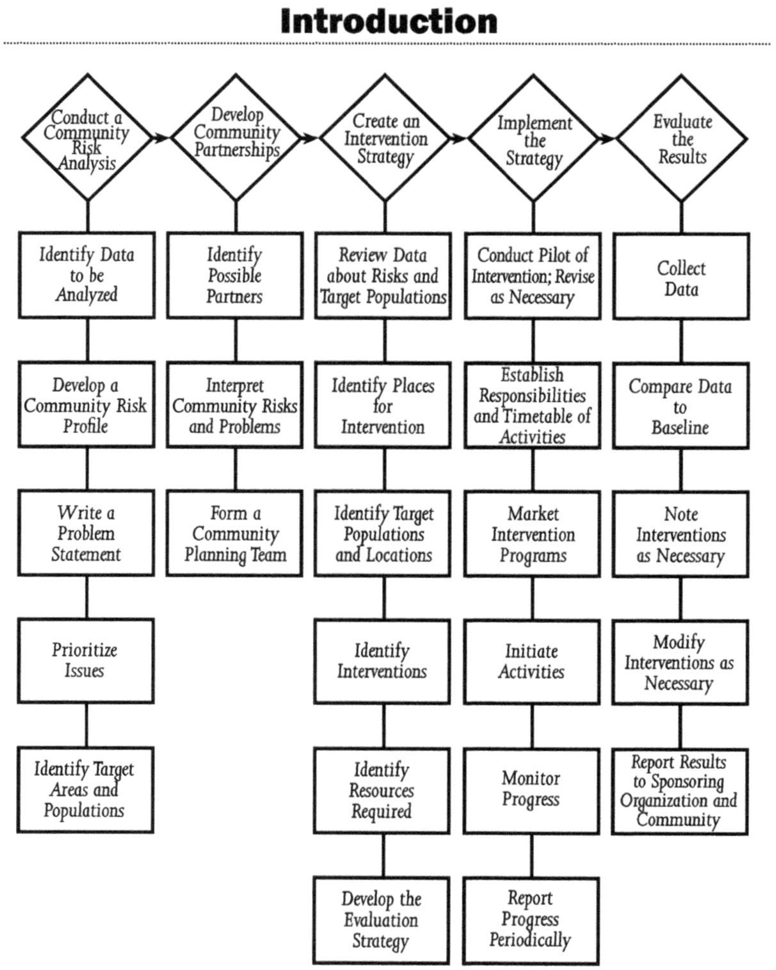

Introduction

Fig. 16.3 The 5-step process. (Source: United States Fire Administration [54])

fully launched. Errors in translation, misunderstood words, unclear artwork, or drawings may all be quickly identified through a pilot test, saving costs for redoing printing and avoiding waste. Once this is done, a project schedule should be developed and the program launched and monitored. Regular periodic reports must be filed, to maintain momentum and identify any problems such as lax recordkeeping or difficulties in reaching certain outlets.

The final step is evaluation of results. This involves a comparison of baseline (pre-intervention) data against current performance. Any changes should be documented, with attention paid to identifying the group that received the intervention as accurately as possible. It is important that results be shared with the community partners.

Of course, a real-world public education program should go through multiple cycles of evaluation and adjustment as necessary.

Another term used to describe education campaigns targeted at behavior change is *social marketing*. Social marketing is a subfield of advertising and grew from the health field. Social marketing is often applied to international contexts, but can be found around topics as varied as promoting covid-19 vaccines, tobacco cessation, and healthy diets [6]. The US Centers for Disease Control maintains significant resources devoted to health communications (https://www.cdc.gov/healthcommunication/index.html).

5 Evaluating Campaign Effectiveness

5.1 *Design with Evaluation in Mind*

One great pitfall of public education campaigns is the failure to begin with a solid understanding of the data. What is the data's origin, is it accurate, complete, and reliable? What steps are in place to control its quality? Where possible, multiple measures may be used to assure that program effects are documented, or that measures selected are sufficiently granular to show results. For example, a program to reduce smoking fires should not rely only on measuring deaths, but include injuries, numbers of fires, and fire severity as additional measures.

A clear process for tracking data on all aspects of the program must be identified in advance, documented, and followed up. Firefighters or community volunteers may be committed to the program, but the importance of collecting data and documenting activity must be instilled in the participants. Data collection forms can be designed, and electronic data collection should be used if possible to streamline collection of information. It is especially critical that someone be designated to receive and check data regularly, so that forms do not go missing, or staff can be questioned while details that weren't properly documented are still fresh in their mind.

5.1.1 Analysis Issues: Know Your Data

Data quality should be a top-level concern. Are rules and definitions developed to guide how data is recorded? What are we counting, what is our program, and what is our intervention? What are we trying to do with our program, and how are we measuring that?

Many campaigns will utilize incident-based data as their basis. Other data sources such as census data on population, income, demographics, or other characteristics are likely to be included in the risk analysis, program design, implementation, and evaluation processes. Local data such as building records and data from other agencies such as education or health departments may also be used. Data may need to be expressed on a per capita or other basis to better identify areas of risk. Multiple years of data may be needed to assemble an accurate portrayal of a community's risk profile if the number of incidents is not high.

5.1.2 Sustain the Effort

On a household level, fires do not occur frequently. This is a good thing. However, it means that to measure the impact or effectiveness of a fire safety education campaign often requires a multiyear effort. Smaller agencies may not experience sufficient incidents to be able to measure impact on a cycle short of a year. Larger agencies may have sufficient incidents to see a measurable change more quickly.

Many agencies begin an ambitious education program and diligently complete their intervention, but fail to document their efforts or lose data or simply stop prematurely. There are many reasons for this, including loss of administrative support, failure to fully embrace the program by personnel assigned, or loss of community partners. The consequence can be an inability to justify continuing the program and diversion of resources to other seemingly more important priorities.

One of the most remarkable and well-documented local public education campaigns is a home fire safety campaign developed and managed by the Surrey, British Columbia (Canada) Fire Service. Surrey, a rapidly growing City, had a significant fire problem and was concerned both for reducing this challenge and also managing the rapid growth of the City without being able to add suppression resources. Following traditional steps for design of fire safety education campaigns, they began with a 20-year analysis of incident data and also studied best practices from the UK fire services based on smoke detector installation and home visits [50].

The intervention consisted of smoke detector installation and home inspections and has been extended for 12 years. Using incident data and including community characteristics related to demographics, income, housing age, and other factors, they targeted neighborhoods. It began in 2008 with a door-to-door campaign by on-duty firefighters. If no one was at home, they left educational materials. In 2009, the program expanded to include home inspections by request (including offers when crews encountered residents at home), and crews began systematically documenting whether smoke detectors in the residence were working when they were out on incidents of all types, and installed detectors when they were missing. Subsequent enhancements to the program included using crime prevention volunteers to distribute literature, and Surrey Fire Service also developed its own cadre of volunteers who not only conducted home visits, but engaged in telemarketing to reinforce safety messaging [50, p. 4].

Surrey was able to achieve a major reduction in fire rate over the 12 years of the program and also doubled the percentage of homes with working smoke detectors from 30% to 60% (Fig. 16.4). Each variation in delivery method was tracked, enabling comparison between approaches. Updated local population estimates and census data were used to adjust targeting throughout the program. The program was

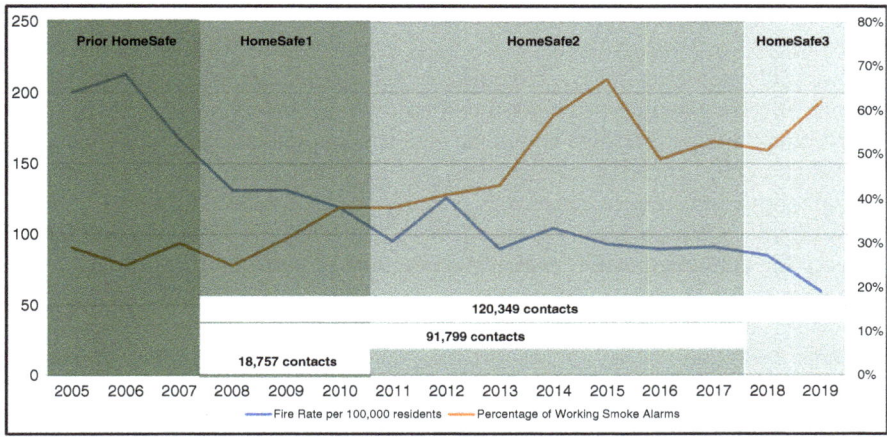

Fig. 16.4 Surrey Fire Service, Fire Rate, and Percent of homes with Working Smoke Detectors 2005–2019

evaluated using a randomized controlled design, the gold standard for social science research [7, 50].

Surrey utilized multiple measures to assess impact of the program. These included:

- City-wide fire rate (decreased).
- Casualty rates (decreased).
- Percentage of working smoke alarms (increased).
- Percentage of fires confined to room of origin (increased).

Their program design, implementation, and evaluation were assisted by partnerships with a local University, a fire researcher, and greatly aided by having an in-house data analyst to manage and oversee the project under direction from the Fire Chiefs. The project was well-accepted by rank and file members of the department, and its results, as well as engagement of the firefighters with the community, were viewed as a point of pride [50].

Many communities operate similar smoke detector distribution campaigns; some funded with grants. Bridgeport, Connecticut, began a smoke detector distribution campaign in 2005, partnering with the local Red Cross Chapter and a government community-service job program. They set up a dedicated phone number for requesting smoke detectors (now expanded to carbon monoxide alarms). Since the program's inception, some 30,000 devices were installed in the City of 144,000 in some 50,000 households. The fire department checks the status of alarms when they are out on incidents and will install them at that time. Installations are performed 7 days per week, and promotional materials including door hangers are available in four languages. The program is credited with alerting 100 residents to evacuate during fires, and additional evaluation is underway [4].

5.1.3 Using Professionals and Advertising Agencies

As we indicated previously, mounting a successful, well-designed campaign requires diverse expertise often not found in fire departments. In addition to grassroots community partnerships within the targeted community, external partnerships for design of the evaluation, data analysis, and design and testing of outreach materials are important areas of concern.

Academic institutions can be an effective resource for identifying specialized support for public education campaigns. Faculty across various disciplines may have expertise in program evaluation, experimental design, marketing, demographic and census analysis, and language skills that may be needed. Identifying such partnerships can make the difference between successful and exemplary programs. Faculty are also likely to have skills in documentation and report writing that will be useful in end-of-project or midterm reviews and evaluations. Disciplines that have played a role in public fire education campaigns include public health, public policy, and statistics or program evaluation programs.

Many academic institutions encourage faculty to be engaged with the community, and some are looking for research projects they can work on or assign students to assist with. A written agreement is best, to set expectations and define roles in the project. The fire service must retain leadership over the effort, and this responsibility cannot be delegated.

Initial design and testing of messages and their presentation and formatting across different media can be a valuable service performed by professionals. While finding a sympathetic local ad agency or person with this expertise, it may be worthwhile to formally pay for such services. Remember that the fire services should be the experts on the fire problem and identifying the specific scenario the program is intended to target.

5.2 Implementation

5.2.1 High-Quality Research and Evaluations

A number of high-quality evaluations of public fire education campaigns have been done over the years. These evaluations have used rigorous methods and observed measurable changes in behavior and losses in numerous settings. They have included smoke detector distribution campaigns alone or as part of broader campaigns [14, 29, 30]; general fire safety injury prevention [27, 28] and some have specifically evaluated interventions led by firefighters [8, 48]. Some are nationally led interventions and evaluations of multiple programs delivered locally, such as the case of an evaluation of both fire and injury prevention [37].

Importantly, DiGuiseppi and collaborators using a cluster randomized controlled trial design found that merely distributing smoke detectors may not be effective in reducing injuries, and that they should be installed as part of the intervention in order to be effective [13]. Another study found that some dwelling residents who received enhanced training along with smoke detector installation had a higher likelihood of maintaining the operational status after 1–3 years following the intervention [19].

Other studies examine characteristics of smoke detector owners and the dwellings they inhabit. These have included national-level studies, such as those done in England [16], and locally based efforts that were tied to local education campaigns [26, 35, 45]. Some studies have focused specifically on selected demographic groups [5, 33] or emphasized methodologies for analysis [15]. Still other evaluations focused on interventions in specific building types, such as high-rise buildings [40].

Systematic reviews have found mixed evidence in several settings. Many reviews found that there were methodological limitations that made interpreting findings difficult. (DiGuiseppi & Higgins, Systematic review of controlled trials of interventions to promote smoke alarms, [12]).

In 2019, a systematic review and meta-analysis of home fire safety programs found that more, larger, and high-quality studies were needed, but that the evidence presented supported the use of home fire safety knowledge and behavior [43]. Their study did not evaluate community-wide programs, but focused only on education programs.

A recent international evaluation of risk factors for residential fire casualties was undertaken with an emphasis on low and middle-income countries, where comparatively less research is undertaken. Nonetheless, the review supported identification of risk factors and areas of intervention that may be effective [44].

5.2.2 Something Is Better Than Nothing

However, each program does not have to be documented in a peer-reviewed scholarly publication. Reports published in trade publications or filed with libraries are very helpful for identifying best practices, as well as documenting the investment of time and resources as well as results in a given community.

Designing a program can be a challenge for smaller agencies. The inability to design an exemplary program should not stop agencies from pursuing their own public education campaign. Basic analysis of incident data, or analyses done in similar nearby communities may suffice to help target efforts.

The goal is to have an intervention where both outreach effort and end results can be measured.

Measures of effectiveness of fire education campaigns – ranked from simplest to most powerful can include [42]:

1. Outreach – distributing educational materials widely.
2. Knowledge gain or refresh – document acquiring information.
3. Behavior change or maintenance – information gained is shown to affect behavior.

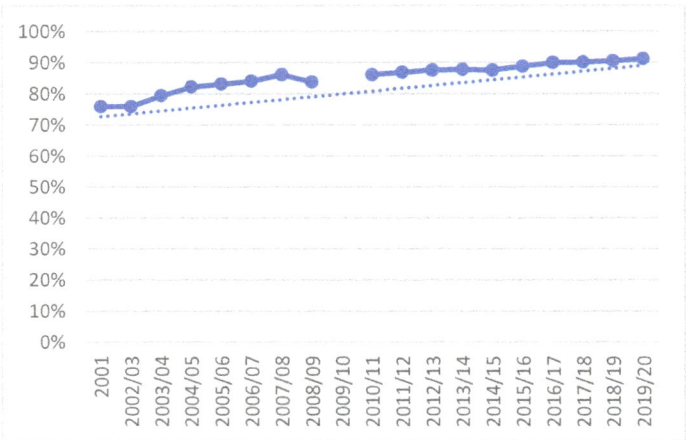

Fig. 16.5 Percentage of Households with working smoke alarms, England and Wales. (Source: https://assets.publishing.service.gov.uk/government/uploads/system/uploads/attachment_data/file/960052/fire-statistics-data-tables-fire0701-110221.xlsx)

4. Environmental change – actions taken to improve the safety of the environment (see Fig. 16.5). An increasing percentage of homes with working smoke detectors is an important measure of environmental change.
5. End impact – measurable change in loss or incidence, attributable to the effort. Source: *Proving Public Fire Education Works.*

5.3 Using National/Regional Campaigns Versus Custom Campaigns

National fire safety education campaigns can have advantages which were discussed previously, but they still require validation that their subject is a concern in the local setting, and that the vulnerable population can be adequately targeted. As national campaigns may rotate topics for year to year, it may be wise to continue a campaign rather than adopt a different message annually based on a national analysis of fire losses. Materials geared to a national audience may need to be adapted to be suitable for a local program.

5.4 Reaching the "Hard to Reach"

Although the term is itself controversial, many elements of society most vulnerable to fires are those that may be marginalized or have limited access to resources and information sources taken for granted by the mainstream population. Reaching such groups takes special attention and increasingly engages people using influencers and social media [22]. Such basic steps as having materials translated into appropriate languages are important, and many metropolitan fire services engage in such efforts. These efforts are formidable, and languages needs can change with migration patterns (Figs. 16.6 and 16.7).

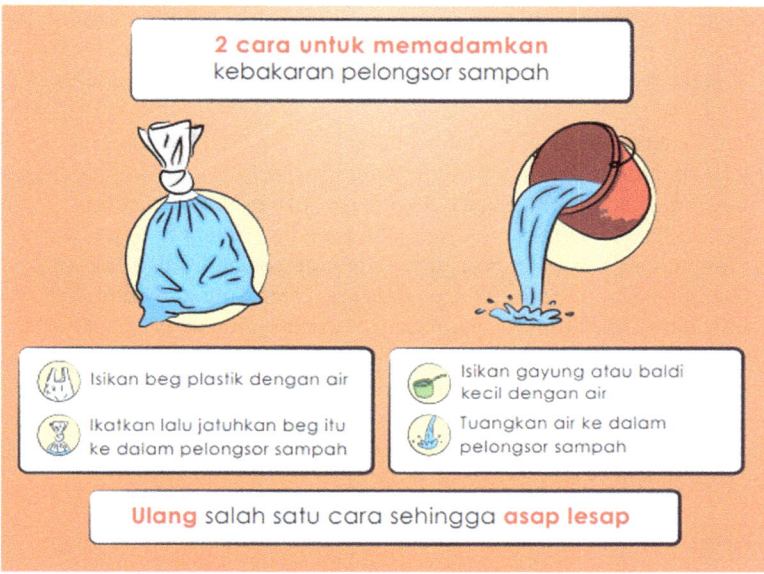

Fig. 16.6 Singapore Civil Defense Force Trash Chute Safety poster (Malay) [46]

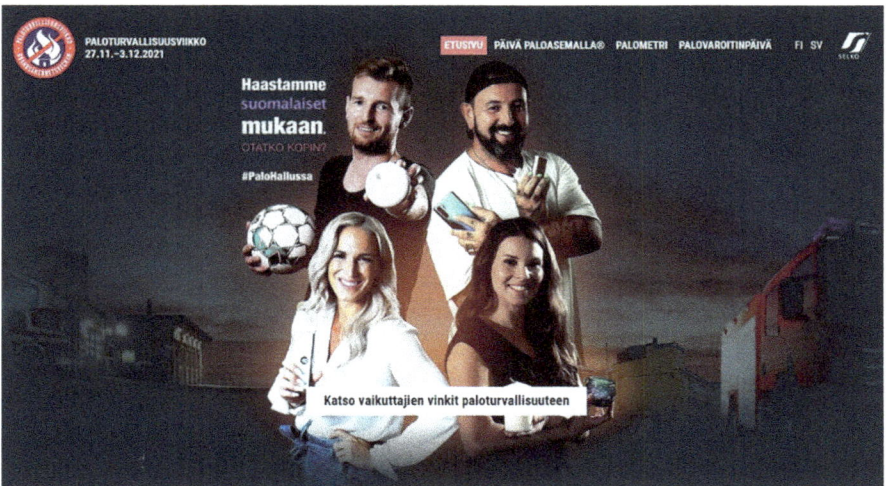

Fig. 16.7 Excerpt of Smoke Alarm Promotion Webpage (Finland) [18]

6 The Future of Social Marketing/Safety Campaigns

Our traditional conception of public education marketing is rooted in face-to-face communication and analog media (posters, flyers, and door hangers). The advertising and social marketing space is increasingly moving to more digital media, as people communicate through cell phones, streaming media, and other channels [1]. This domain is adapting rapidly, and navigating choice about where and how to engage, as well as measure impact, is a specialized area that will require the expertise of an advertising or marketing agency, especially in light of increasing privacy protections [34].

One of the advantages of digital advertising is the ability to potentially identify the target populations in ways that are more precise than can be done with aggregated census data at present. Such outreach can also enable immediate engagement and gathering details on those reached with little investment in a field force of personnel going door-to-door. Importantly, follow-up contact is also possible.

Utilization of digital devices for consuming advertising and outreach varies, but they can be a preferred tool for outreach to certain segments of the "hard to reach" population [2]. Modern advertising campaigns use "multi-touch" approaches, in which multiple formats ad channels are used to reinforce the message. This may include social media, direct mail, email, web sites, and customized web pages tailored to the campaign. Because of the evolving nature of this field, it is recommended that an advertising expert be retained.

7 Conclusion

Fire safety education campaigns have demonstrated success in reducing the toll of fires. Despite emergence of good guidance materials for local fire services, effective, documented programs remain the exception rather than the rule. A shortage of well-documented programs has limited adoption of best practices. A highly decentralized fire service, as found in the United States, also creates additional challenges.

Guidance documents for design of programs exist and are readily available. Nationally directed or regional efforts tend to be better designed, and significant results in terms of driving down fires and deaths were documented in multiple settings. The use of advertising, social media, and best practices in social marketing is evolving with the changing media landscape and offers new opportunities to deliver messages, with a trade-off of greater complexity and need for expertise.

Partnership with academic institutions can be an effective way to acquire capacity for design of measurable programs and can also develop institutional capacity to sustain programs. Documenting and reporting results of public education campaigns is important to develop best practices and to justify resources committed to these programs at the agency level.

References

1. Abromovich G (2021) 15 mind-blowing stats about the future of advertising. Retrieved from Adobe https://www.adobe.com/kr/insights/15-mind-blowing-stats-about-the-future-of-advertising.html
2. Anderson M (2015) Racial and ethnic differences in how people sue mobile technology. Pew Research Center, Washington, DC
3. Beever P (2012) Measuring requirements: quantifying safety from fire. Retrieved from http://static1.1.sqspcdn.com/static/f/1017378/21233282/1355204466473/FA12-Paula_Beever_Final.pdf?token=Y1Z%2B4kpxrjcdZJ7dhz%2B4%2Fgdf6N4%3D
4. Bridgeport Fire Department (2021) Personal communication
5. Cassidy P, McConnell N, Boyce K (2021) The older adult: associated fire risks and current challenges for the development of future fire safety intervention strategies. Fire Mater 45:553–563
6. Centers for DIsease Control (2014) What works: health communication and social marketing. Centers for Disease Control, Atlanta. Retrieved from http://stacks.cdc.gov/view/cdc/25836/cdc_25836_DS1.pdf
7. Clare JL (2012) Reduced frequency and severity of residential fires following delivery of fire prevention education by on-duty firefighters: cluster randomized controlled study. J Saf Res 43(2):123–128
8. Clare J, Garis L, Plecas D, Jennings C (2012) Reduced frequency and severity of residential fires following delivery of fire prevention education by on-duty firefighters: cluster randomized controlled study. J Saf Res 43(2):123–128
9. Crawford J (2015) Comprehensive prevention programs (Vol. Manging fire and emergency services). In: Jennings AT (ed). International City/County Management Association, Washington, DC
10. Department of Communities and Local Government (2010) Evaluation options for fire and rescue services fire safety activities. Department of Communities and Local Government, London
11. Department of Emergency Services (1998) Fire fatalities: who's at risk? Department of Emergency Services, Kedron
12. DiGuiseppi C, Higgins JP (2000) Systematic review of controlled trials of interventions to promote smoke alarms. Arch Dis Child 82(5):341–348
13. DiGuiseppi C, Roberts I, Wade A, Schulper M, Edwards P, Godward C et al (2002) Incidence of fires and related injuries after giving out free smoke alarms: cluster randomised controlled trial. BMJ Br Med J 325(7371):995–997
14. Douglas M, Mallonee S, Istre G (1998) Comparison of community based smoke detector distribution methods in an urban community. Inj Prev 4:28–32
15. Dudley T, Creppage K, Shanahan M, Proescholdbell S (2013) Using GIS to evaluate a fire safety program in North Carolina. J Commnunity Health 38:951–957
16. English Housing Survey (2015) Smoke alarms in English housing 2014/2015. Department for Communities and Local Government, London
17. Evans PE (1913) Official record of the first American national fire prevention convention. Philadelphia. Retrieved from https://catalog.hathitrust.org/Record/006605110
18. Finnish Rescue Association (2021) Smoke alarm day. Retrieved from PALOTURVALLISUUSVIIKKO https://paloturvallisuusviikko.fi/
19. Gielen AC, Sheppard M (2014) Increasing smoke alarm operability through theory-based health education: a randomised trial. J Epidemiol Community Health 68(12):1168–1174
20. Gilbert SW (2021) Estimating smoke alarm effectiveness in homes. Fire Technol 57:1497–1516
21. Goetz BJ (1991) The American fire service and the state. University of California, Berkeley, Berkeley
22. Guo M, Ganz O, Cruse B, Navarro M, Wagner D, Tate B et al (2020) Keeping it fresh with hip-hop teens: promising targeting strategies for delivering public health messages to hard-to-reach audiences. Health Promot Pract 21(1_Suppl):61S–71S

23. Hensler B (2011) Crucible of fire. Potomac Books, Dulles
24. Institution of Fire Engineers (USA Branch) (2008) Vision 20/20: National Strategies for Fire Loss Prevention. Alexandria. Retrieved June 2021 from https://strategicfire.org/wp-content/uploads/2016/08/v2020-2008-report.pdf
25. Jennings C (2015) Evaluating and managing local risks. In: Thiel A, Jennings CR, Jennings AT (eds) Managing fire and emergency services. International City/County Management Association, Washington, DC
26. Jones AR, Thompson C, Davis MK (2001) Smoke alarm ownership and installation: a comparison of a rural and suburban community in Georgia. J Community Health 26(5):307–329
27. Lehna C, Twyman S, Fahey E, Coty M-B, Williams J, Scrivener D et al (2017) An organizational process for promoting home fire safety in two community settings. Burns 43(1):162–168
28. Mallonee S, Istre G, Rosenberg M, Reddish-Douglas M, Jordan F, Silverstein P, Tunell W (1996) Surveillance and prevention of residential fire injuries. N Engl J Med 335(1):27–31
29. McConnell C, Dwyer WO, Leeming F (1996) A behavioral approach to reducing fires in public housing. J Community Psychol 24:201–212
30. Mickalide A, Validzic A (1999) Smoke alarm maintenance in low-income families. Am J Public Health 89(10):1584–1585
31. National Fallen Firefighters Foundation (2019) 17th annual President Harry S. Truman Legacy symposium and the President Truman Fire Forum. National Fallen Firefighters Foundation, Emmetsburg. Retrieved from https://www.everyonegoeshome.com/wp-content/uploads/sites/2/2019/12/2019-Truman-Report-FINAL-022120.pdf
32. National Fire Protection Association (2005) NFPA 1035 professional qualifications for public fire and life safety educator. National Fire Protection Association, Quincy
33. New South Wales Fire and Rescue (2021) Evaluation report: FRNSW's fire safety education programs for children. New South Wales Government, Sydney
34. Nielsen Company (2020) Era of adaptation: forward-thinking strategies for brands of all sizes. Nielsen Company (US) LLC
35. Nilson F, Bonander C (2020) Household fire protection practices in relation to sociodemographic characteristics: evidence from a Swedish National Survey. Fire Technol 56:1077–1098
36. Presidio of Monterey Fire Department (2011) Presidio recognizes fire prevention week Oct. 9–15. Retrieved from US Army https://www.army.mil/article/66776/presidio_recognizes_fire_prevention_week_oct_9_15
37. Public Health England (2016) Evaluation of the impact of Fire and Rescue Service interventions in reducing the harm to vulnerable groups of people from winter-related illnesses. London, England
38. Red Cross (2021) Take action to prevent home fires. Retrieved from Red Cross https://www.redcross.org/get-help/how-to-prepare-for-emergencies/types-of-emergencies/fire/prevent-home-fire.html
39. Rossomando C (1995) The community-based fire safety education handbook. National Association of State Fire Marshals, Washington, DC
40. Safer Scotland (2020) High rise fire safety leaflet 2019/2020 evaluation report. Scottish Government, Edinburgh
41. Schaenman P (2015) Line firefighter attitudes towards fire prevention. Vision 20/20, Warrenton
42. Schaenman P, Stambaugh H, Rossoamando C, Jennings C, Perroni C (1990) Proving public fire education works. TriData Corporation, Arlington
43. Senthilkumaran M, Nazari G, MacDermid J, Roche KS (2019) Effectiveness of home fire safety interventions. A systematic review and meta-analysis. PLoS ONE 14(5):1–17
44. Shokoubi M, Nasirani K, Cheraghi Z, Ardalan A, Knankeh H, Fallahzadeh H, Khourasani-Zavareh D (2019) Preventive measures for fire-related injuries and their risk factors in residential buildings: a systematic review. J Inj Violence Res 11(1):1–14

45. Sidman EA, Grossman DC, Mueller BA (2011) Comprehensive smoke alarm coverage in lower economic status homes: alarm presence, functionality, and placement. J Community Health 36(4):525–533
46. Singapore Civil Defense Force (2021) Publications. Retrieved from Singapore Civil Defense Force https://www.scdf.gov.sg/docs/default-source/scdf-library/publications/publications/chuteflyer_malay%2D%2D-120517.pdf
47. Stamps JE (1980) Public fire education planning. A five step process. Federal Emergency Management Agency, Washington, DC. Retrieved 2021 from https://files.eric.ed.gov/fulltext/ED226184.pdf
48. Sund B, Bonader C, Jakobsson N, Jaldell H (2019) Do home fire and safety checks by on-duty firefighters decrease the number of fires? Quasi-experimental evidence from Sweden. J Saf Res 70:39–47
49. Swedish Rescue Services Agency (n.d.) Prevention of fires and other incidents: report and recommendations. Karlstadt. Retrieved from https://ec.europa.eu/echo/files/civil_protection/civil/prote/pdfdocs/fire_prevention.pdf
50. Thomas L, Garis L, Morris S, Biantoro C (2020) Journey of HomeSafe: community risk reduction in Surrey. University of the Fraser Valley, Abbotsford. Retrieved from https://cjr.ufv.ca/journey-of-homesafe-community-risk-reduction-in-surrey/
51. Tokyo Fire Service (2021) Annual report 2020. Retrieved from Tokyo Fire Department Multilingual Page https://www.tfd.metro.tokyo.lg.jp/hp-soumuka/gyouseigaiyou_e/data/annual_report_2020_04.pdf
52. TriData Corporation (2007) Global concepts in residential fire safety part 1—best practices from England, Scotland, Sweden, and Norway. TriData Corporation, Arlington. Retrieved from https://www.maine.gov/dps/fmo/sites/maine.gov.dps.fmo/files/inline-files/research/documents/global_concepts_1.pdf
53. TriData Corporation (2008) Global concepts in residential fire safety part 2—best practices from Australia, New Zealand and Japan. Arlington. Retrieved from State of Maine, Department of Public Safety https://www.maine.gov/dps/fmo/sites/maine.gov.dps.fmo/files/inline-files/research/documents/global_concepts_2.pdf
54. United States Fire Administration (2008) Public fire education planning: a five step process, vol FA-219. United States Fire Administration, Emmetsburg
55. US Fire Administration and Centers for Disease Control (n.d.) Fire safety program toolkit: a comprehensive resource for fire safety educators. US Fire Administration, Emmetsburg. Retrieved from https://www.usfa.fema.gov/downloads/pdf/publications/fire_safety_program_toolkit.pdf
56. Vision 20/20 (2021) Building CRR acceptance. Retrieved from Community Risk Assessment, A Guide for Conducting Community Risk Assessment http://riskreduction.strategicfire.org/implement-crr-plan/building-crr-acceptance/
57. Walker B (2021) Community risk reduction principles and practices. Jones and Bartlett, Burlington

Dr. Charles Jennings is Associate Professor in the Department of Security, Fire, and Emergency Management at John Jay College of Criminal Justice (CUNY), where he also directs the Christian Regenhard Center for Emergency Response Studies (RaCERS). He has conducted research in community-level fire risk, fire service deployment, tall buildings, and situation awareness in complex emergencies. He has done post-incident analysis and investigations of major incidents. He is a credentialed Chief Fire Officer and has served in operational and administrative roles in fire, Emergency Medical Services (EMS), emergency management, and police organizations.

Chapter 17
Targeted Interventions Towards Risk Groups

Johanna Gustavsson, Gunilla Carlsson, and Margaret S. McNamee

Abstract For a majority of individuals, either severely injured or deceased in residential fires, individual and environmental factors that increase risk are identifiable. Therefore, in order to further reduce injury, there is a need for fire safety programmes that target these individuals and groups. This chapter aims to shed light on how vulnerability to residential fires can be understood and present the basic assumptions for designing programmes targeting these individuals and groups. The problem is complex, requiring knowledge from several fields, and inspiration is drawn from public health, injury prevention and engineering. The chapter presents previous research on the topic, cases that exemplify implementation and the main barriers and facilitators for implementations.

Keywords Vulnerable · Disabilities · Older adults · Individualised fire safety · Residential fire · Implementation

It is apparent from section 1 that certain groups, especially older adults and people with alcohol/drug abuse problems, have a disproportionate risk of dying in fires. How can interventions be targeted towards these groups? Are there any good examples of successful interventions in relation to these groups?

J. Gustavsson (✉)
Risk and Environmental Studies, Centre for Societal Risk Research, Karlstad University, Karlstad, Sweden
e-mail: johanna.gustavsson@kau.se

G. Carlsson
Health Sciences Centre (HSC), Department of Health Sciences, Faculty of Medicine, Lund University, Lund, Sweden

M. S. McNamee
Division of Fire Safety Engineering, Faculty of Engineering, Lund University, Lund, Sweden

1 Individuals with Increased Risk

The risk of injury in residential fires is unevenly distributed in the population, with individuals that can be described as vulnerable found to be over-represented in fire fatalities [5, 12, 24] (see Chap. 2 for further descriptions). There has been a steady decrease of fire fatalities in the developed world over the past decades, and the numbers are now historically low at the level of 5–10 cases/million inhabitants in many developed countries [1, 16, 25]. However, it appears that the downward trend in recent years has reached a plateau and that the decline in fire fatalities has not affected all population groups equally [17]. Thus, while measures of fire protection directed towards the general population are still useful, recent research emphasises that in order to further reduce fatalities, individuals with identified risk factors need to be prioritised in fire prevention [7, 28, 38, 42].

1.1 Determinants of Health

Human behaviour and health are complex and need to be understood from various perspectives. Scientific fields, like sociology, psychology and public health, present models that strive to explain factors that influence individuals' health, so-called determinants of health. The World Health Organisation (WHO) includes the social, economic and physical environment together with an individual's characteristics and behaviours in the determinants of health [41]. By mapping these variables in more detail, we can describe individuals with increased risk for injury or illness and design prevention accordingly. By tailoring preventative action to individual needs, the impact of the prevention is expected to the greater.

The determinants of health, or in the case of residential fires, the risk factors for injury, can be divided into two broad categories that interact with each other: **individual and environmental**, see Table 17.1. Depending on the focus, theoretical models categorise the individual or the population in different ways. The World Health Organization defines *personal factor*s as well as *health and health-related*

Table 17.1 Examples of determinants of health

Individual determinants of health		Environmental determinants of health	
Personal factors	Health and health-related domains	Individual	Societal
Gender Age Lifestyle Habits	Disease Disability Body functions Activity and participation	Living conditions Economic means Family Social network	Support functions, e.g. home care Policy and regulations Economic support

domains as aspects of the individual, in the International Classification of functioning, disability and health (ICF) [40]. The **personal factors** are individual characteristics such as gender, age, lifestyle and habits, which may play a role in the individual's life and affect health and well-being. For example, a person knows that smoking has a negative impact on health, but he or she still might want to continue, because it is part of his or her habits and lifestyle. **Health and health-related domains** include negative aspects such as the prevalence of diseases and disability, but also the positive aspects of functioning in terms of body functions, activities and participation, i.e. what people need or want to do.

Over the course of a life span, the personal factors and health conditions vary, which means that people's risk for injury varies. For example, children develop their physical and cognitive capacities to handle different situations as they grow up. For older adults, the natural degenerative processes might increase the risk for hazardous situations, but above all multimorbidity and impairments place the individuals in vulnerable situations. However, people of all ages can have physical and cognitive impairments, which can be of a more or less permanent nature like acute illness, paralysis, psychiatric symptoms or situational challenges due to intoxication.

The **environmental factors** are associated with a person's living conditions at an individual level, but also at a societal level in terms of formal and informal social structures, services and overarching approaches or systems that have an impact on individuals. The social dimension, including support and relationships, is of utmost importance, where a functioning social network can compensate for individual shortcomings. The economic dimension is another environmental factor, where lack of economic means can increase risk, e.g. lacking means to buy safety equipment or to keep the house in good condition can impact the individual risk. Environmental factors also refer to people's physical surroundings, the natural as well as the built environment [40]. The built physical environment seldom plays a central role in health models, but has a great impact on the risk of injury in residential fires.

> *A common source of for fires causing human injury is cigarettes. Thus, while might not necessarily be a significant risk factor in terms of fire for a healthy person that is well equipped to handle an situation, becomes a significant risk when combined with factors that lower the person's capacity to handle the situation.*

Considering all these factors, and how they interplay, gives us a deeper understanding of the variety in the risk of severe injury outcomes in residential fires, but also how the risks can vary within different groups. A combination of risk factors over an extended period of time can result in a very limited ability to prevent or mitigate risky situations.

Risk factors for fire fatalities are well described, with older adults as the most well-defined risk group [13, 15, 24, 35], an increasing problem given the predictions of an ageing society [32]. Risk factors that have been identified for older adults can be summarised in terms of three main factors; first, a decreased ability to prevent a fire incident; second, a reduced ability to respond to a fire incident and, lastly, a reduced ability to remove themselves from the fire scene. These circumstances exacerbate the situation leading to a fatality [43], and technical systems designed to reduce the risk of fires are compromised due to the natural physical and psychological decline associated with ageing. For example, there are indications that traditional domestic smoke alarms may have reduced efficacy in this group due to impaired hearing [31, 34]. Technical systems can also fail due to misconceptions regarding installation of the system or where the risk might be most likely to manifest itself. After investigating fatality cases among older adults, Cassidy et al. [8] concluded that a smoke alarm was often in place, but not ideally positioned. They suggest that smoke alarms should be placed in the bedroom and living room, as these rooms often are the rooms of ignition.

2 Individualised Fire Prevention Interventions

2.1 Models for Prevention and Promotion

When the field of injury prevention started to emerge, inspiration was drawn from the medical field where measures to promote health and prevent illness have a long history [37]. The assumption that health is not merely the absence of disease or infirmity, but a state of complete physical, mental and social well-being [39], highlights the fact that objective measures are not the only ones of interest, but that the individual's subjective experience is also important in injury prevention.

Prevention and promotion are closely related. **Promotion** refers to increasing a person's ability; in this case, the ability to handle an adverse event. If we think about the individual determinants of health, described in the previous section, some of these factors are modifiable, e.g. habits can change and aids can mitigate a disability. **Prevention,** on the other hand, refers to hindering or moderating the adverse event and its outcomes; in this case, an event with negative health consequences. This relates to the environmental determinants of health where individual and societal aspects can be strengthened. Thus, prevention and promotion are complementary approaches where the desired outcome for both strategies is to increase human health and well-being and to hinder injury and/or illness. Note that prevention is often presented in three stages, primary (before), secondary (during) and tertiary (after), which in the field of injury prevention is often referred to simply as before – during – after.

Traditionally, fire safety engineering has focused more on the environmental factors in terms of technical or technological fire protection rather than interventions directed to specific individuals and their characteristics. Information campaigns are a common intervention when the individuals are addressed, while the use of fire-resistant clothing or the installation of sprinklers represents technical fire protection.

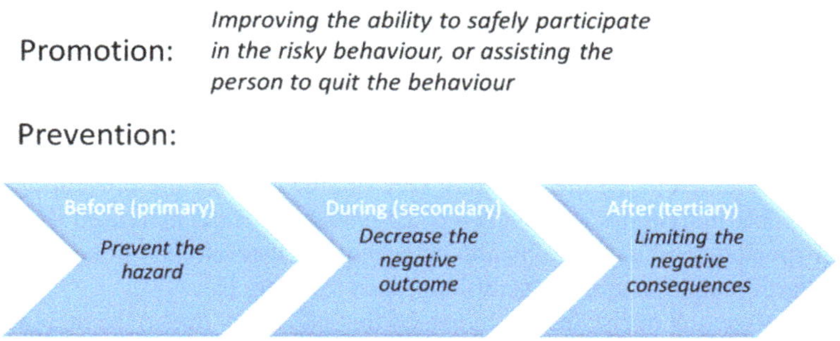

Promotion: *Improving the ability to safely participate in the risky behaviour, or assisting the person to quit the behaviour*

Prevention:

- Before (primary): Prevent the hazard
- During (secondary): Decrease the negative outcome
- After (tertiary): Limiting the negative consequences

Fig. 17.1 Application of promotion and prevention strategies to the scenario of mitigating the fire risk associated with smoking for individuals at risk. Inspired by Andersson [2], Tulchinsky and Varavikova [37]

Let us apply the concept of promotion and prevention to the scenario of a person dropping a cigarette. Prevention and promotion strategies could be illustrated as follows (see also Fig. 17.1): **Promotion** would mean striving to improve the ability to safely use the smoking device. For this to be possible, we need to know what is causing the inability to smoke safely, e.g. illness, intoxication, disability and analyse whether this can be altered in some way, perhaps by assisting the smoker to quit. **Primary prevention** entails preventing the hazardous situation from occurring. For a fire, this could be to remove the source of ignition, in this case, the cigarette. Another solution could be to alter the cigarette in order to decrease the risk, such as switching to an e-cigarette. **Secondary prevention** refers to decreasing the negative outcome during an adverse event. If the person has dropped the cigarette and the fire has, or is about to, occur, a way of preventing injury could be to use ignition-resistant materials and/or devices such as self-extinguishing "fire-safe" cigarettes (see Chap. 10 for further description). In the case of **tertiary prevention,** we strive to limit the negative consequences of the event, through adequate medical care and rehabilitation; relevant measures depend on the severity of the injury.

This example demonstrates how personal and environmental factors interact in the individual situation and must be addressed in order to reduce the risk. Active interventions, which can often be used before the event, include choosing to change risky behaviour, replacing risky material and using suppression systems such as sprinklers; passive interventions must be made before the event, but work during the event includes the choice of ignition-resistant material.

2.2 Targeting Vulnerable Individuals and Groups

The decrease in residential fire fatalities can be attributed to different fire safety improvements, like smoke alarms, as well as to societal changes, with fewer people smoking; but certain vulnerable groups are overrepresented in the fire fatalities that occur. Even though basic general fire protection measures benefit vulnerable groups, interventions need to specifically target vulnerable groups and individuals [18], e.g. people who are unable to react to alarms or who engage in risky smoking behaviour. Cassidy et al. [8], based on data from Northern Ireland, showed that most fire fatalities involving older adults had working smoking alarms; nonetheless, older adults are overrepresented in the fire statistics. Overall, the goal for fire prevention targeting vulnerable individuals or groups is to compensate for the increased risk created by their specific combination of health determinants, theoretically linked to the concept of harm reduction and a systems approach to safety [6].

The combination of risk factors increases the risk, either due to the increased risk of starting a fire, or to increased difficulty in responding to the fire. These are the two starting points for designing interventions; either to prevent the fire from occurring, or to increase the ability to respond to the situation.

> *Imagine a person, living alone, unable to handle ordinary daily situations due to disability or substance abuse and a fire breaks out. What are their options for preventing injury? Essentially two – fire extinction or assisted rescue/. In this case, we are already beyond the phase of promotion and the different levels of prevention are key to facilitating the prevention of injury. Rapid response through active or passive systems and alarm of personnel to assist in rescue and recovery must be facilitated through primary, secondary and tertiary prevention.*

Another way of thinking about how risk can be mitigated is presented in Fig. 17.2. The risk appears in the intersection of individual factors, the activity performed and the environment, here sketched as a triangle perched on its apex. Certain individual factors such as age or gender cannot be changed; assuming that the activity itself is

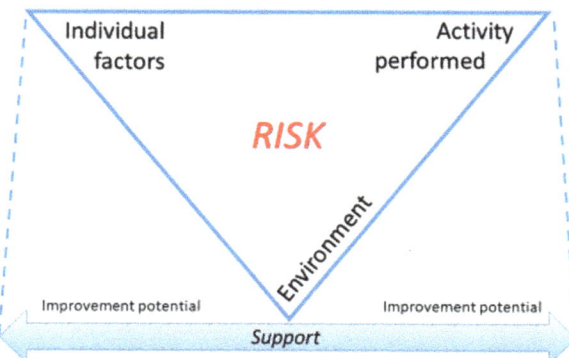

Fig. 17.2 Model for mitigation of risk through the implementation of support systems designed to improve the system stability by broadening the base of the triangle

also not changed, environmental factors become critical. Such environmental factors can be adjusted to mitigate the individual factors and activity performed, e.g. individual habits, prevalence of disability and other determinants of health, which might be changed. In other words, the individual performs various everyday activities, e.g. brewing coffee, cooking and smoking. These activities can be adapted to decrease the risk of injury, e.g. by using another strategy, smoking outside instead of inside the home, or adapting the environmental features, using e-cigarettes instead of incendiary cigarettes. However, an unwanted consequence might be that the value of the activity also changes for the individual due to these changes [14], thereby reducing its value to the individual.

The activities occur in an environment that is more or less supportive. Examples of a supportive environment are reduced presence of flammable material and the installation of a stove guard in the kitchen or a timer on the coffee machine. A stove guard or a timer for the coffee machine might not be necessary for many people, but provide critical support for others. For a person with cognitive decline, these environmental details might be necessary to decrease the risk of fire and associated injury. Figure 17.2 exemplifies how the implementation of mitigation strategies can provide additional support that compensates for individual shortcomings, adding stability to the original risk triangle by broadening the base.

2.3 Intervention Programmes

This section describes the proposed and tested interventions for fire prevention, targeting individuals with heightened risk, which have been presented in the scientific literature. The interventions all include versions of the following three phases: identification of risk groups or individuals, risk assessment and evaluation of needs for fire safety measures. Most intervention programmes include some form of preventative home visit as part of the identification phase. The visits may have a variety of structures and content, but all contain elements of seeking out vulnerable individuals and evaluating the needs for preventative measures. General home visits or canvassing campaigns, which target a broader and more general population, differ from targeted campaigns which approach individuals identified as "at risk" from the outset. In canvassing drives, campaigners knock on doors and offer information and risk evaluations to all who answer, independent of apparent risk. However, there is an overlap between the methods, as canvassing campaigns will identify specifically at-risk individuals and home visits for vulnerable groups can be directed to both at-risk individuals and at-risk communities, where the latter is similar to a canvassing campaign. Thus, while home visits can be effectively targeted at households judged to be at most risk, resources directed to community awareness can help identify these individuals, and information sent to many will also reach at-risk individuals.

In the first step, to detect individuals or households at risk, different registers can be helpful. Arch and Thurston [3] used the general practice registers to detect those older than 65 years of age who might have a heightened risk, such as individuals living alone. One method which has been proposed to identify high-risk communities is through fire incidence rates [9] and household income in a geographical area [4]. It should be noted, however, that it is not clear that areas with the highest number of fires are necessarily those that have the highest number of fire deaths. Nilson and Bonander [30] found that fires occur most often in middle-class households, while these are not those fires that most often result in fatalities or serious injury. Tillett [36] describes another example of how to systematically identify vulnerable communities based on including the proportion of children 14 and under, adults 65 and over, persons with a disability, black and Hispanic populations combined into one minority category, the under-educated, families below the poverty line and the number of multifamily housing structures. These variables were found to be reliable from a US perspective, but it is uncertain whether they are relevant in other national contexts. Regarding the identification of older adults at risk, Cassidy et al. [8] showed that 86% of fire fatalities in this group had regular contact with a person who could have identified the risk. This person was a relative, social worker or health care staff who could be a resource in the preventative work.

The next two steps, risk assessment and evaluation of fire protection needs, are less well described in the literature. In Sweden, the Swedish Civil Contingencies Agency (MSB), the agency responsible for issuing guidance concerning fire emergency management, has provided guidelines for individualised fire safety (IFS) [29]. The guideline suggests ways of assessing risk and needs, including risky behaviour and lack of a serviceable smoke alarm. In this phase, the importance of collecting consent and respecting personal integrity is also emphasised [29]. The importance of contextualisation of interventions is emphasised in the guidelines from MSB, but a methodology recommended by MSB typically includes contact between the municipality and the individual (perhaps through social services or the fire and rescue services (FRS)), assessment of IFS needs, implementation of support, documentation of support, annual review and re-evaluation coupled to potential updates to the IFS needs and support [20].

Applying a social science approach to fire prevention can contribute new perspectives [21]. Gjøsund [19] describe preventing fire for vulnerable groups as a 'wicked problem', i.e. (1) there are challenges that transcend sectoral boundaries; and (2) they span several public agencies, thereby involving different areas of policy across several political-administrative levels [22]. This creates multi-organisational challenges since many barriers or measures are the responsibility of more than one stakeholder. To mitigate this, the institution of one central contact person, who specialises in fire prevention among vulnerable groups, is recommended. Further, it is suggested that the local FRS are ideal partners for implementation [9], but that it can be useful to involve other local actors and volunteers [4].

There are inherent methodological challenges to evaluating community interventions, including economic, ethical and practical aspects [33]. Further, secular trends and general societal changes need to be taken into consideration. Regarding the efficiency of the interventions mentioned here, the results are inconclusive. When evaluating multifaceted programmes, it is difficult to determine causality with regard to which components of the programme were effective. Media and community education showed little benefit in non-randomised trials [11]; smoke alarm installation is included in most programmes [3, 4, 9, 23] and could potentially be the effective component, but we simply do not know for sure. Further, there are signs that individual visits have an initial positive effect and that the effect tends to decrease over time [23]. Indeed, Breslin et al. [7] suggest that repeated visits might be needed. In this chapter, examples and suggestions of how to design prevention programmes are presented. Nonetheless, the effectiveness of fire community risk reduction programmes needs to be further evaluated [18].

2.4 Case Description

Two examples have been selected to exemplify the process of how municipalities in Sweden have chosen to work with and implemented IFS. No single method has been chosen across the board, and as the municipalities themselves are varied, so must the approach be. The first case represents a small municipality which has used home care to leverage expertise in the FRS to evaluate fire risk and develop IFS interventions. The second case represents one of the largest municipalities in Sweden, which has chosen a more general approach with the aim of reaching many, while at the same time identifying those most at risk.

During 2017, a study conducted by the FRS in Northwestern Skåne, a region in the south of Sweden, concluded that 90% of all fire fatalities occur in dwellings and that a number of risk groups, in particular elderly people, are overrepresented among these fatalities. As many of these older individuals particularly at risk for fire fatalities are in contact with local home care providers, a collaboration was initiated between the FRS and home care workers to provide IFS for these citizens. In 2018, a project focusing on one of the smaller municipalities in the region was started to identify the needs of older individuals receiving care in their homes, and where possible to meet those needs through adaptation of the home environment to improve fire safety. The project resulted in education of home care personnel in fire risk assessment of dwellings, the development of a checklist on fire risks which can be used to re-evaluate risk on an annual basis (synchronously with other health evaluations), and the development of a process for evaluating and funding adaptation of private dwellings to improve individual safety. Further, a decision was taken to include fire alarm features in all personal alarm services for older persons in the community. The project was seen to be a resounding success and its expansion is planned to neighbouring municipalities.

The situation for a small municipality is significantly different to that of a large municipality. The number of individuals in risk groups and the scale of home care is significantly larger in a large municipality. The potential to reach more individuals is higher, but the organisational threshold to make decisions concerning changes in routines is also significantly higher. In the case of one of the largest municipalities in Sweden, the approach has been more generalised with a focus on the provision of information and offer of assistance. In the case of individuals with home care, a checklist has been developed with four simple questions to evaluate whether individuals require specialised fire protection. Information concerning the checklist is available through the fire service website but requires active retrieval from the home care providers and is optional rather than incorporated into the annual routine. Further, for individuals who do not receive home care, fire risks are identified only after a fire incident. In this case, a personal letter will be sent to the individual offering support to improve fire safety. There is no follow-up concerning the letter should the individual not choose to contact the fire service as offered. A variety of activities have been attempted in the region where this fire service is active, but it is difficult to maintain momentum when the organisation is geographically distributed and the hierarchical structure is complicated making changes to routines difficult.

3   Implementation Barriers and Facilitators

In the beginning of this chapter, we establish the complexity of IFS. The process of implementation is no exception and, as several barriers have been identified, reflects this complexity ([20], under rev). A programme for IFS needs to incorporate a systematic approach and help identify the actual remediation measures needed.

Individualised fire safety also requires cooperation between municipal sectors, as well as close interaction with the risk-prone individual. Nevertheless, there are some inherent advantages to this type of intervention. Factor working in favour of IFS is that programmes can easily be adapted to local circumstances and tested stepwise, with ample opportunity to make necessary modifications along the way. Another factor that inherently supports IFS is that initiatives that aim to improve fire safety are generally well received.

Two vital stages of implementation that are necessary at the outset as a prerequisite to success are political support for the implementation and the determination of the stakeholder responsible for the implementation. In Sweden, the FRS are responsible for fire protection; but they perceive an uncertainty regarding whether they have a mandate to take action. Designing and implementing fire safety for risk groups often require cooperation between social services, health care and fire and rescue services [19], highlighting the need for establishing roles and responsibilities at an early stage to avoid jurisdictional conflict. Such cross-sectoral cooperation is found to be challenging, both to organise and maintain. Even if fire protection is considered important, it is a relatively a rare problem in that it is difficult for some agencies to prioritise it relative to other pressing needs.

The lack of means, both monetary and other, can also be a significant barrier. This also relates to the question of responsibility, as it related to the integration costs for IFS into the organisational budgets and planning. In cross-sectoral cooperation, differences in norms and traditions can also create a barrier to success. FRS have the expert knowledge about fires, but focusing on IFS can be viewed as an unfamiliar task that differs from their core responsibility (i.e. responding to incidents). As resources in the public sector are seriously strained, interventions need to be designed in a doable way. Instead of adding new tasks, new items can be added to existing tasks, e.g. quality routines and safety rounds. As the target population are often marginalised reflecting underlying social determinants of health [18], fire safety can preferably be combined with other preventative measures. To be able to identify these processes requires substantial knowledge about the organisation and its workflow and a designated position within the FRS has shown to be beneficial in bridging the gap between organisations [27]. Another important factor relates to finding ways to follow up the preventative work. Developing indicators to measure effects can be an effective facilitator, promoting sustainable programmes [26].

An aspect rarely mentioned is the lack of perceived need for fire protection among risk-prone individuals. When overcoming organisational barriers, it is possible that we encounter an individual who has a different agenda, and who is not willing to make adjustments, regarding lifestyle or environment [10]. When looking at fatal fires among older adults, risky behaviour was noted prior to the event in 43.4% of the cases [8], indicating that barriers to motivate behavioural change cannot be neglected.

4 Summary and Conclusions

In this chapter we argue that for fatal fires to continue to decrease, fire prevention needs to specifically target individuals with an increased risk of injury in residential fires. To do this, it is important to understand the underlying mechanisms of vulnerability for such individuals, the so-called determinants of health [33]. These involve the activity itself, individual and environmental factors, as well as the physical environment that all impact the level of risk. Among the identified groups with an increased risk, elderly adults were found to be those best defined. Other identifications of risk groups, however, traditionally include people with mental illness and those with severe substance abuse.

When designing programmes targeting risk individuals, the overall goal is to compensate for the factors that increase the risk and either prevent the fire from occurring or increase the ability of an individual to respond adequately to the situation. In this case, the concepts of promotion and prevention can be useful, and measures to prevent injuries can be applied before, during and after an event.

Experiences from the implementation of individualised fire safety programmes in Sweden, in combination with current research evidence, provide guidance on how to design and implement interventions. Factors that can be leveraged to break down barriers for successful individualised fire safety programme are context-dependent but typically include, although are not limited to:

- Political support and identification of stakeholders.
- Allocation of sufficient economic means in the budget of responsible stakeholders.
- Engagement of the fire and rescue services.
- Activities to mitigate difficulties with inter-sectoral cooperation.

- Identification of risk groups.
- Adaptation of IFS programmes to the specific local setting.
- Integration of the programme into existing procedures (if possible) as a way to ensure programme longevity.

Finally, there is a clear need to tailor any programme to the individuals involved as individual motivation is expected to be key to programme success. Indeed, the motivation or lack thereof for fire protection among risk-prone individuals has been identified as a topic worthy of more focused future research, along with the need of effective evaluation of implemented programmes.

References

1. Ahrens M (2013) Home structure fires. National Fire Protection Association, Fire Analysis and Research Division Quincy, MA
2. Andersson R, Nilsen PER (2015) Personsäkerhet – teori och praktik. Myndigheten för Samhällsskydd och Beredskap, Karlstad
3. Arch BN, Thurston MN (2013) An assessment of the impact of home safety assessments on fires and fire-related injuries: a case study of Cheshire Fire and Rescue Service. J Public Health 35:200–205
4. Ballesteros MF, Jackson ML, Martin MW (2005) Working toward the elimination of residential fire deaths: the Centers for Disease Control and Prevention's Smoke Alarm Installation and Fire Safety Education (SAIFE) program. J Burn Care Res 26:434–439
5. Beaulieu E, Smith J, Zheng A, Pike I (2020) The geographic and demographic distribution of residential fires, related injuries, and deaths in four Canadian provinces. Can J Public Health 111:107–116
6. Belin M-Å, Johansson R, Lindberg J, Tingvall C. The Vision Zero and its Consequences. The 4th international conference on Safety and the Environment in the 21st century, 1997 Tel Aviv, Israel. Roadsafety Sweden
7. Breslin D, Dobson S, Smith N (2019) Improving the effectiveness of fire prevention using the "premonition" agent-based model of domestic fire risk behaviours. Int J Emerg Serv 8:280–291
8. Cassidy P, Mcconnell N, Boyce K (2019) The older adult: associated fire risks and current challenges for the development of future fire safety intervention strategies. Fire Mater 2020:1–11
9. Clare J, Garis L, Plecas D, Jennings C (2012) Reduced frequency and severity of residential fires following delivery of fire prevention education by on-duty fire fighters: cluster randomized controlled study. J Saf Res 43:123–128
10. Damschroder LJ, Aron DC, Keith RE, Kirsh SR, Alexander JA, Lowery JC (2009) Fostering implementation of health services research findings into practice: a consolidated framework for advancing implementation science. Implement Sci 4:50
11. Diguiseppi C, Higgins JPT (2000) Systematic review of controlled trials of interventions to promote smoke alarms. Arch Dis Child 82:341
12. Edelman LS (2007) Social and economic factors associated with the risk of burn injury. Burns 33:958–965
13. Eggert E, Huss F (2017) Medical and biological factors affecting mortality in elderly residential fire victims: a narrative review of the literature. Scars Burns Healing 3:2059513117707686
14. Erlandsson L-K, Persson D (2020) The ValMO model. Occupational therapy for a healthy life by doing. Lund, Studentlitteratur
15. Fernández-Vigil M, Echeverría Trueba B (2019) Elderly at home: a case for the systematic collection and analysis of fire statistics in Spain. Fire Technol 55:2215–2244

16. FRS (2020) Fire prevention & protection statistics England, April 2019 to March 2020. In: Office H (ed). London
17. Garis LBC (2019) Fire risk in senior population analysis of Canadian fire incidents. University of the Fraser Valley School of Criminology & Criminal Justice, Canada
18. Gielen AC, Frattaroli S, Pollack KM, Peek-Asa C, Yang JG (2018) How the science of injury prevention contributes to advancing home fire safety in the USA: successes and opportunities. Inj Prev 24:i7–i13
19. Gjøsund G, Almklov PG, Halvorsen K, Storesund K (2017) Vulnerability and prevention of fatal fires. In: Lesley Walls MR, Bedford T (eds) The 26th European safety and reliability conference ESREL, Glasgow, UK
20. Gustavsson, J., Carlsson, G., Mcnamee, M. S., 2021. Barriers and facilitators for implementation of individualized fire safety (IFS). in Sweden *Fire Technology*
21. Halvorsen K, Almklov PG, Gjøsund G (2017) Fire safety for vulnerable groups: the challenges of cross-sector collaboration in Norwegian municipalities. Fire Saf J 92:1–8
22. Head BW, Alford J (2013) Wicked problems: implications for public policy and management. Adm Soc 47:711–739
23. Istre GR, Mccoy MA, Moore BJ, Roper C, Stephens-Stidham S, Barnard JJ, Carlin DK, Stowe M, Anderson RJ (2014) Preventing deaths and injuries from house fires: an outcome evaluation of a community-based smoke alarm installation programme. Inj Prev 20:97
24. Jonsson A, Bonander C, Nilson F, Huss F (2017) The state of the residential fire fatality problem in Sweden: epidemiology, risk factors, and event typologies. J Saf Res 62:89–100
25. Jonsson A, Runefors M, Särdqvist S, Nilson F (2015) Fire-related mortality in Sweden: temporal trends 1952 to 2013. Fire Technol: 1–11
26. Kerber S (2020) Utilizing research to enhance fire service knowledge. Doctoral University of Lund
27. Kimberly JR, Evanisko MJ (1981) Organizational innovation: the influence of individual, organizational, and contextual factors on hospital adoption of technological and administrative innovations. Acad Manag J 24:689–713
28. Mcnamee M, Meacham B, van Hees P, Bisby L, Chow WK, Coppalle A, Dobashi R, Dlugogorski B, Fahy R, Fleischmann C, Floyd J, Galea ER, Gollner M, Hakkarainen T, Hamins A, Hu L, Johnson P, Karlsson B, Merci B, Ohmiya Y, Rein G, Trouvé A, Wang Y, Weckman B (2019) IAFSS agenda 2030 for a fire safe world. Fire Saf J 110:102889
29. MSB (2020) Brandsäker bostad för alla – Stärkt brandskydd för särskilt riskutsatta individer. Myndigheten för samhällsskydd och beredskap, Karlstad
30. Nilson F, Bonander C (2020) Household fire protection practices in relation to socio-demographic characteristics: evidence from a Swedish National Survey. Fire Technol 56:1077–1098
31. Nilson F, Lundgren L, Bonander C (2020) Living arrangements and fire-related mortality amongst older people in Europe. Int J Inj Control Saf Promot 27:378–384
32. OECD (2003) Emerging risks in the 21st century – an agenda for action. OECD, Paris
33. Robertson LS (2007) Injury epidemiology. Oxford University Press, New York
34. Runefors M, Johansson N, VAN HEES P (2017) The effectiveness of specific fire prevention measures for different population groups. Fire Saf J 91:1044–1050
35. Sesseng C, Storesund K, Steen-Hansen A (2018) Analysis of fatal fires in Norway over a decade, – a retrospective observational study. In: Haugen S, Barros A, van Gulijk C, Kongsvik T, Vinnem JE (eds) Safety and reliability – safe societies in a changing world: proceedings of ESREL 2018. CRC Press, Trondheim, Norway
36. Tillett JL (2019) Residential Fire Impacts on Richmond, Virginia: a plan for identifying and educating our most vulnerable communities. Virginia Commonwealth University, Virginia
37. Tulchinsky TH, Varavikova EA (2014) Chapter 1 – A history of public health. In: Tulchinsky TH, Varavikova EA (eds) The new public health (third edition). Academic Press, San Diego
38. Turner SL, Johnson RD, Weightman AL, Rodgers SE, Arthur G, Bailey R, Lyons RA (2017) Risk factors associated with unintentional house fire incidents, injuries and deaths in high-income countries: a systematic review. Inj Prev 23:131

39. WHO (1986) Ottawa Charter for Health Promotion: First International Conference on Health Promotion Ottawa
40. WHO (2001) International classification of functioning, disability and health: ICF. World Health Organization, Geneva
41. WHO (2017) 10 priorities towards a decade of healthy ageing. Switzerland Department of Ageing and Life Course, World Health Organization
42. Woodrow B (2012) Fire as vulnerability: the value added from adopting a vulnerability approach. World Fire Statistics Bulletin. Geneva The Geneva Association
43. Xiong L, Bruck D, Ball M (2015) Comparative investigation of 'survival'and fatality factors in accidental residential fires. Fire Saf J 73:37–47

Dr. Johanna Gustavsson is a Registered Nurse and has extensive experience in clinical elderly care. She holds an M.A. in Social Risk Management and has since 2010 been employed at Risk- and environmental studies, Karlstad University. Johanna finished her PhD on fall-injury prevention in 2018, and her main research interest is in injury prevention and health promotion for older adults.

Dr. Gunilla Carlsson is an Associate Professor in occupational therapy at Lund University with a focus on how the environment hinder or support activity and participation in an ageing population. Based on clinical experience and many years of research, a specific focus is how to address accessibility problems in the built environment for people with physical and cognitive impairments. Her research is primarily about housing, but also mobility in the public environment.

Prof. Margaret S. McNamee is Professor in Fire Safety Engineering at Lund University in Sweden. She has her technical expertise in sustainable fire safety and has worked in the field of fire and combustion research for more than 30 years. In recent years, she has become interested in the efficiency of the fire services in Sweden. In particular, she has explored the practical implementation of their strategic mission (as defined through governance strategies) in fire service operations.

Chapter 18
Residential Fires in Metropolitan Areas: Living Conditions and Fire Prevention

Nicklas Guldåker, Per-Olof Hallin, Mona Tykesson Klubien, and Jerry Nilsson

Abstract This chapter addresses the benefits of geo-statistical approaches in fire prevention processes, especially in the prevention of residential fires in urban areas. The aim is to demonstrate how residential fire incidents can be theorized and placed in a context where geo-statistical techniques and an area-based approach can support the emergency services fire prevention work. The chapter introduces theoretical concepts such as Fire Risk Environment, Fire Protection Capability, as well as determining factors, types of residential fires, and various hypotheses for further analysis of residential fires in urban contexts. Key themes are the development of residential fire incidents in different metropolitan areas over time, how different types of residential fires can be connected to living conditions, and finally how the emergency services and other actors can work with area-based fire prevention. Examples from Sweden's major cities and especially the city of Gothenburg are used. The results show that variations in spatial residential fire patterns can be explained by a variation of living conditions. The conditions may also look different depending on the residential area and housing conditions, and therefore, preventive strategies and proactive measures should differ between and within cities and be adapted to specific different areas.

N. Guldåker (✉) · M. T. Klubien
Faculty of Social Science, Department of Human Geography, Lund University, Lund, Sweden
e-mail: nicklas.guldaker@keg.lu.se; mona.tykesson_klubien@keg.lu.se

P.-O. Hallin
Faculty of Culture and Society, Department of Urban Studies, Malmö University, Malmö, Sweden
e-mail: olof.hallin@mau.se

J. Nilsson
Region Skåne and Faculty of Culture and Society, Department of Urban Studies, Malmö University, Malmö, Sweden
e-mail: jerry.nilsson@mau.se

© The Author(s), under exclusive license to Springer Nature Switzerland AG 2023
M. Runefors et al. (eds.), *Residential Fire Safety*, The Society of Fire Protection Engineers Series, https://doi.org/10.1007/978-3-031-06325-1_18

Keywords Fire risk · Fire Prevention · Residential fires · GIS · Living conditions · Urban areas

1 Introduction

GIS-based analyses of fire incidents in urban contexts are quite frequent worldwide and in the research literature [1–3]. Different geovisualization methods are used to clarify patterns of residential fires or other incidents in different metropolitan areas [4, 5]. Spatial approaches are also applied for theoretical and practical purposes, such as risk modeling, linking fires to socioeconomic variables, theorizing and developing hypotheses about the causes of fires, and to analyze different types of fire incidents on various geographical scales within a selected area, e.g., a city, region, or nation [6, 7]. The purposes and approaches of different GIS-based methods vary, but they give valuable input to strategic decisions to rescue services and other related authorities and organizations [8].

The spatial dynamics of residential fires are complex and related to a variety of causes. In order to analyze these causes more thoroughly, different spatial, statistical, and theoretical approaches can be applied. An overall challenge is how these approaches actually can be combined and develop the analysis of residential fire incidents on different geographic scales. Another important concern is how these approaches can be useful for both researchers and practitioners in a more organized way.

Although GIS-based methods have been applied extensively to study fire incidents, relatively few examples are found in relation to the rescue services' preventive work on residential fires. Some scientific approaches contain spatial and temporal studies of structural fires for prevention of fires in a planning context and fire response [9], the use of GIS to increase understanding of the relationship between fires and the built environment [10], or the investigation of intentional fires and socioeconomic conditions as a support for fire prevention measures and fire safety policies [11]. Other related studies include development and implementation of spatial models to target services based on risks [12, 13], the exploration of different spatial methods for rescue services [14], and theoretical approaches to fire prevention and the analysis of spatiotemporal patterns of residential structure fires [15]. In several studies, GIS-based methodologies have been applied and implemented in planning processes in order to mitigate fire risks and improve fire safety [6, 16–18]. In this context, geovisualization is an appropriate visual method for presenting and communicating large datasets and the result of spatial analyses [19, 20]. Fire risks or fire incidents are often envisioned through maps, diagrams, and figures, where reliability of these visualizations is affected by the quality of data, accumulated errors in the analysis process, and different settings such as used spatial method, scale, bandwidth, and choice of visualization technique [4, 5, 21].

Thus, there is a need for more comprehensive and validated use of geo-statistical approaches in (residential) fire prevention processes. In this chapter, we aim to demonstrate how residential fire incidents can be theorized and placed in a context where geo-statistical techniques and an area-based approach can support the rescue services fire prevention work. The content of the chapter is based on research and results from a multiyear study on residential fires in metropolitan regions in Sweden [7].

The chapter introduces a theoretical discussion on *Fire Risk Environment, Fire Protection Capability*, as well as determining factors, types of residential fires, and various hypotheses for further analysis of residential fires in urban contexts. Key themes addressed in the chapter are the development of residential fire incidents in different metropolitan areas over time, how different types of residential fires can be connected to living conditions, and finally how the emergency services and other actors can work with area-based fire prevention in metropolitan areas. In the chapter, Sweden's major cities and especially the city of Gothenburg are used as examples.

2 Theoretical Points of Departure

This section presents the theoretical points of departure of the chapter.

2.1 Fire Risk Environment and Fire Protection Capability

Every home and building can be seen as environments where fire can occur. Therefore, the *Fire Risk Environment* can be defined as the individual, social, and technical conditions that affect the probability that a fire incident will occur [22]. People, house types, building structures, technical systems, and possible fire sources vary and therefore constitute different types of fire risk environments. Knowledge, intentions, personal characteristics, people's and group's vulnerability, or overcrowding in an apartment building can affect the probability of a fire incident. Technical deficiencies or poor maintenance can also lead to technically caused fire incidents. Taken together, the building, the dwelling, and the occupants constitute a fire risk environment that can be analyzed on the basis of different scales, such as the dwelling/household, the building, and the residential area.

Individuals, households, and other actors can prevent and manage fire incidents themselves. This can be referred to as *Fire Protection Capability*. With regard to residential fires, *FPC* can be defined as the knowledge and ability of individuals, households, and other actors to prevent and manage fire incidents in residential buildings [22].

In Sweden, it is unclear how large the proportion of unreported fire incidents in some residential buildings and residential areas are compared to others. Perhaps this difference is because the ability to handle fire incidents in different households differs. Some studies indicate that many residential fire incidents are handled without the intervention of the rescue service. In a study of house fires in the UK and Australia, over 75% of the fires were self-extinguished or managed by people [23]. In Sweden, it is stated that about 24,000 residential fires occur annually, of which about 6000 are alerted to the rescue service [24]. Thus, there is an extensive *Fire Protection Capability* in many households and in the general population [25, 26]. Differences between residential areas could in that case depend on how well a fire incident is handled. The *Fire Protection Capability* is normally influenced by different factors, such as individual characteristics and social conditions, socio-technical conditions, and fire conditions [27].

Factors that directly affect the *Fire Risk Environment*, i.e., the probability of a fire incident, may be of a different nature. From an individual and social perspective, fire incidents occur either through an intentional or unintentional act. Intentional fires are likely to occur due to norm-breaking behavior or mental illness. In the latter case, forgetfulness, inattention, handling defects, cooking mistakes, or sleep can lead to fires. Disability, age, addiction, risk behaviors, and also how long periods of time people stay in their homes are all factors that can affect the probability of a fire. During the ongoing pandemic with covid-19, fire incidents may increase in homes where people residing around the clock and possibly become ill. Social factors can be overcrowding and cooking habits. Technical conditions such as the age of the technology or incorrect installations of electrical or heating systems, as well as poor maintenance, are all examples of technical factors that can affect the probability of fire.

2.2 Determination Factors

There are several scientific studies and reviews of determining factors for residential fires [11, 28–32]. For the most part, various statistical correlation or regression analyses are performed. Often no distinction is made between direct and underlying (indirect) determinants. Common direct determinants that show a connection to fire risks are, e.g., mental health, disability, alcohol use, smoking, and the proportion of residents who have installed smoke alarms. The underlying determining factors consist of various types of socioeconomic data such as unemployment, proportion of people with foreign background, single parents, age, income, proportion of empty residents in an area, but also factors such as the building's technology and construction.

2.2.1 Direct Determination Factors

Based on the definition earlier in this section, the *Fire Protection Capability* is very much related to the knowledge and abilities that residents and externals have to prevent and manage fire incidents. This knowledge can be of different kinds. It can be declarative, i.e., expressed verbally or in symbolic form and be tested. An example is that residents know that smoke alarms are useful and that they should have one. Functional knowledge can be translated into action and is often tested by a person who has learned to solve a concrete problem or a task [33]. To take smoke alarms again as an example, it is about knowing how to set up, replace the battery, and test it. Ability is about having the resources to be able to translate declarative and functional knowledge into practical action. If residents do not have access to smoke alarms, tools, or the physical ability to set it up and test it, the knowledge does not do much good.

Proactive Fire Protection Capability is about both declarative and functional knowledge and rely on people's ability to assimilate information. Resident's language skills, their level of education, or own and others' experiences can also influence this capability. *Reactive Fire Protection Capability* is mainly based on functional knowledge and ability, i.e., how to act when different types of fire incidents occur. Individual characteristics such as disability, age, or drug addiction or social conditions such as the number of people in the home are some important factors that affect the reactive *Fire Protection Capability*. *Post-active Fire Protection Capability* is about acquiring knowledge and experience of incidents that have occurred and translating this awareness into a proactive action [22].

2.2.2 Indirect Determination Factors

Behind the direct determination factors for residential fires are other elements that have a more indirect impact on fire risk environments and *Fire Protection Capability*. Below are some important underlying determining factors that can affect people's fire risk environments and the *Fire Protection Capability* they develop.

Having a *job* leads to better financial conditions and opportunities to choose type of accommodation and residential area. *Unemployment* often leads to lower incomes. State and social assistance, financial transfers from others, and accumulated reserves of capital and funds can compensate for reduced earned income from work. However, unemployment and reduced income over a longer period usually means limited choices regarding type of housing but also an increased risk of social stress. It can also lead to more time spent in the homes, having more activities there, and thus the number of fire incidents may increase.

Education is one of the most central factors behind the opportunities to get a job and thus an economic standard with opportunities to choose the form of accommodation and residential area. A low level of education can in itself, and sometimes in combination with a migrant background and shortcomings in language skills, lead to difficulties in assimilating various forms of information about fire safety. Despite the fact that basic fire safety is generally well translated from one cultural context to another, there may be differences in knowledge depending on whether residents migrate from an environment where fire safety is more or less applied.

Low *income* or dependence on income support limits the opportunities to choose housing in the housing market. As indicated above, this factor can be linked to whether residents have jobs or are unemployed. The consequence of low income can be overcrowding and/or that residents are forced to live in homes or residential areas with low or neglected maintenance. Rubbish, damage, and poor cleaning in common areas in apartment buildings can lead to the presence of flammable material in combination with the fact that it signals that no one cares about the residential area.

Overcrowding can increase the probability that a residential fire will occur when cooking, lighting candles, children playing with fire, etc. Homes with many children and adults seem to have a greater fire risk than smaller family units [34]. Overcrowding can also lead to many children and young people staying outside the home, but with lower social control and an increased risk of intentional fire setting both indoors and outdoors [11, 35].

Age and sex can matter in several ways. Older people, and especially those with various disabilities, may be at greater risk of having a fire, but also of having a poorer *Fire Protection Capability* in the event of a fire incident. In addition to the very oldest age group, men are strongly overrepresented compared to women when it comes to fatal fires. In general terms of intentional fires in metropolitan areas, it is often a teenage problem where boys and adolescents are overrepresented [35, 36].

Single parents, and especially in combination with low incomes and shortcomings in language skills, can give rise to social and economic stress [37]. This in turn can lead to difficulties in maintaining attention, parental authority, and setting boundaries for children's behavior.

Various forms of *mental and physical illness* can lead to more fire incidents at the same time as the ability to detect and manage them is lower. High levels of ill health in a residential area may indicate that there is an overrepresentation of people with risk behaviors regarding fire and thus a reduced *Fire Protection Capability*.

Being *born abroad* and moving to a new country can pose major challenges that affect fire protection capabilities. The level of knowledge of the official language of the new country can affect the ability to communicate and assimilate information about fire safety. It also affects the opportunities to acquire knowledge of how to act in the event of a fire, or when a fire develops, and the ability to communicate with others including rescue services. Traditions and habits from the original home country can also affect the *Fire Protection Capability*. For example, high use of cooking oil or spending a lot of time cooking can increase the risk of accidents connected to the stove.

Low incomes among residents mean that the choices in the *housing market* are limited and that there is a concentration of low-income earners in certain residential areas, preferably with rental apartments. This in combination with the fact that many with low incomes have a foreign background that leads to ethnically segregated areas where fewer residents speak the official language of the country. However, not speaking the official language of the country does not have to be a barrier to fire safety in homes in these areas, especially if information about fire safety is available in different languages. But it can lead to fire prevention not being given priority because of, e.g., stressful living conditions, experiences from previous types of housing (informal and formal), or varying trust in authorities.

2.3 Geo-Statistical Approach on Residential Fires

In a socially fragmented city, the underlying determining factors often are unevenly spatially distributed. In order to determine the extent to which they affect the occurrence of different types of residential fires in different residential areas, statistical analyses need to be carried out. In addition, residential fires need to be analyzed and mapped in GIS in different ways to show how they vary within and between cities. Later in the chapter, a GIS-based approach is applied in the city of Gothenburg in Sweden as an example. The purpose of the geo-statistical approach is to show possible socio-spatial differences, but also to develop proactive proposals on how to work fire prevention in different residential areas.

2.4 Types of Residential Fires

Residential fires can be categorized in several ways, for example by fire ignition or fire losses, or by human or nonhuman action [38–40]. In this study, the residential fires registered by the rescue services in Swedish metropolitan areas are classified into three main groups or types depending on their causes [22].

1. *Intentional fires* can be seen as an expression of norm-breaking behaviors or mental illness. The intentional act of setting things on fire can be related to a conflict or to hide other crimes. In many cases, there are other motives behind, such as thrill seeking, boredom, or serious play with fire [35]. Intentional fires in buildings often take place in common areas in apartment buildings, e.g., stairwells, basements, and attics [41].
2. *Unintentional (accidental) fires due to human behavior* can occur due to various activities and where the ability to prevent, detect, and prevent them is insufficient. Stress, forgetfulness, inattention, disability, decreased level of consciousness due to intake of alcohol, drugs, or medication, or accidents can lead to fire incidents [27]. Common causes or activities are cooking, smoking, using candles, etc.
3. *Residential fires caused by technical errors,* e.g., *electrical faults, work processes, or other causes* can occur as a result of defects in technical equipment or neglected maintenance. They can also take place during maintenance work in a residential building or be related to the heating system such as chimney fires

[42]. Residential fires with other causes are also fires where the rescue services cannot determine the underlying causes. Residential fires that occur because of children playing with fire or fireworks have also been placed in this category. Children's play with fire can be said to be a form of intentional fire, but which cannot be directly linked to pronounced motives and can moreover be due to trill-seeking, ignorance of the individual, and lack of control from adults [36]. The categories of other and unknown fires are treated overall in this context and not as specific types of residential fire in the geographical reporting and analysis below.

2.5 Modeling of Causes of Residential Fires

Although it is possible to demonstrate statistical correlations between the occurrence of different types of residential fires and the underlying determining factors, it is not the same as having a causal relationship. As an intermediary, different hypothetical arguments can be applied and tested to highlight the dynamics between direct and indirect determining factors. Following hypotheses exemplify possible causal links between different types of fires and underlying determining factors. The hypotheses are also spatially valid in that they can be linked to residential areas with specific socioeconomic and demographic conditions [22].

Hypothesis 1 Inattention and forgetfulness lead to an increased risk of fire in a home. Unintentional residential fires can affect most people. Fire incidents are most often handled by household members and rarely require support form rescue services. *There should be an overrepresentation in residential areas with many single elderly people (reduced mobility) or young people living alone (outdoor life and alcohol).*

Hypothesis 2 Abuse of alcohol and drugs, mental illness, or disability lead to an increased risk of fire in the home. These accidental fires can affect most people but above all risk groups. Fire incidents are handled less often by the individual and usually give rise to operations from the rescue service. *There should be an overrepresentation in residential areas with many people with risk behaviors, e.g., people with substance abuse, mental illness, physical disability, and people who over fill their homes with things (so-called collectors). In this group, there is a higher risk of fatal fires.*

Hypothesis 3 Overcrowding, specific cooking habits, and difficulties in assimilating information in the prevailing language can lead to an increased risk of fire in the home. This applies to residential fires that occur in living environments where people live crowded and use a lot of oil in their cooking. Fire incidents can be handled by residents but often require operations from the rescue service. *There should be* *an overrepresentation in residential areas where many families have a foreign background, live cramped in their homes, and use a lot of oil in their cooking.*

Hypothesis 4 Behaviors that lead to an increased risk of intentional fire setting in and around residential buildings. This type applies to residential fires that occur in residential areas with low social control and many young people with norm-breaking behaviors or where there are people with mental illness. In most cases, intentional fires occur in common areas such as basements, laundry rooms, garbage rooms, and attics. Intentional fires usually cause a rescue service operation. *There should be an overrepresentation of this type of residential fires in residential areas with unstable family conditions, overcrowding, neglected care, and maintenance.*

The analysis examples below relate only to a limited extent to how these hypotheses can be applied, but they can, based on previous research results [22, 43], work as a point of departure for further analyses of residential fires in metropolitan areas. The hypotheses are particularly important in the area-based fire prevention work, which is exemplified at the end of this chapter.

3 Data and Methods

This section presents the datasets and methods used in this chapter. There are also references to more detailed descriptions in previous research.

3.1 Data

The dataset used in this chapter has its origin in several Swedish agencies and organizations. The statistical dataset on residential fire incidents and socioeconomics from 2007 to 2015 is based on 853 subareas from 16 municipalities and 5 different Emergency services in Sweden covering the three largest metropolitan areas in Sweden [44].

The fire dataset provided by the Emergency Services Gothenburg over the city of Gothenburg consists of 2797 residential fire incidents from 2007 to 2015. The dataset includes positions (X- and Y-coordinates) of residential fire incidents as well as a diversity of information about assessed causes of fire, addresses, starting places, and starting times of fires. Residential data and additional geodata are collected from the city of Gothenburg and Statistics Sweden. ESRI's basemap *Human geography Map* (without labels) is used as background.

3.2 GIS and Statistics

In this chapter, the statistical approach in Sect. 4.2 is based on an indexation (social index) of the variables, education level, employment rate, and disposable average income. In previous studies, these variables have been linked to analyses and explanations of differences in living conditions between different areas within and between cities [7, 37]. These variables have also been shown to correlate with residential fires in various major Swedish cities [44].

Different methods for geovisualization – *point data*, *kernel density*, and *choropleth mapping* – have been applied to increase the possibility for spatial analysis of residential fires (Sect. 4.3). Earlier studies show that each method itself has limitations regarding analytical depth and visualization of fires, but that, in combination, they can improve the possibilities of targeting different forms of area-based fire preventive measures [5]. The kernel density map is combined with a map layer over living conditions, which is an indexation based on eight socioeconomic and demographic variables from 2016 to 2018. This index has been applied in previous research in order to analyze the geo-statistical relationship between living conditions and crime [37, 45]. The index is based on the variables, marital status (single parents), number of children between ages of 0–15, number of adolescents between the ages of 16–19, population per square kilometer, descent, employment rate, and income. Many of these variables have been presented above as indirect determinants of residential fires. Populated areas in Gothenburg are mapped in 250 × 250 meter grids.

3.3 Study Area

In this chapter, the GIS-based visualizations of residential fire data are demonstrated using the municipality of Gothenburg as an example. Gothenburg is the second largest city in Sweden, with more than 1300 inhabitants per km². The municipality have about 582,500 inhabitants (2020) and more than 286,000 residences. Over 81% of the residences are rented or cooperative apartments in apartment buildings [46]. The city of Gothenburg is characterized by a social, economic, and spatial division spread over a large surface (447.76 km²). Between 2008 and 2020, the population has increased by over 7000 people per year, a total of over 86,000 inhabitants for these years [46]. This continuous influx of new residents, especially to apartment buildings, has probably contributed to increasing the number of reported residential fires in the city.

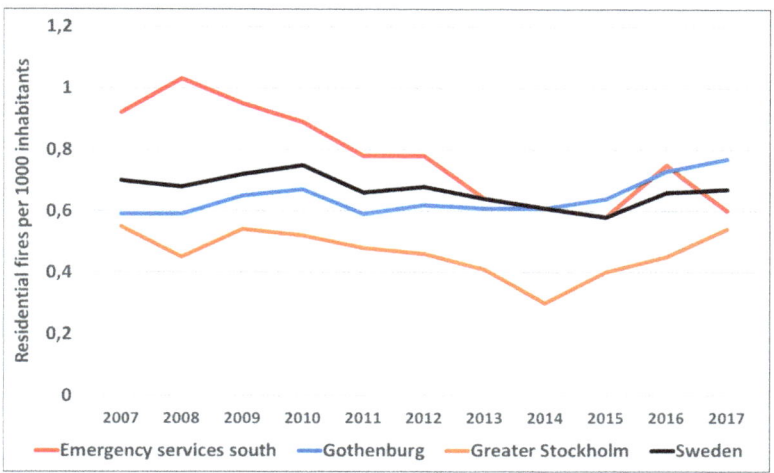

Fig. 18.1 Residential fires per 1000 inhabitants in four emergency services organizations in Sweden 2007–2017

4 Residential Fires and Living Conditions

This section addresses how residential fire incidents in different (Swedish) metropolitan areas have developed between the years 2007–2017. The section also exemplifies how different GIS-based methods can be applied effectively to present, analyze, and help explain the spatial patterns of residential fires in the city of Gothenburg. In the section, the geo-statistical relationship between different types of residential fires and underlying indexed determining factors/living conditions is presented and analyzed more deeply.

4.1 Fire Statistics in Sweden and Gothenburg

The number of interventions from the rescue services to residential fires has gradually decreased in Sweden 2007–2017 (Fig. 18.1). Differences between major cities are particularly interesting. The average number of residential fires per inhabitant in the year of 2008 differs by a factor of two between the highest and lowest value. Not least, the differences between Stockholm, Gothenburg, and Malmö (Emergency Services South) are unanticipated (Fig. 18.1). The differences between the cities are much lower in 2017. Even within these metropolitan areas, there are large differences. A study from 2013 on outdoor fires 2007–2013 in Malmö identified clear concentrations in socioeconomically vulnerable areas. In several of these areas, there was also a high concentration of residential fires [11, 35].

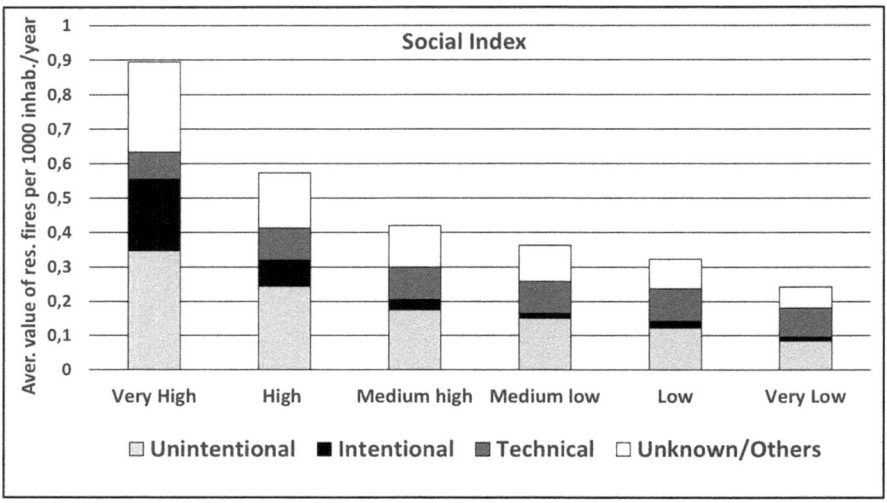

Fig. 18.2 Number of fires per 1000 inhabitants by social index class

Statistics on residential fires from 2007 to 2017 show an upward trend for the city of Gothenburg, which goes from 0.59 residential fires per 1000 inhabitants in 2007 to 0.77 in 2017. As shown in Fig. 18.1, Gothenburg also goes from having lower average than all of Sweden and the other metropolitan areas of Malmö and Stockholm in 2007, to increase above the national average in 2017. The main reason for the upward trend is a slightly increase of unintentional residential fires from 2007 to 2017. Gothenburg City is the largest out of five municipalities within the Emergency Services Gothenburg's geographical district of responsibility.

4.2 Statistical Relationship: Living Conditions and Residential Fires

Figure 18.2 shows the relationship between living conditions and the occurrence of house fires in 853 subareas from three metropolitan areas divided into six groups. These groups have been ranked after level of living conditions and frequency of residential fires. A chi^2 test verifies a significant relationship between the categories [44]. The social index goes from very exposed to good living conditions, from left to right. Subareas with the most exposed living conditions (the bar on the far left) have a much higher number of residential fires per 1000 inhabitants than those with the most advantageous living conditions (the bar on the far right). The number of residential fires that give rise to rescue service operations are four times higher in areas with the most exposed living conditions than in areas with the good living conditions. The bar on the left also shows an exceptional high number of residential fires. There are more unintentional and intentional, and unknown/other residential fires compared to other groups. This indicate that a large part of the rescue operations are carried out in densely populated areas with poorer living conditions, and where there are many apartment buildings.

Living conditions are thus of great importance for the number and type of residential fires that cause rescue service operations, which are also shown in the GIS analysis in Sect. 4.3. In residential areas with very exposed living conditions, the probability of a residential fire incident is four times as high compared with those areas with very good living conditions. There is also a significantly higher risk the incident developing into a fire. On the other hand, the probability that the residential fire is unintentional or has an unknown reason is approximately equal in all types of residential areas. In residential areas with better living conditions, the proportion of fires caused by technical faults, including chimney fires and soot fires, is higher. An explanation is that in these areas there are more villas and detached houses.

There seems to be a spatial and statistical correlation between different living conditions and residential fire incidents that lead to rescue service operations. An indicator of this is that many intentional fires appear to occur in socially exposed residential areas [11, 41]. A second possible explanation lies in the already introduced concepts of *Fire Risk Environment* and *Fire Protection Capability*. Different individual, social, and technical conditions in residents may affect the probability of a fire incident to occur. However, some studies indicate that fire risk environments may not differ between households, and that fire incidents occur at least as often in households with high average incomes [25]. A possible explanation is that residents' Fire Protection Capability is higher in residential areas with good living conditions. If these citizens handle many of their own fire incidents, the rescue service is not alerted, nor is an event report written. This is also consistent with studies that show that households have more fires than can be seen in the statistics [47]. A hypothesis based on this reasoning is therefore that households and residential areas with poorer living conditions have lower *Fire Protection Capability*. Another hypothesis is that residents in apartment buildings more often call the emergency center.

4.3 Geographical Distribution of Residential Fires in Gothenburg

Figures 18.3 and 18.4 show all residential fires in Gothenburg between 2007 and 2015 as well as living conditions. In map 1 in Fig. 18.3, there are 2797 coordinated residential fires. This map gives an overall representation of residential fire incidents in Gothenburg.

Map 2 in Fig. 18.3 presents residential fires per 1000 inhabitants and year distributed over subareas in Gothenburg. The average value for mapped subareas in

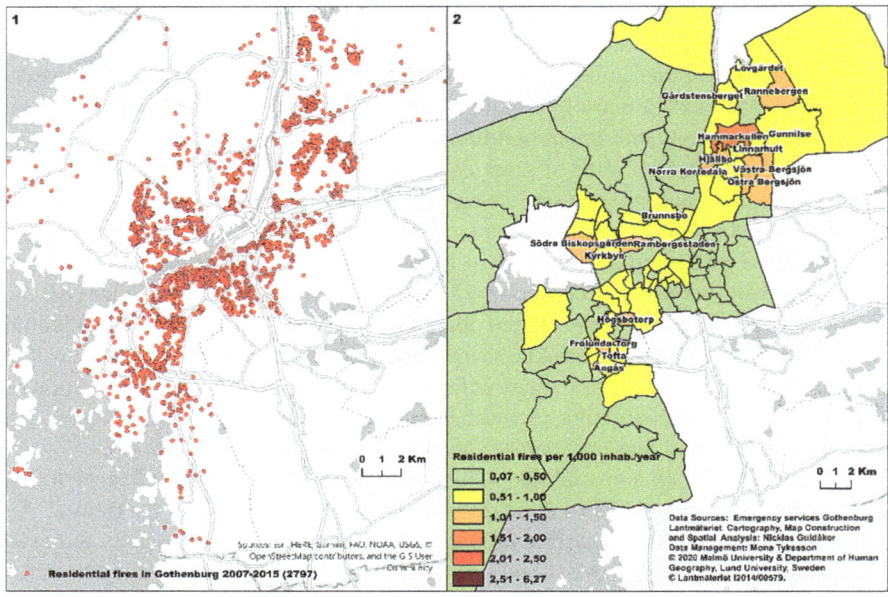

Fig. 18.3 Positions of residential fires and residential fires per 1000 inhabitants and year 2007–2015

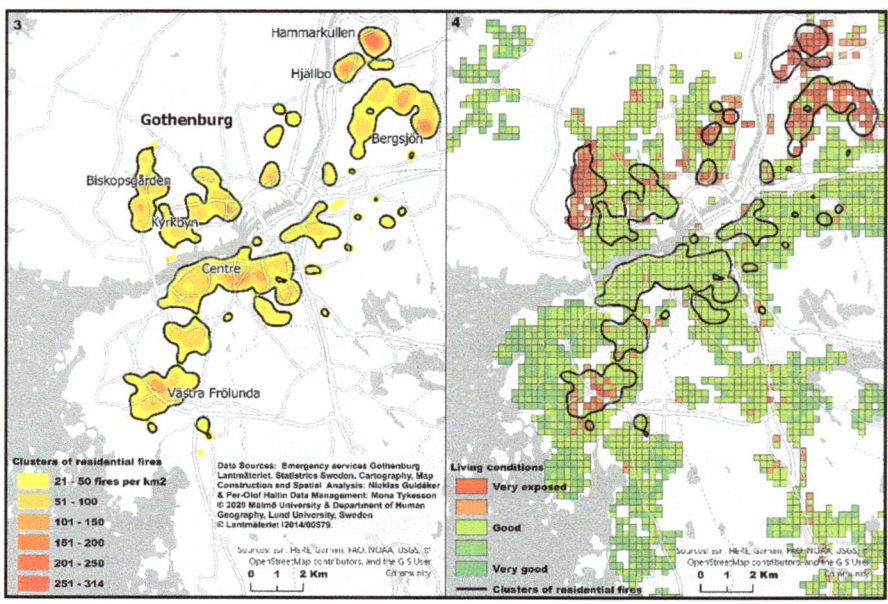

Fig. 18.4 Clusters of residential fires and living conditions in Gothenburg

Gothenburg is 0.60 residential fires per 1000 inhabitants and year. This is lower than, e.g., the City of Malmö (0.88), but higher than the average for Sweden's metropolitan areas (0.49). In Gothenburg, Hammarkullen has the highest value with 1.86 residential fires per 1000 inhabitants and year. Other subareas with higher values than the average are Östra Bergsjön, Frölunda Torg, Rannebergen, Västra Bergsjön, Rambergsstaden, Hjällbo, Södra Biskopsgården, and Högsbotorp.

The surface-based cluster map 3 in Fig. 18.4 of residential fires coincides to a large extent with population-normalized map 2 in Fig. 18.3 over Gothenburg's populated areas. The strongest surface-cluster is again to be found in Hammarkullen with 314 residential fires per km^2. Some other subareas with high concentrations of residential fires are Hjällbo and Rannebergen, Östra and Västra Bergsjön, Norra and Södra biskopsgården, Kyrkbyn, Rambergstaden, and Frölunda torg.

Map 4 in Fig. 18.4 combines the most clustered fire areas with living conditions. As can be seen in the map, there are strong concentrations of residential fires in several areas with very exposed living conditions, mainly in relatively fire dense areas such as Hammarkullen Hjälbo, Biskopsgården, Östra and Västra Bergsjöns, and Västra Frölunda. This result states that spatial clusters of residential fires are probably related to social and demographic causes. The types of residential fires that dominate areas with exposed living conditions are both intentional and unintentional, but also fires with unknown causes (see Sects. 2.4 and 4.1). There are also concentrations of residential fires in other parts of Gothenburg, e.g., in the city center where living conditions are normally good. This pattern is expected because the population density, which is a fundamental determinant to residential fires, is usually high in central urban environments. A frequent cause of residential fire in urban areas with good living conditions is accidental fire, with the kitchen as the most common starting point for the fire [41].

5 Prevention of Residential Fires

This last section addresses how an area-based systematic fire prevention work in metropolitan environments can be carried out and evaluated within an emergency service organization.

5.1 Area-Based and Systematic Fire Prevention Work

Research results from the multiyear study on residential fires in Swedish metropolitan cities show that both general and specific measures are implemented to reduce the number of residential fires and limit the consequences of these fires when they occur. In order for the rescue services to reach different target groups, physical objects, and residential areas, different types of activities are conducted, such as home visits, targeted campaigns, supervision, and fire security-creating projects

[43]. Studies from Canada and the UK show that several of these preventive activities can help reduce the number of fires over time [18]. As the Swedish multiyear study also shows, conditions may vary in different residential areas, and there are large differences regarding the type of residential fire that occurs, and the number of residential fires that give rise to rescue service operations [41]. As stated earlier in this chapter, differences in spatial residential fire patterns can be explained by a variation of living conditions over an urban area [44]. Various individual, structural, building-based, and area-based factors affect residents' fire protection capability and residents can be seen as fire risk environments [22]. Thus, the conditions may look different depending on the residential area, building stock, housing conditions, and socioeconomic conditions, and therefore, preventive strategies and preventive measures must differ [10, 18].

The proposed working method for area-based and systematic fire prevention work takes spatial variations of fires into account and includes activities such as *fire prevention work for both general and specific target groups, selection of areas, creation of area profiles, area analyses, creation of an action plan, and evaluation.*

Fire prevention strategies can be aimed at the entire population, certain risk groups, building types, or in residential area where there is an increased probability of fire. Important activities are information campaigns, home visits, and personalized fire prevention. Collaboration between the rescue service, social services, and the municipality is important for identifying residents, risk individuals, and groups with special fire protection needs.

Starting points for *selection of areas* should relate to statistics and time series on residential fire data and socioeconomic data [44]. To support this selection process,

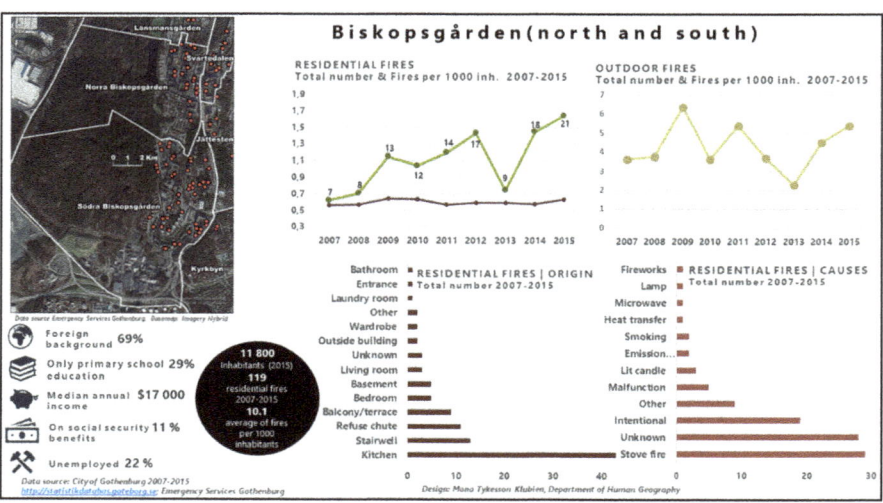

Fig. 18.5 Example of area profile of the subareas: Norra (Northern) and Södra (Southern) Biskopsgården in Gothenburg

the GIS-based methods, analyses, and map visualizations presented above can be applied [41].

Area profiles can help understand underlying trends and causes of residential fires. Such a profile should include fire development over time, different types of fire, causes of fire, starting points for fires, and socioeconomic data. Figure 18.5 presents an area profile for two subareas within Emergency Services Gothenburg.

In the *area analysis*, it is clear that the variety of information over time and space provides the rescue services with additional support in selecting areas as well as establishing different strategies for more targeted fire safety work to different areas. Depending on available resources, hypotheses and statistical analyses can be performed and tested. In the area example in Fig. 18.5, residential fires in kitchens in apartment buildings seem to be a problem. It is clear that many fire incidents in these two subareas start during cooking. In this context, the hypothesis about overrepresentation of many families having a foreign background, living cramped in their homes, and using a lot of oil in their cooking seems appropriate to test and evaluate (see Sect. 2.5). The Northern and Southern Biskopsgården have also had problems with intentional fire setting related to criminal activities, riots, and other forms of social unrest during the period 2007–2015 [48]. Here, hypothesis about overrepresentation of this type of residential fires in residential areas with unstable family conditions, overcrowding, neglected care, and maintenance should also be tested and evaluated.

The *action plan* is thus based on geographical patterns, area profiles, and the causal analysis. The plan also describes the preventive activities that need to be implemented in the residential areas. In the case of Northern and Southern Biskopsgården, preventive measures in order to try to reduce the number of kitchen fires and intentional fires are priority. There are several challenges for the emergency services, including trying to reach a heterogeneous and multilingual population and cooperating with other societal key actors, such as the police, municipality social services, property owners, schools, security companies, leisure centers, etc.

The *evaluation* should be carried out in accordance with the action plan. This can be done by assessing expected effects in the short and long term, as well as assessing the outcomes. Insurance companies may also be important actors in this process. Furthermore, it is important that the fire prevention work is well-documented in a digital operating system, and that the rescue service's organization and members receive clear feedback. An emergency service organization should also preserve special functions that work with learning and evaluation of the fire prevention work. This work should also take into account key aspects such as social sustainability, diversity, gender equality, behaviors, and attitudes.

Acknowledgments The chapter is based on results from research project *Residential Fires in Metropolitan Areas: Spatial Differences and Fire Safety Work in the Socially Fragmented city, 2014–2018*. Special thanks to the funder, the Swedish Civil Contingencies Agency (grant number Dnr 2013-2657). Special thanks also to the Emergency Services Gothenburg, Emergency Services South (Malmö), and Emergency Services Stockholm for their supply of data and valuable input.

References

1. Corcoran J, Higgs G, Higginson A (2011) Fire incidence in metropolitan areas: a comparative study of Brisbane (Australia) and Cardiff (United Kingdom). Appl Geogr 31(1):65–75. https://doi.org/10.1016/j.apgeog.2010.02.003
2. Kiran K, Corcoran J (2017) Modelling residential fire incident response times: a spatial analytic approach. Appl Geogr 84:64–74. https://doi.org/10.1016/j.apgeog.2017.03.004
3. Yang C-H, 楊奇樺 The Study of Spatial and Temporal Distribution of Fire Events in Tainan City from 2004 to 2013. 臺南市2004至2013年火災案件時空分佈之研究
4. Špatenková O, Virrantaus K (2013) Discovering spatio-temporal relationships in the distribution of building fires. Fire Saf J 62 (Part A):49-63. https://doi.org/10.1016/j.firesaf.2013.07.001
5. Guldåker N (2020) Geovisualization and geographical analysis for fire prevention. ISPRS Int J Geo Inf 9(355):355–355. https://doi.org/10.3390/ijgi9060355
6. Martín-Gómez C, Vergara-Falces J, Elvira-Zalduegui A (2015) Geographic information system software application developed by a regional emergency agency. Case Stud Fire Saf 4:19–27. https://doi.org/10.1016/j.csfs.2015.06.002
7. Guldåker N, Hallin P-O, Nilsson J, Tykesson M (2018) Bostadsbränder i storstadsområden, MSB1171 edn. Myndigheten för samhällsskydd och beredskap, Karlstad
8. Taylor M, Higgins E, Lisboa P (2012) Testing geographical information systems: a case study in a fire prevention support system. J Syst Inf Technol 14(3):184. https://doi.org/10.1108/13287261211255310
9. Asgary A, Ghaffari A, Levy J (2010) Spatial and temporal analyses of structural fire incidents and their causes: a case of Toronto. Can Fire Saf J 45(1):44–57. https://doi.org/10.1016/j.firesaf.2009.10.002
10. Jennings CR (1998) Urban fire risk: using GIS to connect fire, census, and assessor's data. Reg Sci Rev 17:105–112
11. Guldåker N, Hallin P-O (2014) Spatio-temporal patterns of intentional fires, social stress and socio-economic determinants: a case study of Malmö, Sweden. Fire Saf J 70:71–80. https://doi.org/10.1016/j.firesaf.2014.08.015
12. Higgins E, Taylor M, Jones M, Lisboa PJG (2013) Understanding community fire risk—a spatial model for targeting fire prevention activities. Fire Saf J 62(Part A):20–29. https://doi.org/10.1016/j.firesaf.2013.02.006
13. Taylor M, Higgins E, Lisboa P, Jarman I, Hussain A (2016) Community fire prevention via population segmentation modelling. Community Dev J 51(2):229–247. https://doi.org/10.1093/cdj/bsv006
14. Krisp JM, Virrantaus K, Jolma A (2005) In: Oosterom P, Zlatanova S, Fendel EM (eds) Using explorative spatial analysis to improve fire and rescue services. Geo-information for Disaster Management. Springer, Berlin, pp 1283–1296. https://doi.org/10.1007/3-540-27468-5_89
15. Wuschke K, Clare J, Garis L (2013) Temporal and geographic clustering of residential structure fires: a theoretical platform for targeted fire prevention. Fire Saf J 62(Part A):3–12. https://doi.org/10.1016/j.firesaf.2013.07.003
16. Zhang X, Yao J, Jin Y, Sila-Nowicka K (2020) Urban fire dynamics and its association with urban growth: evidence from Nanjing. China ISPRS Int J Geo-Info 9(4). https://doi.org/10.3390/ijgi9040218
17. Ferreira TM, Vicente R, Mendes R, da Silva JA, Varum H, Costa A, Maio R (2016) Urban fire risk: evaluation and emergency planning. J Cult Herit 20:739–745. https://doi.org/10.1016/j.culher.2016.01.011
18. Thomas L, Garis L, Morris S, Biantoro C (2020) Journey of home safe: community risk reduction in surrey analyses from surrey historical data. Surrey Fire services and University of the Fraser Valley, British Columbia
19. MacEachren AM, Gahegan M, Pike W (2004) Visualization for constructing and sharing geo-scientific concepts. Proc Natl Acad Sci U S A 101:5279. https://doi.org/10.1073/pnas.0307755101

20. MacEachren AM, Gahegan M, Pike W, Brewer I, Cai G, Lengerich E, Hardistry F (2004) Geovisualization for knowledge construction and decision support. IEEE Computer Graphics and Applications, Computer Graphics and Applications, IEEE, IEEE Comput Grap Appl 24(1):13–17. https://doi.org/10.1109/MCG.2004.1255801
21. Tykesson Klubien M, Nilsson J, Guldåker N, Hallin P-O (2018) Bostadsbränder i storstadsområden – Kvalitetsgranskning av insatsrapportering av bostadsbränder – Storstadsområdena Malmö. Department of Human Geography, Lund University. Urban studies, Malmö University, Göteborg, Södertörn och Stockholm. https://doi.org/10.13140/RG.2.2.14809.67687
22. Hallin P-O, Guldåker N, Nilsson J, Tykesson Klubien M (2018) Bostadsbränder i storstadsområden – teoretiska utgångspunkter. Department of Human Geography, Lund University. Urban studies, Malmö University. https://doi.org/10.13140/RG.2.2.13736.11527
23. Barnett M, Bruck D, Jago A (2007) Mean annual probability of having a residential fire experience throughout a lifetime: development and application of a methodology. Melbourne
24. Hallin P-O, Andersson R, Andersson P (2018) Brand i bostäder – så ska färre skadas och dö. Myndigheten för samhällsskydd och beredskap (MSB) och Brandforsk, Karlstad
25. Nilson F, Bonander C, Jonsson A (2015) Differences in determinants amongst individuals reporting residential fires in Sweden: results from a cross-sectional study. Fire Technol 51(3):615–626. https://doi.org/10.1007/s10694-015-0459-0
26. Nilson F, Bonander C (2020) Household fire protection practices in relation to sociodemographic characteristics: evidence from a Swedish National Survey. Fire Technol 56(3):1077–1098. https://doi.org/10.1007/s10694-019-00921-w
27. Kobes M, Post JG, Helsloot I, de Vries B (2010) Building safety and human behaviour in fire: a literature review. Fire Saf J 45(1):1–11. https://doi.org/10.1016/j.firesaf.2009.08.005
28. Jennings CR (2013) Social and economic characteristics as determinants of residential fire risk in urban neighborhoods: a review of the literature. Fire Saf J 62 (Part A):13-19. https://doi.org/10.1016/j.firesaf.2013.07.002
29. Taylor MJ, Higgins E, Lisboa PJG, Kwasnica V (2012) An exploration of causal factors in unintentional dwelling fires. Risk Manag (14603799) 14(2):109. https://doi.org/10.1057/rm.2011.9
30. Jonsson A, Jaldell H (2020) Identifying sociodemographic risk factors associated with residential fire fatalities: a matched case control study. Inj Prev 26(2):147–152. https://doi.org/10.1136/injuryprev-2018-043062
31. Špatenková O, Stein A (2010) Identifying factors of influence in the spatial distribution of domestic fires. Int J Geogr Inf Sci 24(6):841–858. https://doi.org/10.1080/13658810903143634
32. Jonsson A, Bonander C, Nilson F, Huss F (2017) The state of the residential fire fatality problem in Sweden: epidemiology, risk factors, and event typologies. J Safety Res 62:89–100. https://doi.org/10.1016/j.jsr.2017.06.008
33. Biggs JB, Tang CS-K, Society for Research into Higher E (2011) Teaching for quality learning at university: what the student does, vol, 4th edn. McGraw-Hill Education, Maidenhead
34. Goodsman RW, Mason F, Blythe A (1987) Housing factors and fires in two metropolitan boroughs. Fire Saf J 12(1):37–50. https://doi.org/10.1016/0379-7112(87)90014-2
35. Guldåker N, Hallin P-O (2013) Stadens Bränder Del 1 – Anlagda bränder och Malmös sociala geografi. Malmö University publications in urban studies (MAPIUS). Malmö University, Malmö, p 9
36. Lindgren S-Å, Björk M, Ekbrand H, Persson S, Uhnoo S (2013) Barn/ungdomar som anlägger brand – orsaker och motåtgärder – Slutrapport. The Department of Sociology and Work Science, University of Gothenburg
37. Hallin P-O, Westerdahl S (2020) Utsatta livsvillkor. In: Gerell M, Hallin P-O, Nilvall K, Westerdahl S (eds) Att vända utvecklingen: från utsatta områden till trygghet och delaktighet, Malmö University publications in urban studies (MAPIUS), vol 26. Malmö University, Malmö, pp 24–40
38. FEMA (1997) Socioeconomic factors and the incidence of fire. Federal Emergency Management Agency United States Fire Administration National Fire Data Center (U.S.)

39. Higgins E, Taylor M, Francis H, Jones M, Appleton D (2015) Transforming fire prevention: a case study. Transform Gov 9(2):223. https://doi.org/10.1108/TG-05-2014-0017
40. Taylor M, Higgins E, Francis M, Lisboa P (2011) Managing unintentional dwelling fire risk. J Risk Res 14(10):1207–1218. https://doi.org/10.1080/13669877.2011.587884
41. Guldåker N, Tykesson Klubien M, Hallin P-O, Nilsson J (2018) Rumsliga skillnader i den socialt fragmenterade staden. Department of Human Geography, Lund University and department of Urban Studies, Malmö University. https://doi.org/10.13140/RG.2.2.24876.00649
42. Bengtsson L-G (2013) Inomhusbrand, vol MSB595, 4th edn. Myndigheten för samhällsskydd och beredskap, Karlstad
43. Guldåker N, Hallin P-O, Tykesson Klubien M, Nilsson J (2018) Brandsäkerhetsarbete i den socialt fragmenterade staden. Department of Human Geography, Lund University. Urban studies, Malmö University. https://doi.org/10.13140/RG.2.2.13011.94241
44. Nilsson J, Hallin P-O, Tykesson Klubien M, Guldåker N (2018) Skillnader i brandförekomst inom och mellan olika storstadsområden – en statistisk analys. Department of Human Geography, Lund University. Urban studies, Malmö University. https://doi.org/10.13140/RG.2.2.23399.39846
45. Guldåker N, Hallin P-O (2020) Livsvillkor och strategisk lägesbild. In: Gerell MH, Nilvall K, Westerdahl S (eds) Att vända utvecklingen – Från utsatta områden till trygghet och delaktighet, vol 26. Malmö University publications in urban studies (MAPIUS) 26. Malmö University, Malmö, pp 181–188
46. Göteborgs Stad Statistik och analys (2020) Available via Göteborgs stad. Göteborgs Stad https://goteborgse/wps/portal/enhetssida/statistik-och-analys/demografi-och-analys/korta-kommentarer/befolkningsutveckling-20192?uri=gbglnk%3A20200302112859772. Accessed 1 April 2021
47. Sandqvist A, Holmberg, H (1997) Vill du bidra till ett säkrare samhälle? – resultat från en undersökning om bränder och brandskydd i hemmet. Statistiska centralbyrån (SCB)
48. Weirup L (2020) Gangsterparadiset: Så blev Sverige arena för gängkriminalitet, skjutningar och sprängdåd. Bokförlaget Forum, Stockholm

Assoc. Prof. Nicklas Guldåker is a senior lecturer and associate professor in Human geography at Lund University. His research interest are in the fields of fires and fire prevention, but also more broadly in the fields of risk and crisis management, risk and vulnerability analysis, critical infrastructure, urban studies of crime, social unrest and social risks, data driven analysis, geostatistics, geovisualization and geographical information systems (GIS).

Prof. Per-Olof Hallin is a senior professor in Human geography at the Department of Urban Studies at Malmö University. His main research interest is different aspects of urban sustainable development. In later years, his research has focused on risk- and vulnerable analysis, residential fires, and crime development in urban areas.

Ms. Mona Tykesson Klubien has a Master in physical geography at Lund University. Mona is a lecturer in GIS at the Department of Human Geography, Lund University. Mona has been involved in several projects on residential and intentional fires, primarily as an expert in GIS and data management.

Dr. Jerry Nilsson has a Master in human geography at Lund University and finished his PhD in 2010 at the Division of Fire Safety Engineering. He was employed at Malmö University from 2010 to 2018 where he, apart from lecturing in GIS and statistics, has conducted research on residential fires. His research expertise also covers the field of risk and vulnerability analysis.

Chapter 19
Early Responders as a Resource for Effective Response

Björn Sund and Sofie Pilemalm

Abstract The public sector and emergency response worldwide face budget constraints and lack of resources while having to respond to an increasing number of emergenices. In this chapter, we will describe how the Swedish municipal fire services have addressed this challenge by initiating a first response with new ways of organizing their response units and through collaborations with other societal sectors, i.e., semiprofessionals and with citizen volunteers. This, by using experience from a ten years period and analyzing it in terms of cross-sector collaboration and coproduction. The chapter includes different emergency types the new resources can be dispatched to, with a specific focus on residential fires. The results show that the major benefit for all three forms of reorganization is a shorter response time, which can lead to more saved lives, reduced human suffering, and less material damage. When using semiprofessionals and volunteers, identified challenges include, e.g., prioritization of tasks, making the engagement collective, the dispatch technology, and avoiding risky situations. We discuss the implications of the results and provide some suggestions for future work.

Keywords First response · Co-production · Semi-professionals · Volunteers · Dispatch technology · Response time

1 Introduction

The public sector faces substantial and increasing challenges in terms of having to address complex societal challenges like, e.g., climate change and increased proportion of the elderly population while having scarce financial and personnel resources. Some of the ways to deal with the challenges are either to organize existing resources

---

B. Sund (✉)
Swedish Civil Contingencies Agency, Karlstad, Sweden
e-mail: Bjorn.Sund@msb.se

S. Pilemalm
Linköping University, Linköping, Sweden

in a different way or to create new collaboration forms that stretch over traditional organization and sector boundaries. Two of the latter forms are cross-sector collaboration and coproduction of public services with civil citizen volunteers [1, 9].

All of the above become crucial in emergency response which have to respond to frequent routine emergencies (such as residential fires) at the same time as being prepared to handle extraordinary events, large-scale crises, and catastrophes. The time from incident to emergency work starts (response time) is often crucial to limit the consequences of an emergency. Here, for instance, smaller fire response units may be nearer the emergency site than the fire station and/or have shorter reaction time (time from emergency services are alerted to first vehicle is departed). Also, other societal groups and sectors like local community associations or private security officers can collaborate with the municipal fire services in certain first response tasks, if they have sufficient training and equipment. In this chapter, we will focus on the Swedish municipal fire services possibilities to initiate a first response with new ways of organizing their response units and through collaborations with other societal sectors, i.e., semiprofessionals and with citizen volunteers (Fig. 19.1). The chapter will include various incidents the new resources can be dispatched to, but with a specific focus on residential fires.

The chapter will be disposed as follows. First, emerging ways of organizing first response will be presented, including dynamic fire response units, cross-sector collaboration, and coproduction. Then, the range of tasks they can potentially perform with perceived effects and benefits are described. This is followed by a presentation of empirical data on the various groups/collaborations. These data include tasks actually performed and estimated effects, but also identified challenges and future

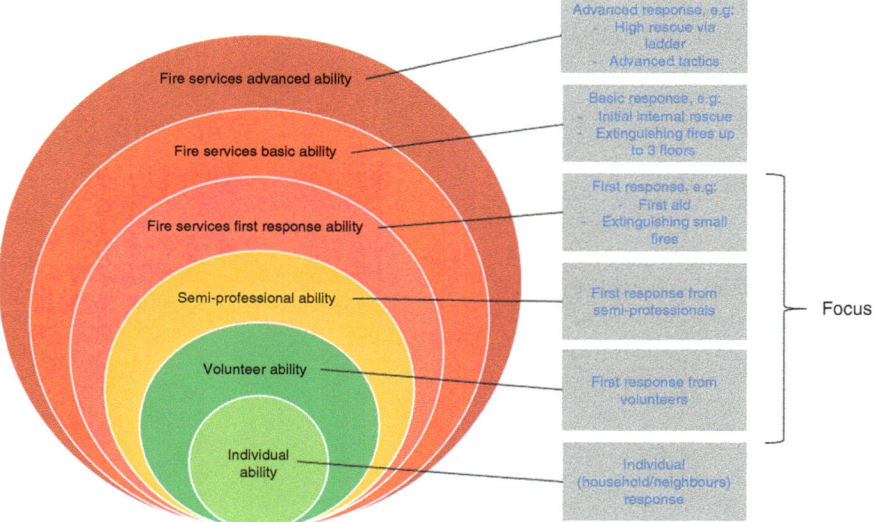

Fig. 19.1 Society's ability to respond to a residential fire. (Source: Adapted from Fire Services West)

needs. The chapter ends with a discussion of the main results, general conclusions, and future work. The chapter is based on a Swedish setting, but the results should have clear international relevance, since the public sector challenges a global and many basic first response the same across countries.

2 Reorganizing Swedish Emergency Response: Dynamic Resource Allocation, Cross-Sector Collaboration, and Coproduction

The Swedish fire rescue services have traditionally been organized in a statice manner according to the 4 + 1 principle. This implies that the fire team (usually residing at the fire station) includes four firefighters and a fire-chief in command that were dispatched to any emergency (e.g., residential fire) regardless of type, size, and complexity. Beginning in the early 2000s, initiatives started to emerge that leaned on *dynamic resource allocation*, i.e., more flexible fire units, including first response units [6, 19]. A fire service's first response unit is a resource from the rescue services organization consisting of at least one person and one vehicle (Fig. 19.2). This person, normally the fire-chief in command, has own vehicle at home or at the current workplace.[1] This means that he/she quickly can get to the accident site without

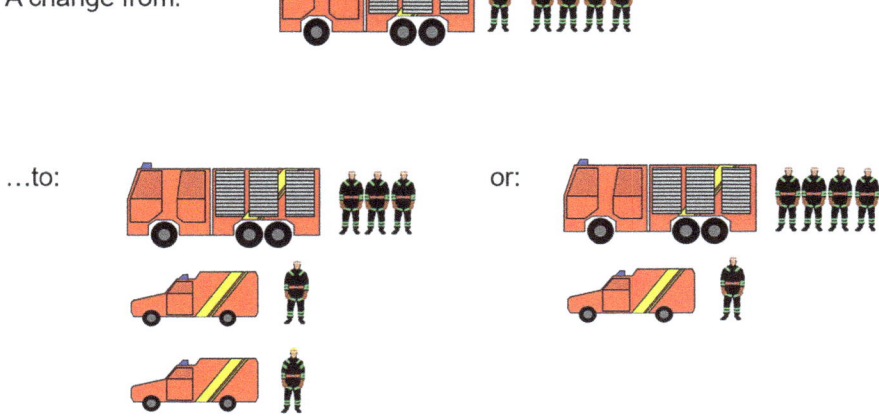

Fig. 19.2 Introducing a fire services first response unit (FIP)

---

[1] The current workplace can be at the fire station, but can also be at, e.g., the regular workplace (for a part-time fire-fighter) or a company's facilities in case of a fire inspection.

having to go past the fire station (or wait for the rest of the group).[2] Faster response and earlier lifesaving, delimiting property and enivonmental damage, and earlier existential support can be achieved. The Swedish abbreviation for first response units is often referred to as *FIP*, and we will use this abbriviation in the chapter.

Cross-sector and coproduction trends can be seen in many areas, e.g., in public health, health care, education, and emergency management [1]. In the past decade, an increasing number of Swedish municipal rescue services have also engaged in this by either engaging semiprofessionals or volunteers as first responders. *Cross-sector collaboration* simply refers to partnerships or network among different sectors, aimed to jointly address a common societal phenomenon. They can be both public-public and private-public [13]. Swedish emergency response has used the term *semiprofessionals* referring to individuals who do not have first response as their primary occupation but have competence and/or equipment that can be used in first response. Often are they on the move or on patrol in society, which imply that they can be near an emergency site. Common examples are security guards, home care personnel, and janitors.

Coproduction was first defined by Ostrom (described, e.g., in [9]) as the notion that society cannot maintain public service delivery without the active participation of its citizens. Coproduction implies a shift in how this delivery is seen where civil citizens become coproducers of services, rather than only receivers. In Swedish emergency response, volunteers are civil citizens who collaborate with the rescue services, receive basic equipment and training, and are alerted on certain predefined incidents, using apps installed on their own mobile phones. In Swedish, they are often referred to as *CIP* (civil first responder).

Sweden is seen as progressive both in using semiprofessionals and CIP in response to frequent emergencies including residential fires. This is perhaps due to the Swedish decentralized emergency response system leaving the local municipal rescue services with own mandate to decide on these matters. It is important to note that in both cases, as compared to a FIP, response is always voluntary. When you receive the alert, you can choose to go or not to go. As a semiprofessional, you are supposed to always prioritize your ordinary job, if a conflict of interest arises. Also, semiprofessionals and CIP act as first responders, while waiting for the professional resources to arrive; they never replace them.

The results in this chapter are based on various studies on FIP, semiprofessionals, and CIP in Swedish emergency response and spanning over a time period of 10 years (2010–2020). During this decade, the concepts have emerged, developed, and spread. For instance, using CIP first emerged in remote, sparsely populated areas in north Sweden, spread to rural areas and small municipalities, and finally, to cities, suburbs, and socioeconomically vulnerable areas [11].

---

[2] The reorganization to first response units is most applicable to part-time fire stations, but greater flexibility can also be achieved in full-time organizations, where, e.g., the fire-chief in command can be at a fire inspection or education without the rest of the group.

3 What Are the Effects of a First Response?

Compared to a basic or advanced fire response unit, the abilities of a first responder of all the above types are limited. However, the experience is that first responders can perform several important steps in the initial rescue work. FIP is generally more able to extinguish fires and might have mandate to scale up or scale down the rescue operation, while a semiprofessional from the home care might be better able to perform CPR or first aid. CIP may be successful in backing crowds in their own neighborhoods, and so on. Examples of tasks for first responders in case of a residential fire are:

- Briefing and assessment of accident site, submit status report to alarm center
- Report to following units (location/directions and overview of accident site)
- Plan rescue operation
- Scale up (request reinforcement) or scale down (return following units or report that the situation is not urgent) the rescue operation
- Review premises in case of automatic alarm
- open gates or doors to premises
- Warn people and inform[3]
- Extinguish minor fires with, e.g., a handheld fire extinguisher
- Take initial necessary lifesaving actions, e.g., CPR, first aid
- Provide early existential support for injured victims and bystanders

The opportunities of combining different tasks for first responders are many and sometimes they are not delimited to residential fires. A FIP also performs tasks in case of traffic accidents, drownings, etc. The main positive consequence is the shortened response time that leads to an earlier start of a selection of the possible tasks. This time saving should lead to less lost values in the form of lives, injuries, property damages, and environmental damages (Fig. 19.3). Of course, the ability is lower than for a basic or advanced response unit arriving at the same time.

To assess the efficiency of a first response initiative, it is necessary to identify both the additional benefits and costs (Table 19.1). The costs of introducing a first response unit are often straightforward to quantify. Benefits are more complicated to establish. Three general questions need to be answered: (1) what is the time difference, (2) what is the share of total rescue effort (ability) carried out by the unit, (3) what is the value of response time in case of a residential fire? E.g., if the time difference is five minutes, the ability is 25% and the value of time reduction is SEK 100,000, and the monetary benefit is SEK 25,000. Practical examples and experiences from the response categories will be discussed below.

One complication of evaluating residential fire first response is that the relatively low incidence rate and variation in characteristics of the fire and outcome,

---

[3] Information may be extra crucial in areas where people speak different languages, e.g., to explain why an individual who has been exposed to smoke needs to be taken to hospital even if he/she feels fine.

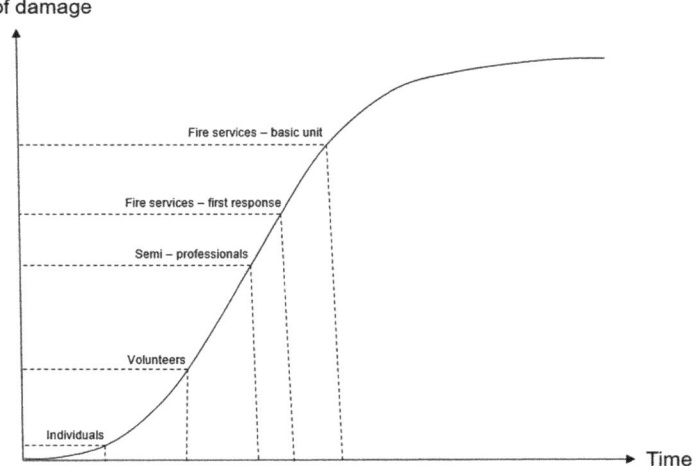

Fig. 19.3 Relation between response time for different resources and lost value

Table 19.1 Evaluation of first response units (example of benefits and costs)

Benefits (benefits are directly generated by a faster response time and an earlier start of possible tasks)	Costs
Saved lives	Equipment
Less injuries	Training (introduction and repetition)
Saved property values	Call-outs
Less environmental damages	Dispatch center
Earlier existential support (Elmqvist et al. [3] and Svensson et al. [17])	Hospitalization and health care
	Overhead

especially at municipal level, would not allow any estimation of the effect in many years. Another circumstance is that it often is interesting to make an effect estimation before the implementation. In this case, geographic information system (GIS) simulations can be one useful tool to estimate the reduced response times [16]. GIS can simulate the number of persons reached earlier by different sets of response resources.

4 Empirical Results

In the following sections, we describe the practical experience of using FIP, semi-professionals, and CIP, based on a number of Sweden initiatives and corresponding research studies. It should be noted that experience from the different groups is not described exactly in the same way. This is due to different perspecives in different studies and also to the time period the various initiatives have existed. For instance, the use of FIP has been established for more than one decade and much real estimations/quantitative data exist. For semiprofessionals and volunteers, initiatives are newer and still under development. CIP is also a different form of organization (of unaffiliated volunteers) and initiatives in the early phases in the cities/suburb. A related challenges is, thus, that the capacity of these two groups is not yet identified and thereby not quantified. In other words, what they can handle and what value they add to first response are still mostly on a predictive level. It has been necessary to first identify capacity by developing the collaboration forms, in some cases from scratch. Therefore, the available data regarding these two groups is in the main qualitative and based on action research [8]. However, some real estimations and experimental quantitative data exist.

Also, the FIP studies have been more targeted to residential fires, while studies on the latter groups are broader. This is simply because most common alerts here relate to other incidents. However, the residential fire aspect is taken when possible, and many of the tasks they perform can be used in residentital fires as well.

5 FIP

FIP was introduced in Sweden in the beginning of the 2000s. The most common FIP is a part-time firefighter who can directly get to the accident site in own emergency vehicle. FIP does not first go to the emergency station and therefore arrive earlier than the other part-time firefighters. The tasks that FIP normally can perform in case of a residential fire are listed in Sect. 3.

Perceived Benefits
What do we know about the effects of a FIP introduction? A cost-benefit analysis of introducing FIP in the municipality of Jönköping shows that the first response unit was first on accident site in 80% of the alarms [6]. Mean time difference was 2.5 min, and the first unit was able to manage *34% of the total rescue work* in 171 cases of structural fires.[4] The benefit-cost ratio is between 3 and 8.5, implying that introduction and use of FIP are economically beneficial to society.

Results from a project in Mälardalen (west of Stockholm) between 2008 and 2011 confirm the change in response time from introducing FIP units.[5] Measurement of the vehicles response times showed that the mean difference was about 3.5 min (889 accidents), which mainly corresponds to the *differences in the unit reaction time*. Only a marginal share of the time gain derives from driving time to incidence site. The observations are based on automatic time reports on department and arrival

---
[4] Structural fires include residential houses, but also industrial buildings, hospitals, hotels, etc.
[5] The results are not published and differences in response ability were not evaluated. Time measurements are for all types of accidents.

of emergency vehicles, which leads to high validity. A smaller scale quantitative data analysis (182 accidents) shows similar time gain, 3:51 min, and in 23% of the assignments, FIP was able to resolve the situation completely [17].

Challenges and Needs
FIP is now an established and widespread organization form in Sweden. One development that is taking place is that municipalities are expanding the number of FIP units to two or three units per emergency station. Depending on where, e.g., part-time firefighters are located, this can lead to a significant decrease in response times. The challenges of FIP are usually that personnel needs relevant training and a more strategic approach is sometimes requested. Another aspect is that the contact with the rest of the group can be lost or disturbed, which makes it more difficult to have a complete tactical plan on arrival to incident site. The need for support after a severe assignment is also raised [17].

6 Semiprofessionals

There are different groups of semiprofessionals currently active in Sweden, the most common being home care personnel and security guards which consequently are in focus in this chapter. Semiprofessionals act on a range of incidents including heart failure, single-vehicle traffic accidents, drownings, and outdoor fires (e.g., vehicles). Of specific relevance to this study are unintentional and intentional fires in residences. In relation to the above general list of potential tasks that first responders can perform (Sect. 3), the semiprofessionals report that they mainly carry out the following tasks:

- Extinguish small fires (both residential, other buildings and cars and both intentional and unintentional)
- Check if the fire has spread, and in this case inform the fire services
- First aid (e.g., CPR)
- Provide early existential support for injured victims and bystanders
- Keep bystanders at a distance when the response organizations arrive
- Break into buildings (security guards)
- Cut up cars with victims in them (security guards who have the equipment)

All incidents and tasks are predefined and regulated in formal agreements with the fire rescue services and their own employer.

Dispatch
To receive alerts, the semiprofessionals have to be within a certain radius from the emergency site. There is thus the hope of a more effective response if an emergency arises, even if the initiative is taking place in an urban area, where the response times for professional response organizations are relatively short. The semiprofessionals can also bring their own equipment to the emergency site. For instance, security guards have uniforms, fire extinguishers, and body armor. They also have

their own vehicles, provided by the security company and used in their ordinary occupation, and have their own training programs in addition to the first-response training provided by the fire association. They also have access to their own debriefing activities, are insured by their own employer, and are also provided with vaccination programs, e.g., for Hepatitis B [11].

The dispatching is achieved using handheld RAKEL terminals. RAKEL is the national radio communication system used in Sweden, used by all the blue-light response organizations, e.g., the fire services, the ambulance services, the police, and the public safety answering point (PSAP). This means that they use the same system as the rescue services and can communicate with all of them, in real-time. RAKEL is primarily for audio communication [11].

Perceived Benefits

The major benefit of using semiprofessionals is *shorter response times* since they are continually on patrol in the subareas, so they have no reaction time (the time it takes from alarm to leaving the fire station). As an example, the estimated mean time to reach the incident site is 3 min and 56 s[6] for an entire Södertälje municipality south of Stockholm (with about 300,000 inhabitants), including the most remote areas. For the central municipality, the average time is even shorter, as reported by a security guard in Pilemalm [11]. In another study in Norrköping municipality of about 100,000 inhabitants, there was no access to real response times since it was a development project. However, predictive quantifications and modeling were performed in parallel to developing the concept of semiprofessionals, in part based on how they could contribute to decrease of response times, in part based on their expected contributions at the incident site. The results showed that for Norrköping and Linköping municipalities, a few (3–4) semiprofessionals could decrease costs for accidents and acute illness with about 700,000–5,000,000 SEK per year, depending on station reaction time [2].

A study in a municipality in the south of Sweden (Helsingborg with about 140,000 inhabitants 2016) evaluates a potential agreement between the fire services and a private security officers' firm in responding to residential fires [16]. A geographic information system (GIS) simulation is used to estimate the response times and the results show that the reduction is 52 s on average. The potential initiation has positive economic effects with the benefits estimated to be 1.4 (saved lives) and 2.3 (saved lives and property damage) times higher than the costs.

Weinholt et al. [19] have also analyzed the effects of using security officers for fire response in a municipality in Sweden (Söderköping with about 15,000 inhabitants 2019). They found that, out of 60 alarms, the security officers were first on the incident site in 34 cases. In seven of these, the security officers were able to suppress the fire on their own. In two of these fires, there was a risk of the fire spreading and causing damage. The benefits were estimated to exceed the costs, so although the incidents were few, an economic evaluation indicated that the collaboration was socially beneficial.

---

[6] Including emergency call handling time, station reaction time, and driving time to incident site.

Using the qualitative data, we have seen several examples of home care personnel extinguishing fires before they spread. As mentioned, a major difference as compared to FIP is that semiprofessional must not go on the alerts (it is voluntary). However, it seems both security guards and home care personnel are used to acting in acute situations (e.g., medical alarms, small fires) and do not seem afraid to act upon them, either alone or together (e.g., [11]).

Another benefit is *preventive* to create a sense of presence, security, and social relations and thereby decrease the incidence of, e.g., intentional fires, assaults, and vandalism. Direct removal of flammable objects is another preventive effect.

Challenges and Needs

The associated challenges are perceived somewhat different depending on occupation group. The agreements regulating the semiprofessionals' first-response missions and tasks are sometimes seen as a challenge. It has happened that security guards are dispatched to types of incidents for which they are not prepared (e.g., drownings), since this is stipulated in their contracts. Conversely, they sometimes go to incident types that they should not attend based on personal judgements, e.g., suicide or traffic accidents on the highway. Also, in Sweden, the Public Procurement Act currently stipulates that the Swedish municipalities that want to use security guards must in the future perform procurement processes. The security guard company's project leader argues that this may lead to a situation in which those companies providing the service for the lowest price will receive the assignment since no other quality indicators currently exist: There is thus a fear that the Procurement Act will not only lead to a lower-quality response; but also that the preventive work, i.e., patrolling the area and talking to young people, preventing them from engaging in crime, and creating social relations perhaps leading to recruitment as security guard, will diminish. The perceived need for quality indicators and clear regulations is repeatedly stated by project manager [11]. As regards home care personnel, the major challenge seems to be prioritization between first response and ordinary tasks since their ordinary work schedule is tight [20]. Evening and night personnel have easier to take on first response tasks than daytime personnel.

As for information and communications technology (ICT), the security guards seem content with being able to audiocommunicate with the other response organizations through RAKEL but still describe it as heavy, old-fashioned, and clumsy. There have been requests on Android-based mobile solutions through which text-based information, pictures, and even video recordings from the incident site can be sent, in order to prepare the arriving response organizations better.

7 Volunteers

Civil volunteers (CIP) in Sweden are currently active in remote, rural, and urban areas. They are usually provided with one day of basic training in such areas as first aid, cardiopulmonary resuscitation (CPR), extinguishing small fires, and acting in single-vehicle traffic accidents. They also receive a backpack containing a first-aid kit, reflective vests, pocket masks, and handheld fire extinguishers. They are then dispatched to the following types of emergency: outdoor fires (e.g., vehicle), residential fires and certain fires in other buildings (e.g., shools), heart failure, single-vehicle traffic accidents, and drownings. The emergency should not be risky for them (e.g., uncontrolled fires or a shooting) [11].

Relating to the general list, a first responder can perform (see Sect. 3.) a range of tasks at the emergency site. Those reported as most frequent are:

- Extinguish small fires (both residential, other buildings and cars and both intentional and unintentional)
- Check if the fire has spread, and in this case inform the fire services
- First aid (e.g., CPR, band aid, stopping major bleeding)
- Provide early existential support for injured victims and bystanders
- Keep bystanders at a distance when the response organizations arrive
- Act as interpreters in urbans areas where many people do not speak Swedish

The collaboration with the fire services is generally much less formalized than for semiprofessionals. For instance, they receive a debriefing from fire service personnel immediately after a response operation, but no follow-ups. The civil volunteers are collectively insured by the fire association.

Dispatch
The principle for dispatch is the same as for the semiprofessionals, i.e., they have to be within a certain radius (e.g., 5 km) from the incident site to receive an alert. However, CIPs are most often dispatched by means of commercial apps connected to their own mobile phone GPS functions which in their turn are connected to the fire services' system for handling incoming alerts. The apps can, e.g., display the position coordinates, the address (road, but not specific number), municipality, and type of emergency, giving basic information. It sometimes also includes a map, and when the alert is triggered, a red button appears on the map, indicating the emergency site. Through this button, the volunteers (receivers of the alert) can also communicate with the rescue services and each other, to some extent, and provide updated information about the emergency. It is the fire services' back-office systems that provide the GPS coordinates, the addresses, and the information about the emergency, i.e., CIP receives the same basic information as FIP [11] (Fig. 19.4).

Perceived Benefits
The major perceived benefit is also the same as for semiprofessionals: a more effective response (shorter response times). In remote and rural areas, CIP close to always arrive at the incident site before the professional response organizations [14]. In urban areas, they sometimes do [11]. It has occurred also in urban areas that the CIPs have extinguished fires before they spread, e.g., cars or even an intentional fire threatening to burn down a school. As mentioned before, for CIPs, in the qualitative data, are the main source, due to the newness of the related initiatives. However, there are several studies that have produced general prediction models for optimal dispatch of the CIPs including estimations of response times and how

increased efficiency and use can be reached (e.g., [7]). Also, there are similar initiatives in Sweden focusing only on dispatching volunteers to out-of-hospital cardiac arrests (SMS-life-rescuers). Here, studies have had access to real data and performed economic evaluations for the regions in Sweden in applying the concept. For each region, expected saved lives and costs for quality-adjusted lifeyears (QALYs) were calculated. The results indicate that SMS life rescue saver is a cost-efficient intervention for prehospital acute care of heart failure patients outside hospitals [4]. Even if this is a specialized form of volunteers not including residential fires, it is possible that cost-efficiency could apply in the latter case as well.

There are also perceived qualitative benefits relating to, e.g., restoring services and vitality in rural areas and to increase security in urban areas. In the latter, in socioeconomically vulnerable areas, it has also been shown beneficial that CIPs who are active in a certain area speak its dominant language and can act as interpreters, since many people in these areas do not speak Swedish. In Pilemalm [11], a respondent, for instance, describes a residential fire where an apartment building was on fire and the residents wanted to jump, due to language barriers where they could not communicate with the fire association personnel. The respondents also describe how they can inform people, e.g., about risks being exposed to smoke and the need for a hospital checkup.

Challenges and Needs

The major perceived challenge in urban areas, especially in those socioeconomically vulnerable, is to ensure that the CIPs actually respond to alerts and go to the incident site. There are a few enthusiasts who respond to many alerts, but they are often the only ones responding to that particular alert, making the first response an individual task [11]. In remote and rural areas, the perceived challenges are the other way round. The first response becomes a highly collective task where many CIPs act jointly, which is positive, but can also create difficulties, e.g., if they block

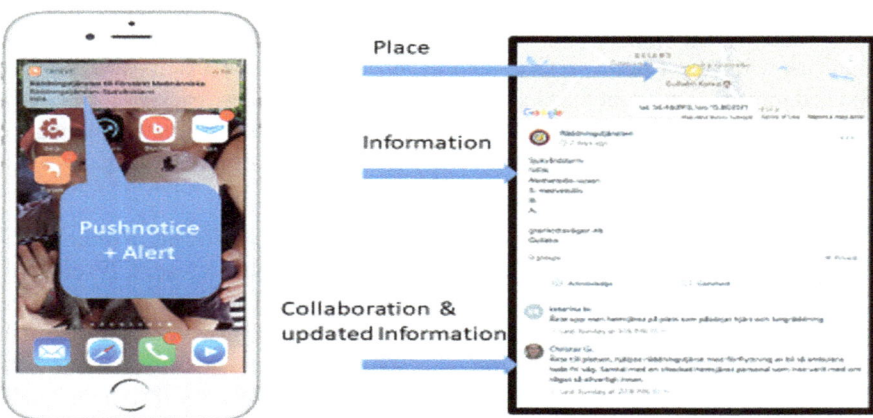

Fig. 19.4 Dispatching of volunteers through the app. The type of incident here is a single-vehicle traffic accident in which the victim is unconscious

the way for the professional response organizations. A related challenge/difference concerns gender aspects. In socioeconomically vulnerable areas, all the active volunteers are men. In rural areas with dominating Swedish ethnicity, gender distribution is equal [12].

Another perceived challenge in the former is language (which thus is both perceived as a benefit and a challenge). It is not optimal to send just any volunteer, but rather one who knows the particular language of those involved in an emergency or the dominant language in the given subarea. An organizational challenge is to make all rescue services take on CIP the concept at management level. Even though most rescue services are positive, others are resistant mostly in urban settings. This might have to do with the higher level of risk CIPs are exposed to in these settings. An identified challenge which mainly relates to urban settings is if a situation escalates into something dangerous, e.g., an explosion or a shooting. Then there is currently no way of withdrawing the CIPs [12].

Concrete needs concern mostly the ICT solution and include, e.g., better GPS positioning (exact coordinates, information indicating roads, and GPS guidance (incorrect positioning has sometimes delayed response time)) and calibration. Also, a withdrawal function seems necessary if an emergency turns into something dangerous. The latter implies that some structure, templates, and matching are needed to send the "right" CIP to the "right" site, reaching different roles, competences, and language groups. It is also notable that in rural areas CIPs are much more active in "equipping themselves", e.g., in jointly buying flashlights and powder extinguishers [14, 15].

8 Discussion

In this section, we first discuss the identified values of reorganization, cross-collaboration, and coproduction in emergency response. We compare the groups of FIP, semiprofessional, and CIP, identifying similarities and differences. Second, we discuss the importance of digitalization and proper ICT for dispatch. Finally, we make some general conclusions on cross-sector collaboration and coproduction trends, in emergency response and in public service delivery.

Reorganizing Emergency Response: The Perceived Value
Initiating different categories of first response resources is generally economically beneficial to society [6, 16]. One important reason for this is that the marginal cost is very low. The direct costs consist only of a relatively short training and limited equipment. In the case of FIP, the cost can also imply a vehicle. No time for preparedness is initiated in either case, so the only alternative cost of time (after education) is the short time spent on callouts. Resources are generally "back at work" within one hour. The benefits are potentially very large, and even though the time gains generally are larger in rural areas, the number of fires and the steeper slope of

the survival curve at short response times (reference to this in the book) provide relevant arguments for first response in urban areas.

Our research involving various groups acting as early responders confirms the above. Regardless of if they are FIPs, semiprofessionals, and CIPs, and work in remote, rural, and urban areas, in various municipalities and/or socioeconomically vulnerable areas, they have one thing in common: *they can contribute to a more effective first response* where they have saved lives and reduced injuries, property, and environmental damages. The response time is of course crucial, but from our experience there are also other perceived benefits such as improving security and social relations in communities, inclusion of vulnerable groups, and preventing crime and accidents (e.g., intentional and unintentional fires). This above all applies to cross-sector collaboration and coproduction.

There are also perceived differences between various groups of early responders. As indicated in Sect. 3, the groups can perform a range of tasks, but FIPs (that are firefighters) can naturally perform a wider range than semiprofessionals and CIPs. On the other hand, semiprofessionals can perform other tasks, for instance if they have keys to apartments in residential fires and CIPs in socially vulnerable areas may communicate with residents that the fire services would otherwise not reach efficiently.

In relation, perceived differences include that formalization is much more present in, of course, FIPs, but also in the case of semiprofessionals/cross-sector collaboration. This gives them a more secure position than volunteers, protected by agreements and training provided by their own employer. As to volunteers, in rural areas the response time is more affected since the volunteers almost always arrive before the professionals as compared to the same in urban areas. Also, to have the concept working in urban areas requires more investment in time and resources. Acting in residential fires is more common in urban areas since there are more apartments and so on. Within the semiprofessional groups, daytime firefighters and security guards seem to have more possibilities to prioritize between first response and "ordinary" tasks than home care personnel, etc.

In summary, various groups should be seen as complements and reinforcements of each other, not competitors. It should also be noted that even though we in this chapter have included more types of incidents than residential fires (especially for semiprofessionals and CIPs), most of the tasks carried out as reported by our respondents are highly applicable to a residential fire as well. Moreover, and for the future, it is important to evaluate the marginal effects of first responders, but also to study the possibility to take on extra tasks for the individual category of responders. In the latter case, society needs to provide better support for prioritizing different tasks and be more coordinated in distributing the alarms.

Digitalization and ICT for Dynamic Resource Dispatch
In relation to the above need for improved coordination of, above all, semiprofessionals and volunteers, it is interesting to observe that they, though being different groups, have similar requirements on the ICT artefact. Ramsell et al. [15] let the groups put requirements on an app prototype for alert and both groups identified

similar basic requirements (needed to solve the task) and additional functionality (not necessarily needed but which would improve the assignment). Differences rather related to how they prioritized certain requirements. In Pilemalm [11], the semiprofessionals express that their RAKEL terminals are clumsy and the audio-based communication limits them, requesting text-based alternatives, android-based solutions, and the possibility to send pictures from the incident site. The authors also argue that it is likely that the semiprofessional volunteers would benefit from the same calibrations of ICT solutions as the civil-citizen volunteers. By matching competence with situation, semiprofessionals might avoid potential risky situations they sometimes encounter today. As for volunteers in rural and urban areas, there are similar needs to calibrate the ICT artifact to optimize dispatch and response, e.g., by matching incident with competence, training, and equipment. In socioeconomically vulnerable areas, language constitutes another factor. There is also a need for alarm strategies, however, in urban areas to enable collective enactment of volunteers on an alert and in rural areas, the other way round, to hinder too many volunteers showing up at the incident site at the same time. This, by alerting in descending order based on their closeness to the incident site. There are also a common need for a withdrawal function if the incident should turn into something dangerous for the volunteers (e.g., explosion, gunfire) [11]. All in all, this would contribute to the dynamic resource dispatch – and optimized response – that the reorganization and new collaboration forms aim at.

Global Increasing Trends of Collaboration and Coproduction: International Transferability
Taking a general perspective, the need for cross-sector collaboration and coproduction will likely continue to grow, in Sweden and internationally. This, since challenges relating to increased crises, pandemics, and the simultaneous need to simultaneously handle frequent accidents (sometimes in growing populations) with strained public sector resources are global (e.g., [1, 18]). To our knowledge, Sweden is progressive in using semiprofessionals as early responders. As for volunteers, international research and practice tend to focus on large-scale crises and crowdsourcing, not on organized long-term collaborations in relation to accidents of smaller scale. Here, the Swedish experience pan paves the way and be used as a source of inspiration for similar research and initiatives in other countries. From a digitalization perspective, our experience confirms previous research (e.g., [5]), pointing out the need to pay larger attention to the ICT artefact as an enabler of digitalized cross-sector collaboration and coproduction.

9 Future Work

In the future, it is a need to further develop the various concepts of early responders from various perspectives, including policy aspects and ICT support. As for residential fires, steering models including the fire services and the real estate companies, and in socioeconomically vulnerable areas, the social services, are deemed of particular importance [12]. Also, for residential fires, it would be possible to connect the ICT dispatch artifact to smoke detectors in selected real estates, for an even faster response. From an international research perspective, it would be of great interest to explore similar initiatives in other countries, to enable comparisons and transfer experience. Also, one of the most urgent societal developments for fire safety work in Sweden is the dramatic growth of the absolute number of elderly single people. The number of inhabitants older than 80 years will increase with 50% within the next 10 years. Although old age and living alone are not risk factors for dying in a residential fire in itself, these factors indicate increased difficulty perceiving or evacuating in the event of a fire. In these cases, proximity to early responders becomes even more important in the future. Particularly when these vulnerable individuals continue to live in their residences instead of moving to retirement homes.

References

1. Alford JA, O'Flynn J (2012) Rethinking public service delivery: managing with external providers. Macmillan, Hampshire
2. Andersson Granberg T, Pilemalm S (2020) Evaluation of new first response initiatives in emergency services. Socioecon Plann Sci 71. https://doi.org/10.1016/j.seps.2020.100829
3. Elmqvist C, Fridlund B, Ekebergh M (2008) More than medical treatment: the patient's first encounter with prehospital emergency care. Int Emerg Nurs 16:185–192
4. Ennab Vogel N, Levin L-Å (2020) Sms-livräddare vid akut omhändertagande av patient med hjärtstopp utanför sjukhus - en kostnadseffektivitetsanalys. English title: Sms-livesavers in acute care for out-of hospital cardiac arrest
5. Gil-Garcia R, Dawes SS, Pardo TA (2008) Digital government and public management research: finding the crossroads. Public Manag Rev 20(5):633–646
6. Lång E (2012) Är införande av förstainsatsperson samhällsekonomiskt lönsamt? En kostnadsnyttoanalys av FIP-verksamheten i Jönköpings kommun. English title: is introduction of first responders economically beneficial to society? A cost-benefit analysis of the project of first responders in the municipality of Jönköping. Karlstad Business School. Economics. Master thesis. (In Swedish, abstract in English)
7. Matinrad N, Andersson Granberg T, Andelakis V (2021) Modeling uncertain task compliance in dispatch of volunteers to out-of-hospital cardiac arrest patients. Comput Ind Eng 159. https://doi.org/10.1016/j.cie.2021.107515
8. Myers M (2009) Qualitative research in business and management. Sage Publications, Thousand Oaks
9. Ostrom E (2016) Crossing the great divide: coproduction, synergy, and development. World Dev 24(6):1073–1087
10. Pilemalm S (2020) Volunteer co-production in emergency management in excluded areas – using civil citizens and semi-professionals as first responders. E-journal of E-democracy and E-participation. JEDEM 12(1). https://doi.org/10.29379/jedem.v12i1.583
11. Pilemalm S (2021) Digitalized co-production: using volunteers as first responders. Proceedings of Eigth International Conference on eDemocracy & eGovernment (IceDeg), in Press
12. Pilemalm S, Yousefi Mojir K (2020) ICT enabled cross-sector collaboration in emergency response: emerging forms of public-sector network governance. Int J Emerg Manag 16(3):249–280

13. Ramsell E, Pilemalm S, Andersson Granberg T (2017) Using volunteers for emergency response in rural areas – network collaboration factors and IT support in the case of enhanced neighbors. Proceedings of 14th international conference on Information Systems for Crisis Response and Management (ISCRAM), Albi, pp 2411–3387
14. Ramsell E, Andersson Granberg T, Pilemalm S (2019) A smartphone application for volunteers in emergency response. Proceedings of the 15th international conference on Information Systems for Crisis Response and Management (ISCRAM), Valencia, pp 1044–1056
15. Sund B, Jaldell H (2018) Security officers responding to residential fire alarms: estimating the effect on survival and property damage. Fire Saf J 97:1–11
16. Svensson A, Almerud Österberg S, Fridlund B, Stening K, Elmqvist C (2018) Firefighters as first incident persons: breaking the chain of events and becoming a new link in the chain of survival. International Journal of Emergency Services 7(2):120–133
17. Voorberg WH, Bekkers VJM, Tummers LG (2015) A systematic review of co-creation and co-production: embarking on the social innovation journey. Public Adm Rev 17(9):1333–1357
18. Weinholt Å (2015) Exploring collaboration between the fire and rescue service and new actors cost-efficiency and adaptation. Linköping University. Linköping Studies in Science and Technology. Thesis No. 1710. Licentiate Thesis
19. Yousefi Mojir K, Pilemalm S, Andersson Granberg T (2018) Semi-professionals: emergency response as an additional task in current occupations. Int J Emerg Serv 8(2):86–107

Dr. Björn Sund holds a PhD in Economics from Örebro University. Björn started as a project assistant and researcher in the field of Fire and Rescue Services in 1996. Since 2011 he has been employed as an analyst at the Learning from Accidents Section at the Swedish Civil Contingencies Agency. Research focus has been valuation of statistical life, stated preference methodology, cost-benefit analysis regarding faster emergency response to cardiac arrests, demographic determinants of incident experience and risk perception, willingness to pay for a quality-adjusted life-year (QALY) and residential fires. From 2018 he has been involved in evaluation and revision of the Swedish national strategy for strengthened fire protection. He is also a lecturer in economic evaluation at Karlstad University.

Prof. Sofie Pilemalm is a Professor in informatics at Linköping university. Since 2011, she is Director of the Centre for Advanced Research in Emergency Response (CARER), financed by the Swedish Civil Contingencies Agency and runs a related research programme. Her research interests include information systems development with focus on user participation, organizational learning and co-production, all taking place within the emergency response domain. She has supervised several Ph. D. students with focus on semi-professionals and volunteerism in emergency response. Since 2021, she also holds a part-time adjunct professorship in information systems at University of Agder, at the Centre for Integrated Research in Emergency Management (CIEM).

Chapter 20
Swedish Strategies for Prevention of Residential Fires: The Case of the Swedish Fire Protection Association and the Swedish Civil Contingencies Agency

Mattias Delin, Maya Stål Söndergaard, and Björn Sund

Abstract The chapters above and the research they are based on point towards a viable strategy to reduce the consequences of fire in dwellings, regarding mortality, injury, loss of residence and property. How can this be put into practice? In this chapter, two synchronised and complementary strategies from the Swedish Fire Protection Association and the Swedish Civil Contingencies Agency are presented as models, and the processes connected to the strategies are discussed.

The two organisations strive towards a common goal on paths that sometimes differ because of their differences in characteristics. Collaborations between the two are seen as a way to make that a strength. Together, they can influence many different parties with many different tools. The scope can also be widened based on the collaboration when the Swedish Civil Contingencies Agency weighs more towards the safety of lives and the Swedish Fire Protection Association therefore can weigh more towards the safety of the environment and property.

The chapter takes the perspectives of the two organisations and is based on their experiences and policies, which may not always be results of academic research.

Keywords Residential fires · Fire strategy · Fire safety strategy · Vision-zero implementation · Fire indicators · Prioritized fire measures · Sustainable residences

---

M. Delin (✉) · M. S. Söndergaard
The Swedish Fire Research Foundation (Brandforsk), Stockholm, Sweden
e-mail: mattias.delin@brandforsk.se

B. Sund
The Swedish Civil Contingencies Agency, Karlstad, Sweden

1 A National Fire Protection Strategy

In many countries, the prime responsibility for the Fire and Rescue Services and, consequently, for the bulk of the fire prevention work falls upon the local municipalities. In Sweden, this responsibility is regulated in the Law on Protection Against Accidents [1]. According to this Law, municipalities shall plan and organise its prevention activities in order to effectively prevent fires. Special emphasis shall be put on the prevention of fatalities and other serious injuries. To achieve this, the municipalities shall have a goal-oriented action programme describing its preventive activities. The factual situation is, however, that in most municipalities, even in the bigger cities, fatal fires will not occur with such a frequency that a local statistical analysis or goal-oriented follow-up of occurrences will be meaningful. Therefore, the need for a national goal-setting regime and strategy, combined with a nation-wide surveillance system, will be evident.

There exist several such strategies in other countries. For example, in Norway the parliament set a strategy for fire prevention in 2009 [2], later followed up with a communication strategy [3]. In Europe, initiatives for common strategies on EU level have been put forward more recently [4].

In the United States, the Vision 20/20 [5] was founded in 2008 by the US branch of the Institution of Fire Engineers with the support of a number of public and private organisations.

In Sweden, more people than usual died in connection with residential fires 2009 (124 people).

During the autumn, three notable fires occurred in which a total of 15 people lost their lives. The three tragic events became an eye-opener for society and a symbol of the problem of fatal residential fires. Sufficient knowledge on how one should act in the case of a fire was lacking as well as functioning fire alarms which could have warned those in danger at an early stage. In one of the fires, those who died were also restricted in their ability to move and could not evacuate without help.

In November the same year, the Swedish government gave the state authority, the Swedish Civil Contingencies Agency (MSB), the task of producing a national strategy on how fire protection could be improved through support to individuals. A national vision zero inspired by the national vision zero for transport safety was formed: "No one should die or be seriously injured as the result of a fire" (see Chap. 15). Concrete goals were also established which would lead towards the vision. The number of deaths and serious injuries would reduce by a third by the year 2020. Furthermore, awareness among individuals with regard to fire risks and how to act in the case of a fire should be increased as well as the number of functioning fire alarms and fire protection equipment in residences. From the start, it was clear that this must be a long-term commitment and that it would need to be carried out together with many different parties.

In 2010, a national group for fire protection was formed by MSB with the task of coordinating, managing in the long-term and, when necessary, develop the national strategy. The identification of the need for support and guidance for the implementation of the strategy and assistance with resources in order to produce these guidance documents is very important. The parties participating in the group are state authorities with responsibility in the area, representatives from the municipalities as well as interest groups for the municipalities and regions, property owners, insurance companies, chimney sweeps, fire chiefs and the Swedish Fire Protection Association (SFPA).

Since the national strategy was adopted in 2010, the available knowledge has changed considerably. A large research undertaking was launched in 2013, and in the years following, researchers have mapped different aspects of residential fires: in which residences fires take place; where the fires start; who is affected and how; as well as which efforts and technical systems can prevent a fire from starting or reduce its effects.

At the start of 2019, a review of the focus of the strategy was begun in which the goal was to establish new milestones up to 2030 and to prioritise measures in order to achieve the established goals. MSB gathered stakeholders together in several workshops in which issues connected to the setting of goals and development within the fire protection field up to 2030 were discussed. In the same year, SFPA initiated its work on a new strategy for residential fires, a project that is similar to MSB's in many ways but done from the perspective of a non-profit organisation.

In order to make long-term improvements to fire safety possible, many parties must come together, and a strategic plan is an important element in the leadership of this project. The creation of a national fire protection strategy sends an important message and can help to bring the issue to the fore. If important stakeholders choose to support it, society can gather the strength to achieve the desired result. The great challenge then lies in the implementation of the strategy, to get those involved to go from nice words to concrete action which will lead to the common goal.

A strategic plan also lays the groundwork for long-term work which can encompass many different operational plans and can be adjusted when needed without changing the strategic plan. In addition to their own organisation, other organisations can easily connect to the strategic plan with their own operational plans. In that regard, the strategy can serve as guidance and support. By helping to build a network from a national perspective, stakeholders can be inspired by each other and good examples can be set. Local involvement and champions of the project can function as catalysts (Fig. 20.1).

> The strategy should be a long-term plan that leads to a (long-term) goal. Simply, where are we today? Where do we want to be? How do we get there?

2 A Strategy for the Whole Society

In order for a national fire protection strategy to be able to take real effect, broad participation is needed from those involved at different levels. All parties concerned should be included early on in the process and they should also get the opportunity

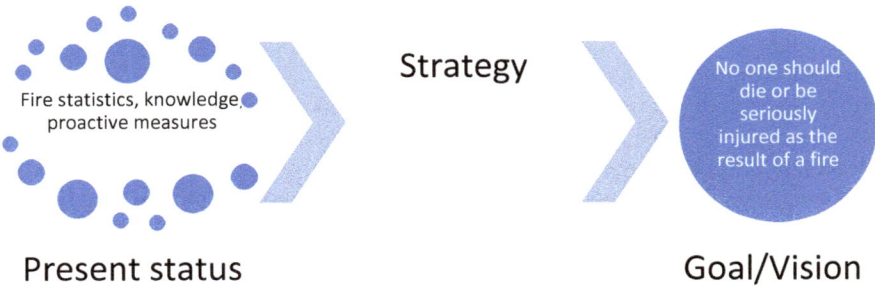

Fig. 20.1 The strategy forms the overall journey from present status to desired status but needs to be supplemented by operational plans

to comment on the final strategy before a decision is made. Those involved must feel a sense of 'ownership' for the content in order to be able to take responsibility for the implementation in the next stage. It must also be clear in which way the different parties can contribute and how they can work together. When the strategy is implemented, it will be advantageous for other parties to be involved through their own operational plans that connect to the strategic plan.

At a *national level*, a central authority or organisation should be given a clearly designated responsibility in order to coordinate and drive the project forwards. However, it is also important to note that the work must be done in close collaboration with other authorities and interest groups. At a national level, it is important to focus on developing the system and creating the conditions needed for the project on a local/regional level. This can happen by, for example, revising and clarifying regulations and legislation, creating support and guidance for the project on a local/regional level and setting good examples, etc.

At a *local/regional level*, the municipal rescue services can be a driving force for the project, but it is important that this happens in close collaboration with other authorities and organisations. There are several examples of successful collaborations with property owners of multi-residential buildings. For example, with respect to spreading knowledge to the residents and ensuring that there are functioning fire alarms in the residences. In order to improve fire protection for vulnerable individuals in society, authorities such as social services and health care in the municipality must work together. The staff in these organisations can best identify which individuals require improved fire protection and can also identify risks and carry out measures in the home environment.

It is also important to involve *academic representation* (researchers) in the project. From a national perspective, it is possible to create incentives and stimulate different initiatives in order to increase knowledge of the challenges and of the best way to work to reduce the number of residential fires and their consequences.

The reasoning behind involving many different parties in the strategy project is to achieve a greater impact and to reach a wider audience. As the parties involved possess different competencies, the quality of the work will most likely be better.

However, those involved have different incentives and different conditions that they must adhere to. In certain cases, an authority can have the right to demand things from certain parties, for example through legislation. At the same time, there are constitutional restrictions on what can be asked of other parties. In contrast, non-governmental organisations, for example, a non-profit organisation, cannot demand anything from anyone, but there are also no limitations on whom they can try to influence.

3 The Process to an Established Strategy

Broad participation is a success factor in reaching the goal and in the success of the strategy. This means that important parties need to be involved with both the development of the strategy and continually during the implementation.

The process of developing a new strategy can begin once a decision to do so has been made at the necessary level. That decision should be proceeded by a pilot study which should at least include a needs analysis, goal setting and resource allocation, as well as which resources in society should be covered by the strategy. One very important part of the preparatory work is to describe the challenges and the knowledge that exist in the area. The result of the most recent research must lay the basis for the needs analysis, which is a part of the preparatory work, so that the strategy goes in the right direction in order to achieve the goals.

A presentation of the results of the pilot study should also be conducted in conjunction with other stakeholders in order to ensure that all involved understand the conditions of the project. Thus, forming an important basis for good leadership for the project leader. The project needs to find a balance between, on the one hand, taking ownership for their own process in order to achieve the goal within the framework set out, and on the other hand, fostering a project that allows other parties involved to feel a sense of "ownership" for the end product. The process can take form in many ways, but it must include many occasions for dialogue in order for agreements to be made, similar to the Delphi method. It cannot be expected that all parties will be in complete consensus from the start; however, with a good process, this can be achieved in the end, and it is of the utmost importance for the success of the strategy that this happens (Fig. 20.2).

4 From Strategy to Practice

When the strategy is determined, the real work will begin, namely creating results and thereby achieving the goals of the strategy. The project can be likened to a cyclic process where the different steps repeat in order to constantly evaluate and improve the strategy (plan, carry out, follow up and provide feedback of results), see Fig. 20.3.

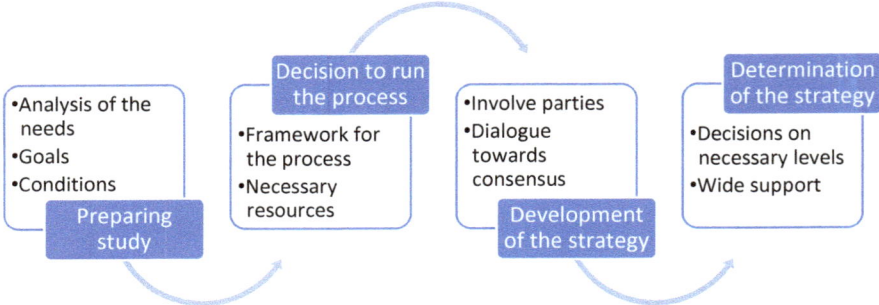

Fig. 20.2 Four stages through the process: Preparing study – Decision to run the process – Development of the strategy – Determination of the strategy

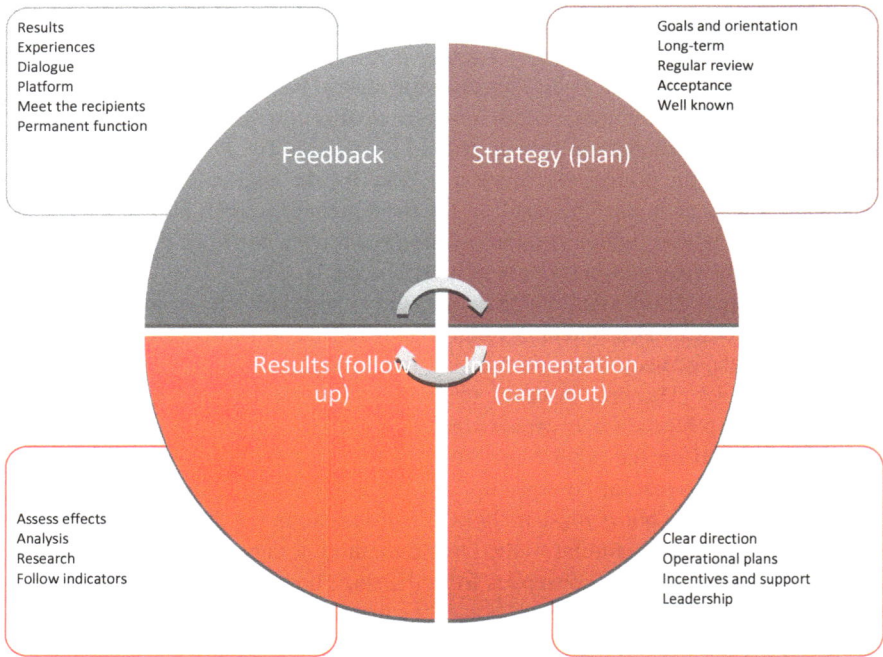

Fig. 20.3 The process from strategy, through implementation to results will need regular feedback loops followed by adjustments of the strategy/operations

4.1 Strategy (Plan)

As mentioned before, the strategy should set out the long-term plan that leads toward a long-term goal. In order to take real effect, it needs to be clear to all parties where we are going and why, as well as what needs to be done. Over time, the results will show if we are going in the right direction, or if the strategy needs to change. Therefore, a regular review of the strategy is necessary.

An advantage of the strategic plan is that it can be supplemented with operational plans which are adapted for each party and do not need to correspond with the whole strategic plan. Thus, operational puzzle pieces from the different stakeholders are created. The implementation must be based on the incentive and abilities of the different parties involved. Some of those involved have a liability to work towards better fire safety, while others work voluntarily towards the goal. To be successful, every stakeholder must be willing and able to contribute, based on their respective circumstances. The strategy's project leader will also need to assume responsibility to take the lead and show the way.

> The implementation of the strategy is a process in which the feedback of results is an important component. Regular review of both the strategic plan and operational plans needs to be carried out as the state of knowledge changes.

4.2 Implementation (Carry Out)

The strategic plan must be supplemented with operational plans which are adapted to each party and its capabilities. To help those involved, examples of things that can be implemented are needed and help with incentives may also be required sometimes so that their efforts can be motivated in their own organisation. In other words, the project leaders need to be able to help with both motivation and ability in order to do what is required. "Early adaptors" are often valuable when it comes to the effort put into the initial stages as they are often both willing and able and can contribute to getting living examples off the ground.

The incentive for the project can vary for the different parties involved. For some, it could be a matter of strengthening their own brand through showing that they believe the matter to be important or for others there could be a political dimension which is driven by prevailing public opinion. Policy instruments at national or regional level can be financial incentives, knowledge-driven or regulatory, enforced through inspections of the participating organisations. Knowledge is an important driving force in order to be able to answer the question *why* we should work on this matter and also *how* we should do so to best achieve the goal.

Clear goals and a clear focus will contribute to the different parties going in the same direction, even if it is in different ways. The goals must be sufficiently broken down and concretised so that those involved will be able to assimilate them and follow up on them over time. It can be good to focus on several areas so that the project is not spread out too much, but at the same time can be given the necessary scope for some flexibility and adjustment.

In order for the implementation of the strategy to be successful, the parties involved need to seek support for the project from within their own organisations. Senior management should not only back the strategy, but also take responsibility for the implementation and ensure that sufficient resources are set aside for the project. With regard to politically controlled organisations, the operational plan should be established in the political assembly with clear expectations for feedback and results.

To facilitate the implementation for the different parties involved, concrete support and guidance is needed from a national level/system level. This could take the form of handbooks, communication material, digital support, skills development, support with evaluations/research, etc. The purpose of this is partly to facilitate the process of going from words to actions for those involved and partly to gather strength and align the project in order to have a greater effect. It is preferable that the different parties are involved in the implementation of this support so that it will be appropriately designed and fill the required needs. Those involved can also be helped to set good examples and support each other.

To successfully implement a strategy, important factors are:

- Clear direction.
- Operational plans.
- Incentives and support.
- Leadership.

4.3 Results (Follow Up)

"What gets measured gets managed" – an expression that has been around for a long time and which is often accepted as a truth, even if not everything that means something *can* be measured and not everything that can be measured is *important*. In order for a strategy to be carried out systematically and for the long term, we believe that the follow-up of results within the area of fire safety is important. Therefore, we must also regularly follow results which can be measured and which are meaningful. At a national level, this can be done, for instance, by following and analysing a number of indicators which show the direction that the development is going in and indicate how the measures should be designed. The indicators can also function as a driving force and motivation in the implementation.

> The purpose of the indicators is to give an idea of whether fire safety for the individual has been strengthened and whether developments in the fire safety area are moving towards the targets set.

How should the indicators be chosen? A logical 'map' is needed which comprehensively describes how the organisations are interrelated – what affects what. We can call this a logic model or program theory. It stretches from goals and resources to the project itself and performance and finally to the results/effects. The effects can often be achieved in the short term or in the longer term. The indicators can be measured along the whole chain and measure the performance of individual parties as well as the long-term effects. In Fig. 20.4, an example is given of what a logic model in the area of fire safety can look like and which indicators can be connected to it.

Resources	Activities	Achievements	Short term effects	Medium term effects	Long term effects
Examples: • Budget • Personnel • Competence • Equipment	Examples: • Regularly review the direction of the strategy • Involve actors • Be active in innovation processes	Examples: • Knowledge based reports • Communication efforts • Guidance on at-risk individuals • Investigation of responsibilities • Financial contributions • Review of general advice (e.g. smoke alarms) • ...	Municipalities prevent and manage residential fires better Indicators: - Proportion of municipalities that carry out home fire and safety checks - Proportion of municipalities with developed cooperation between several administrations	The fire protection of the individual increases Indicators: - Proportion of households with smoke alarms - Proportion of households with fire extinguishers - Proportion of households with fire blankets	Fires cause fewer deaths and injuries, property and environmental damage is reduced Indicators: - Number of fatalities - Number of injured - Costs for property damage - Number of developed fires

Fig. 20.4 Examples of impact relationships and indicators for a national strategy

After the logic model has been mapped, appropriate indicators will need to be specified. The first step is to "brainstorm" possible candidates. Then every indicator suggestion will need to be judged based on the specified requirements. For example, that the indicator must be clear, relevant, available at a reasonable cost and sustainable over time. An indicator also needs to be related to something else. For example, a goal, in order to contribute in the end to increased knowledge and to judge if the measures carried out have had an effect. In-depth analysis of the development of the indicators and what affects them is also needed. Research can also be a tool for mapping these chains of effect. Revision of the indicators and how they are measured should be ongoing.

4.4 Feedback

Perseverance and feedback are often important factors when it comes to implementations. The participants need feedback on their work and need to see results. They also need knowledge of how they can undertake and develop their work. The message must be consistent over the duration and providing feedback of efforts and effect is important in order for those stakeholders to maintain the work and to motivate others to become involved. Within this project, there are also good opportunities for feedback to the project leader to assist with continual development of methods and eventual adjustments of the strategies.

The implementation of the activities in the strategy will be carried out by different parties at a local, regional and national level. In order for the project to be successful, the content and aim of the strategy must be well communicated. The same applies to new knowledge which is generated while the project is in progress and feedback of experiences. Thus, regular communication of results, new knowledge and experiences must be ensured to involve and inspire all parties involved.

Communication to all stakeholders needs to be retained and organised based on different needs. More simplified and comprehensive reporting and more in-depth follow-up research are useful for different purposes. Large information platforms with different channels are an effective way of having a collective communication system which is both comprehensive and easily accessible. For example, a homepage can constitute the central platform where different information is collected and organised into different parts and where all communication can be linked.

Communication and dialogue can take place both when gathered, for example, at yearly conferences or webinars, and successively in various forums. Digital possibilities which can reach many are important so that communication is not restricted to face-to-face meetings as these often have a smaller number of participants.

To make a developing dialogue possible while the project is in progress, it is of great importance to have permanent underlying functions which spread information and good examples to the local stakeholders. This can ensure a long-term perspective in the activities by communicating the results of the work and channel-gained experiences. Temporary ad hoc efforts tend to lose engagement and energy and fail in the long run.

4.5 Review of the Strategy

Gradually as the results are followed up while those involved work with the implementation of the operational plans, it will become more apparent if the strategy has had the intended effect. Are we moving in the direction of the goal or are we focusing on the wrong things? It will take time before the effect can be seen and patience and perseverance are necessary for the project to produce results. At the same time, it is important to review critically the strategic focus regularly and consider if anything should be done differently. It is especially important to remember that the knowledge available will change over time.

The best time to review the strategy can vary depending on how much has happened in the field. On a strategic level, goals and focus should be reviewed around every ten years. Measures and activities which have a direct link to the operational plans should, therefore, be reviewed more often, approximately every three years. The aim is to keep the strategy alive and relevant.

5 Examples of Two Strategies

MSB is responsible for issues concerning civil protection, public safety, emergency management and civil defence as long as no other authority has responsibility. Responsibility refers to measures taken before, during and after an emergency or crisis.

SFPA is a non-profit public utility association that works for a fire-safe Sweden since 1919. The national association is complemented by 20 local associations in Sweden and cooperates closely with the CFPA (the international Confederation of Fire Protection Associations).

Having two strategies written by two different organisations can seem strange but they can have their advantages. In Sweden, MSB and SFPA have different roles and different capabilities, and thanks to the interface between them, they can have slightly different but complementary focuses. MSB, as a government authority, can act with legal support within its jurisdiction but also has restrictions with regard to what can be asked of whom. SFPA does not have the same capabilities, but it is free from the governmental restraints.

5.1 MSB: A National Strategy for Improved Fire Protection

The vision "No one should die or be seriously injured as the result of a fire" is a guiding star for the national project, and in 2010, four strategic areas were identified: knowledge and communication, technical solutions, local cooperation, as well as evaluation and research. Within the area of evaluation and research, a number of indicators were developed in order to be able to follow up on development within the area in the long term. Three goals were formulated up to 2020: (1) the number of deaths and serious injuries as a result of fires in residential environments will be reduced by at least a third, (2) individual awareness of the risks of fires and how one should react in the event of a fire will increase and (3) the amount of functioning fire alarms and fire protection equipment in residences will increase.

The goals for the indicators will be followed up continually. For example, it can be stated that the number of deaths in residential fires reduced by 20% and the number of serious injuries by 25% between the years 2010 and 2018 (see Table 20.1). Now new goals have been set for the next ten-year period (2020–2030) [6]. The work has been based on the historic trend of the indicators and relevant external factors (collected through literature and workshops). Based on this, new goals were established using the keywords: Achievable and Challenging.

What measures should be taken in order to achieve the goals for 2030? Based on previous strategy projects, research within the field and workshops has been used and evaluated according to which measures are judged to have the greatest effect on the origin of residential fires and their consequences. Fatal fires and fires which lead to serious injuries are incidents which must be especially prioritised, but measures with a broad approach should be included in a national strategy.

Risk groups have been identified for incidents with different consequences (fatalities, fires with response from the emergency services and self-reported fires) and prioritised measures have been chosen based on the desired specific effect. In general, the measures have been categorised in five areas, and within these areas, activities can be found which the different parties involved can relate to. The most important measures can be found at a local level where other parties such as regions, property owners, interest groups, non-governmental organisations (NGOs) or insurance companies can get connected and receive guidance. Within the prioritised areas, supportive activities can also be found at a systems level which concern, for example, legislative reviews, guidance or participation in innovations and standardisations. The prioritised measure areas are:

Table 20.1 Indicators and milestones from 2010 to 2030

Indicator	Start 2010	2020	Goal 2030	Measure of effect
Number of fatalities in residential fires	102	79	Below 60	Personal injuries
Number of persons to hospital care	–	626	Below 600	
Number of persons in institutional care	630	470	Below 400	
Insurance payments regarding fires and thunderstorms (MSEK)	1870	1629	Decreasing trend	Property damages
Number of rescue service interventions in developed residential fires	2569	2695	Below 2500	
Percentage of households with functional smoke detectors	79%	88%	At least 95%	Protective measures (performance of the individual)
Percentage of households with fire extinguishers	36%	68%	At least 80%	
Percentage of households with fire blankets	4%	44%	At least 70%	
Percentage of municipalities with developed collaboration	–	48%	–	Protection production (performance of the municipality)
Percentage of municipalities carrying out home visits	–	40%	–	

To improve fire protection in the home environment of particularly at-risk individuals. Examples:

To deepen the cooperation between those involved at a municipal level as well as municipal rescue services and social services and health care.

To identify individuals who require improved fire protection due to an increased risk behaviour and/or limited ability to react and act in the event of a fire.

To suggest and offer adapted risk reducing measures.

The investigation of responsibilities based on legislation connected to improved fire protection for at-risk individuals, e.g. those receiving home care.

Improved knowledge to prevent and act. Examples:

To map and identify different groups with a high risk of residential fires, e.g. specific residential areas. Based on the developed area profiles, directed target-group-adapted communication efforts can be carried out such as home visits, fire protection education within language courses for those who have recently come to the country or recruitment, and training of fire ambassadors in order to spread knowledge and the message of fire protection in society.

To educate primary school students on fire protection and safety, coordinated with other parties in the municipality (e.g. the police).

The development of support for the analysis of area profiles.

The updating of training material and national recommendations.

To increase the number of functioning fire alarms. Examples:

The municipality should actively follow up on the property owner's responsibility for the fire protection in multi-residential properties. Both technical and systematic fire protection in multi-residential properties should be monitored. It is appropriate to particularly follow up on fire protection in areas where home visits show that the number of functioning fire alarms is low.

To review the standardisation around fire alarms in residences. For example, analyses, building regulations and general advice.

To work to carry out a first response within a short response time. Examples:

To analyse and plan in order to reduce the response time of a first response based on local conditions. Society's collective resources should be considered and involved to the greatest extent possible.[1]

To develop knowledge through research, learning and innovation. Examples:

To work for innovation in the welfare sector and join digital initiatives by creating collaboration between health care parties who aim to reduce accidents and unwanted incidents among users of welfare services, for example.

Inventory of the need for research.

Coordination and financing of development investments and innovation processes.

To work towards the implementation of the knowledge of the future development of society in standardisations.

The measures have been identified as especially prioritised over the next 3–4 years in order to achieve the goals in the national strategy. They should not be viewed as comprehensive, but instead as guidance for those parties who work within the area on where focus should be put in order to achieve the greatest effect. The measures complement other measures which are already in use or planned. We hope that, with the participation of many parties, the goals for 2030 will be achieved, e.g. the goal for reduced fatalities (see Fig. 20.5).

5.2 *The Swedish Fire Protection Association Strategy: A Fire-Safe Residence for Everyone*

SFPA's strategy "A fire-safe residence for everyone" [7] encompasses all residential fires regardless of the size of the damage, even if efforts can then be prioritised and dimensioned with respect to size and cost/benefit. An important starting point for the position taken by SFPA is the certainty with which MSB's strategy places emphasis on fires which result in fatalities or serious injuries, which means that

---

[1] See Chap. 18 for a description of capabilities and experience in relation to achieving a faster response time.

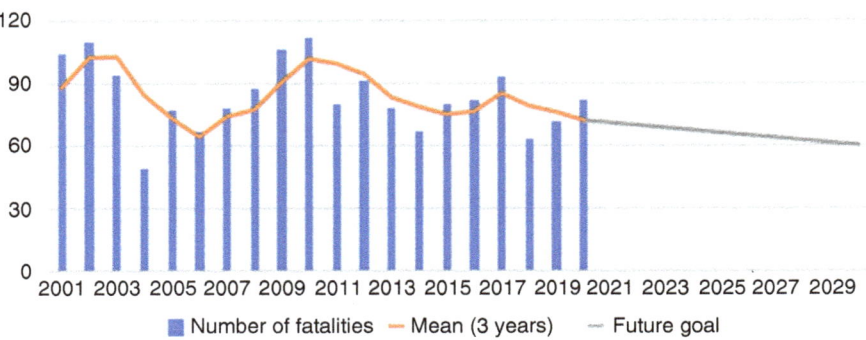

Fig. 20.5 Fatalities in residential fires in Sweden between 2001 and 2020 and future goal to 2030

SFPA can focus more on other fires. Thus, the design of the two strategies provides a resource for both parties in which they both overlap and complement each other.

The process was given two main focuses: Strategies to influence individuals to act towards the goals and strategies to work through other organisations towards the goals.

SFPA's strategy consists of four sub-areas: Sustainable residences; Safe care at home; Civil society's involvement; A strategy for everyone. The final sub-area is perhaps the most important as it clearly demonstrates that success requires the help of many. The problems surrounding residential fires cannot be solved by anyone individually and SFPA has clearly taken the position to support MSB's strategy as part of their own strategy. SFPA's role as a non-profit is also valuable in offering a hub in the joint efforts. The sub-areas have the following focuses.

Sustainable Residences:

To gather the parties concerned in order to establish goals, knowledge acquisition, collaboration and the follow-up of the consequences of residential fires.

Ecological sustainability work is focused on reducing the environmental and climate impact of repairs and rebuilding after fires by reducing the extent of the damage. Primarily, with measures on how the buildings are constructed and what fire protection is used and then through residual value saving work.

Social sustainability work must utilise the importance of a residence as a place for well-being. Work relating to fires in socially vulnerable areas must also be addressed with special measures. Deaths and injuries are of course also included in this.

Economic sustainability work focuses on the costs of fires.

Resilient multi-residential buildings are an important issue which can be quantified by measuring in: the number of residences that need to be evacuated as a result of a fire; the time which evacuated residences are uninhabitable; the economic and ecological costs of damages after a fire. Timber buildings are considered to have the greatest need for measures and the goal is that they should have at least the same resilience as concrete buildings.

Renewable energy and the technology built around it require fire safety. In this area, work is focused towards new knowledge and ensuring that the knowledge reaches where it is needed.

Safe Care at Home:

Knowledge in this area is insufficient and research is primarily needed in both practical and legal aspects.

The development of an injury prevention concept which systematically helps all parties to give residences a good quality of fire safety.

To work towards *customised fire protection for equal fire safety*. This forms an important approach which facilitates the work for those who want to help and aim to make a big difference for those who require help.

The groups have been mapped, in respect to personal risk, through research and appropriate help and relevant parties that can work to introduce this help are identified for each group.

Civil Society's Involvement:

Involvement from civil society is growing in order to support society in crises and to ensure safety in the local area. SFPA invests in utilising such resources by first response volunteers (Swedish abbreviation: CIP), enabling the upscaling of this resource.

A Strategy for the whole society:

Many of us must help if we are to succeed and there are many who can make a difference.

The Swedish Fire Protection Association, together with the 20 local organisations, operates a nationwide operation in which we reach all the different levels of society across the whole country.

We are experienced and collaborate well with big parts of society and we want to contribute where we can together with those who wish to be involved.

We have long worked to support MSB's zero vision – *No one should die or be seriously injured as the result of a fire* – and we will continue to do so.

References

1. Swedish Law on Protection against Accidents 2003:778. Swedish Government Sweden 2003
2. Stortingsmelding nr 35 (2008–2009) Brannsikerhet. Norwegian Government Norway 2008–2009
3. Nasjonal kommunikasjonsstrategi for brannsikerhet. Direktoratet for samfunnssikkerhet og beredskap. Norway 2015
4. European Fire Safety Action Plan. European fire safety Allience. Europe 2018
5. Vision 20/20 National Strategies for Fire Loss Prevention. Institution of Fire Engineers. USA 2008

6. A National Strategy for Improved Fire Protection. Swedish Civil Contingencies Agency Sweden 2020
7. A fire-safe residence for everyone. Swedish fire protection association. Sweden 2020

Mr. Mattias Delin holds a Bachelor of Science degree in Fire Safety Engineering from Lund University. For more than 20 years, starting 1998, he worked as a fire safety consultant focusing on fire safety in buildings, before he joined the Swedish Fire Protection Association and the Swedish Fire Research Foundation – Brandforsk as Research Director in 2019. Since 2021 Mattias is working full time with Brandforsk only. Mattias has also been member of the board and president for the Swedish chapter of SFPE, Society of Fire Protection Engineers.

Mrs. Maya Stål Söndergaard holds a BSc in Fire Safety Engineering from Lund University. Maya has worked 18 years at the Swedish Rescue Services and is now employed as a fire and risk consultant at Brandskyddslaget. She has extensive experience from working with fire prevention and residential fires and has since 2010 participated in the development and implementation of the national fire protection strategy. Most recently, she has been part of the project group that has worked to review the strategy and its goals and activities.

Dr. Björn Sund holds a PhD in Economics from Örebro University. Björn started as a project assistant and researcher in the field of Fire and Rescue Services in 1996. Since 2011 he has been employed as an analyst at the Learning from Accidents Section at the Swedish Civil Contingencies Agency. Research focus has been valuation of statistical life, stated preference methodology, cost-benefit analysis regarding faster emergency response to cardiac arrests, demographic determinants of incident experience and risk perception, willingness to pay for a quality-adjusted life-year (QALY) and residential fires. From 2018 he has been involved in evaluation and revision of the Swedish national strategy for strengthened fire protection. He is also a lecturer in economic evaluation at Karlstad University.

Part IV
Conclusion

Chapter 21
The Road Ahead

Marcus Runefors, Ragnar Andersson, Mattias Delin, and Thomas Gell

Abstract This chapter sums up some major findings and draws conclusions on desirable future directions for fire safety practices and research. Like in parallel fields of safety where human life is at stake, there is a need for a broadened systems-oriented approach, and towards preventing adverse consequences rather than preventing their preceding events. Due to demographic transitions, the residential fire safety problem is increasingly to be seen as a matter of human vulnerability, thus raising new challenges for all actors involved in designing and providing living environments.

A **resident** is anyone from zero to hundred years or more. Regardless of age, abilities and health, everyone deserves safe housing conditions. This matter is a shared responsibility across sectors. Relevant **actors** need to be identified and ascribed roles in a more systematized multi-sectoral fire safety work. Fire safety **technology** already offers significant protection if fully employed. Yet, new challenges appear ahead in the wake of ageing populations, shifting lifestyles and household structures and changing housing policies for residents with special needs.

A major concern relates to the **governance** of fire safety at local, national and international levels with regard to leadership, monitoring, accountability, implementation, learning and sharing in order to ensure continuous improvements.

Keywords Risk governance · Actors · Global perspective · Innovation · Strategy · Fire prevention

---

M. Runefors (✉)
Division of Fire Safety Engineering, Lund University, Lund, Sweden
e-mail: marcus.runefors@brand.lth.se

R. Andersson
Risk and Environmental Studies, Centre for Societal Risk Research, Karlstad University, Karlstad, Sweden

M. Delin · T. Gell
The Swedish Fire Research Foundation (Brandforsk), Stockholm, Sweden

© The Author(s), under exclusive license to Springer Nature Switzerland AG 2023
M. Runefors et al. (eds.), *Residential Fire Safety*, The Society of Fire Protection Engineers Series, https://doi.org/10.1007/978-3-031-06325-1_21

1 Introduction

Like other adverse events, fires do not occur randomly, even if it sometimes may seem so. They always result from latent conditions (technical, social and organizational), allowing them to happen and influencing their likelihood and severity. Moreover, frequent adverse events like fires tend to appear with strong regularity. They tend to reoccur with similar frequency and patterns year by year, implying a resembling continuation in the future as long as nothing is done to really alter the situation.

These regularities and environmental latencies constitute the rationale for applying a holistic systems approach when addressing human risk problems. Human risks and their adverse manifestations reflect design features of human environments for housing, working life, transportation, etc., which are usually man-shaped and thus also usually modifiable. Historically, accidents and other adverse events were often blamed on the individual or seen as acts of God. Today, we know better and realize that it is by designing our human environments we also determine our human risks, and that it is a societal responsibility to continuously strive for safer environments.

Residential fire is a type of adverse event occurring in the home environment. The home as a system, or rather the "housing system" to include its users as well, constitutes in its inner core of the physical home plus its occupants and visitors. This core is surrounded by a spectrum of actors who, in various ways and to various degrees, influence the design of our housing system in its broadest sense: Who lives where and under which socio-technical conditions? What do we do, and what do we store in our homes? etc. The housing system is also located in a broader context in the form of built environments, business activities, infrastructure, climate and so on, bringing further actors into the scene.

In this final chapter, we wish to reflect on some major challenges and related potentials, based on the aggregate knowledge as presented in previous chapters of this book. These challenges and potentials are structured according to the above-mentioned system components, plus one overarching perspective intended to meet the need of continuous improvements (Fig. 21.1).

The remaining of this chapter is structured around the components in the figure above.

2 The Resident(s)

"Resident" includes human beings in ages from zero to a hundred years or even more. Over a long age span, human capabilities and associated needs of support and environmental adaption vary within wide frames. In periods of life, such as in early childhood, we are helpless and fully dependent on others, and in periods we might be well functioning and supposed to care for both ourselves and others in need. At

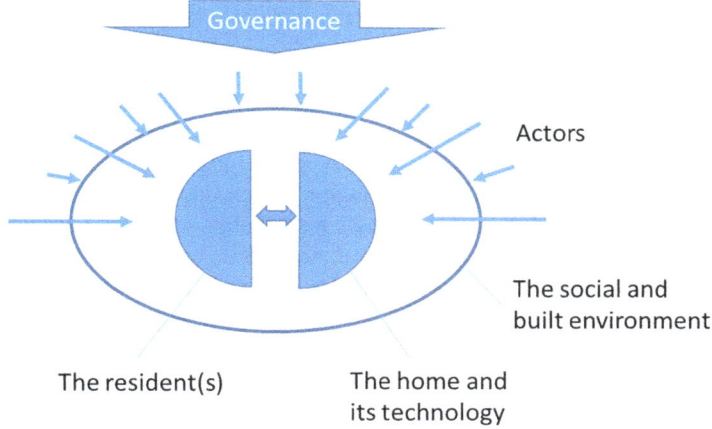

Fig. 21.1 The components of the housing system

older age, many of our capabilities often diminish, making us once again dependent on the care of others. The way this collective responsibility is organized varies between societies and over time; historically within family structures and more recently through institutionalized welfare systems. Modern societies tend to move towards larger proportions of single households with older residents, often with multiple health impairments and less resilient to injuries caused by fire (Chap. 4). This makes way for excessive vulnerabilities with regard to a number of residential hazards, not least fire (Chap. 5). There are also younger groups, typically without impairments, that have a high risk since addiction to alcohol and drugs limits their abilities to respond in case of fire.

As clearly shown in several chapters in Part I, human life and health in case of fire are increasingly related to vulnerability characteristics. This fundamental observation implies important needs for further developments in fire safety:

Even though the risk groups of fires have been rather well known for quite some time (see Chap. 2), further efforts are needed to deepen our understanding of why certain groups are at elevated risk. The literature, which is almost exclusively from western countries, clearly points at the elderly as the main group of concern. However, "the elderly" constitutes a very heterogeneous group with regard to capacities, vulnerabilities and lifestyles, calling for more detailed studies on this matter in the future. Smoking and alcohol are well-known risk factors, but in addition prescribed drug consumption combined with functional and medical impairments may play increasing roles. In other parts of the world, children still stand out as a group of major concern from a fire safety perspective (see Chap. 1). Why is that, and which developments in richer countries contributed to the significant reduction of fire fatalities in this group over time? In yet other parts of the world, women in younger adulthood represent the most exposed group in terms of fire-related mortality. This phenomenon still remains largely unexplained, although handful studies exist suggesting a spectrum of causes including dressing style, cooking habits and various types of family violence. Further analysis and clarification are very much needed.

Expected future developments of fire-related mortality need to be better modelled and projected, as input for elaborated and more realistic strategic planning at national and international levels. Such projections presuppose accuracy in historical data, both with regard to fire-related mortality and demography. Major determinants of fire-related mortality, as identified through research, such as health and disability status among residents, proportion of single households, prescribed drug consumption, smoking and alcohol habits and so on, need to be taken into account as well. Parallel political trends in housing policy for frail and service-demanding elderly are other factors of concern.

Strategical conclusions must be reached in each country separately, based on national conditions, but some generic implications can be outlined. These include:

- Ageing populations and deinstitutionalization in health and social care raise new challenges for the fire safety community. A growing share of frail residents, often living in single households, with considerable health and functional impairments and often under incapacitating medication, tends to remain living in their original homes without continuous assistance and surveillance. The challenges include installation (and sometimes development) of new technology to compensate the reduced abilities, e.g. new alarms for the hard of hearing and extinguishing systems for those unable to evacuate themselves in case of fire.
- Groups at risk in case of fire are characterized by elevated risks in many other respects, such as falls, suffocation, poisoning, suicide and cardiovascular issues. Fire safety professionals should seek collaboration with health and social sectors to provide broader safety solutions, taking all these problems into account. Addressing each risk one by one implies serious suboptimization of public resources and substandard solutions for those in need.

3 The Technology

Even though future technological innovation provides large opportunities to reduce the risk from fires, there is also a lot of currently available technology that should not be overseen. The most prominent example is the smoke alarm described in Chap. 8. This device has been instrumental in reducing the number of fatalities from fires and has received a wide adoption. Regulatory requirements on smoke alarms in many building codes have been vital to achieve this level of adoption, but also widespread give-away programmes, which have shown to often be cost-effective (Chap. 13).

Other available technologies, such as sprinklers and stove guards (see Chap. 11), have not yet received the wide implementation of the smoke alarm. There are a few countries that mandate sprinkler in certain residential structures, but there is often a conflict with the interest to not increase the cost of new housing. The time span needed for wide implementation is also substantial given that the lifetime of a buildings is many decades. Also, since the risk of fire for the general public is relatively low, it is not obvious that the investment in sprinklers can be motivated from a cost-benefit perspective (Chap. 13).

Stove guard is a newer innovation, tailored to handle cooking top fires, which is one of the leading causes of fire injuries in many countries. Despite this, the adoption rate is quite low, which might be due to the rather high price and, possibly, reliability issues related to early products. However, given the rapid development of new sensors, it is not difficult to foresee that the stoves of the future will have the inherent ability to detect and prevent the ignition of materials on the stove.

A well-known fire problem, especially pronounced after the transition to petroleum-based materials, is upholstered furniture. In many countries, a large proportion of the fire victims die before the fire has spread from the furniture first ignited. This requires measures to be implemented that influence the fire very early in the development. The most common way to address this is by fire-retardant treatment of the materials (Chap. 10) which has been implemented in several codes in the US and in the UK some decades ago. However, environmental concerns about the substances being used have led to a partial roll-back of the requirements. This is despite the more environmentally friendly alternatives that have been lately developed [e.g. 1]. In parallel, there has been an effort to modify the most prominent ignition source in these fires, the cigarette, through the implementation of the RIP-cigarettes in many countries in the last decade. Unfortunately, this has been found not to be effective in reducing the risk of ignition (Chap. 10).

Other available sophisticated fire protection systems such as the detector-activated sprinkler system can hardly be motivated for all housing, but is very cost-effective for the high-risk groups previously described. This clearly illustrates the necessary link between the understanding of the resident and the specific technology.

Except for incremental improvements of available technologies, such as interconnected and/or multi-sensor smoke detectors or smoke detectors that are less sensitive to user errors, it is difficult to foresee where new innovations that reduce the risk of residential fires will emerge. It can, however, be speculated that the surge of new technologies in the area known as Internet-of-Things (IoT) will provide huge opportunities as well as the increased installation of home surveillance cameras. What is clear, however, is that effective innovations will only be possible when the innovators have deep knowledge about the actual problem as presented in this anthology. Almand [2] has asked 14 global leaders in fire safety about where innovation is most needed, and they primarily named cooking and upholstered furniture as key areas of concern.

Turning to generally technological development in society, this can provide both opportunities and challenges from a fire safety perspective. Exploiting potential synergies between fire safety and more generic developments can be both faster and cheaper than the development of stand-alone fire safety technologies. Several such synergies can be identified. One example is the reduced energy consumption in many consumer products, which decreases heat development both in the product and in potential bad connections in the fixed wiring system. Also, the introduction of induction stoves, which results in both lower temperatures and that only metallic materials will heat up, is likely to reduce the risk of stove-related fires.

Although much of the technological development in the electrical system is likely to be positive from a fire safety perspective, there is also reason to closely monitor other developments such as charging of electric cars, solar panels, DC-circuits as well as energy storage in batteries or hydrogen. Although neither of those has so far proved themselves as major hazards in this respect, the development needs to be thoroughly investigated [3, 4].

Other developments in the building sector, such as increased use of wood as building material in large structures as well as the use of flammable claddings, cannot be expected to have a large influence of the general mortality rates since the victims typically die early in the fire development. However, they do introduce the risk of large catastrophic fires such as the Grenfell tower fire. Another pronounced development in the building sector is low energy housing which requires very airtight buildings, which might cause very large pressures in case of fires, potentially hindering evacuation (Chap. 9).

4 The Actors

By tradition, fire safety in dwellings has been regarded as mainly the responsibility of the resident. In the days when people built their own houses/furniture and mainly depended on their family for support when in need, this was a natural view. But today, our houses are designed by architects, built by building companies, and we buy our furniture and household appliances from resourceful multinational companies. In case of unemployment or illness, we depend on others such as the society to provide support. It seems rational to put forward the idea that all those organizations, having a profound influence on the preconditions for a safe system, also take on the responsibility to make it safer beyond minimum standards.

The National Fire Protection Association in the United States has formulated the notion of the "Fire & Life Safety Eco-System" [5] presented in Fig. 21.2. This idea of an ecosystem with a plethora of actors having a significant impact in different phases of a process aiming at creating fire safety is quite useful and underlines to a large extent the same idea of the importance of the responsibility of the "system designers" as put forward in the Vision Zero philosophy (see Chap. 15).

The Vision Zero target statement can, at least initially, be difficult to grasp as it seems to have an air of unrealistic or wishful thinking. However, behind the ethically motivated statement itself, as described in Chap. 15, there is a consistent underlying systemic safety philosophy that is truly goal-oriented and pinpoints responsibilities and driving forces necessary to create a safer system.

The mobilization of the entire system of actors, striving in the same direction, would benefit from better structures of incentives. Today, it is not rare that the saving of one actor becomes another actor's cost, or a resident's fatality. The national

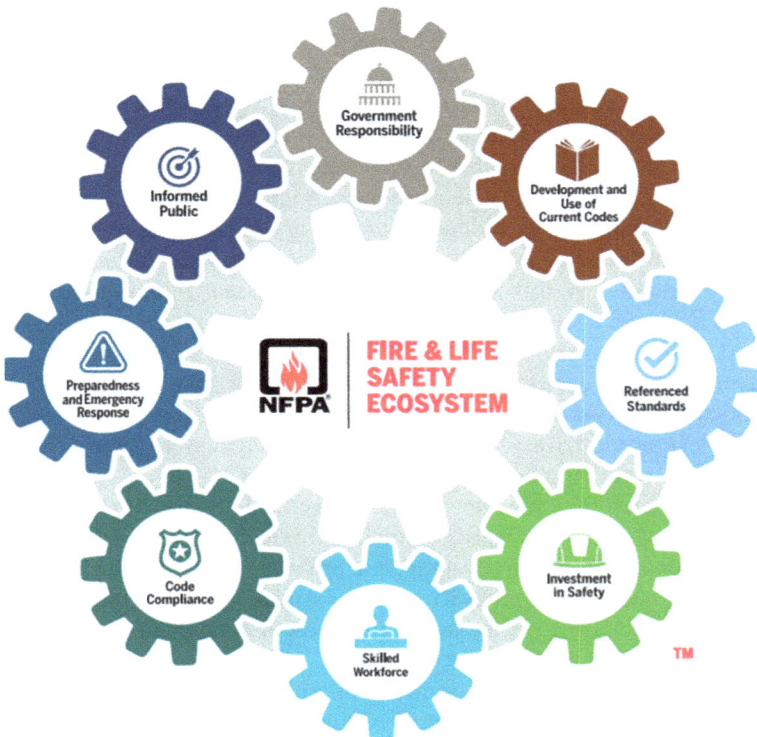

Fig. 21.2 The NFPA Fire & Life Safety Eco-System. (Source: Reproduced with permission from the National Fire Protection Association, Copyright© 2020, NFPA, Quincy, MA. All rights reserved. For a more information on the referenced subject, please go to www.nfpa.org)

strategies presented in Chap. 20 invite and encourage all actors to participate based on existing frameworks of legislation, altruism and own decisions, e.g. responsibility in line with Agenda 2030, but better incentives, e.g. economic, are needed in the future, and we need to monitor a broader spectrum of values of a resilient residence and correlate incentives to that.

Much of the programmatic activities and campaigns that have been directed towards the residential fire problem have been performed by local fire services, often with support from the national level. Some of the efforts have been very successful, such as the campaigns to increase the share of households with working smoke alarms. However, in most cases, campaigns and other interventions within the fire safety area are poorly measured and evaluated, making it difficult to judge their effectiveness. As suggested in Chap. 16, partnering with academic institutions can be an effective way to acquire a capacity for the design of measurable programmes and can also develop institutional capacity to sustain such programmes.

The community of involved actors, however, stretch far beyond "the usual suspects" – i.e. the organizations that we normally understand as the Fire safety professionals; the fires services, the fire appliance industry, fire engineering consultants, the building inspectors, etc. As described in, e.g. Chap. 2, the population most at risk for not surviving a residential fire is a very selected group of people, whose vulnerabilities render them unable to manage even a trivial fire situation. In this respect, caregivers and domestic help providers might be the key actors for identifying at-risk individuals and as well as for providing additional safety measures. The establishment of broad efforts, involving fire, social, health and other experts, is therefore a natural way forward. Such programmes and initiatives exist, but as pointed out in Chap. 17, preventing fire for vulnerable groups can in part be seen as a 'wicked problem', as there are challenges that transcend sectoral boundaries; and span several public agencies, thereby involving different areas of policy across several political-administrative levels. A major obstacle is, in many cases, regulations on data protection and privacy, making it difficult to share information as needed for cross-sector cooperation to be meaningful and effective.

Another aspect of stretching beyond the actors mainly present today is the use of volunteers and semi-professionals to gain time for the first response to a residential fire, perhaps a neighbour intervening in case of fire, as described in Chap. 19. This is still a novel strategy, but is probably a safety measure worth to expand and develop further to save lives. Perhaps it can be optimized in combination with the rescue service with the use of the model in Chap. 12.

One systemic problem when it comes to housing is that the building industry in general hardly works according to industrial principles and also has a very low level of standardization. Even in cases where the production is partly industrialized, as in the case of buildings constructed of prefabricated modules, the assembly of these modules into complete buildings might fail due to lack of quality control and an educated workforce. Further, the non-uniform and 'bushy' nature of the building industry are also making it difficult to get it to take on its responsibility as a key actor in the fire safety ecosystem. Fire safety, albeit included in material standards, in building codes and normally subject to some type of inspection, is seldom regarded as a true value in the finished building. It is rather seen as a burden or costly add-on, generally leading to migration towards minimum legislative requirements.

A relevant question is thus: how can fire safety become a core value in residential buildings – for the building industry as well as for the residents? One role-model is undoubtedly the automotive industry, where safety has become a key characteristic, valued by the car-buyers and something the car manufacturers must relate to if they want to stay in business. A way forward could possibly be to try to make the fire safety characteristics an inherent value in the rating systems that already exist for "green" or "sustainable" buildings.

5   Governance: Leading, Learning and Sharing

As presented in Chap. 2, much is known about the characteristics of victims of fatal fires and the risk factors associated. The chapter also clearly demonstrates the striking similarities among those factors across the investigated countries, which is instrumental for cooperation. It should, however, be noted that the studies are almost exclusively performed in Western countries and, given the differences in age- and sex patterns for some countries found in Chap. 1, more variation on a global scale can be expected compared to what is apparent in the published literature.

There are also still some issues on data collection with the lack of consistent global data on fire fatalities, which causes difficulties in comparing countries and injury patterns. Some efforts are underway to develop joint criteria in the European Union [6], and a new ISO-standard has also recently been released [7]. However, there is still a long way until a coherent definition and coding of fire fatalities have been implemented globally.

Systematic safety work relies to a large extent on access to data. Data on the adverse events themselves – the fires – is normally collected by the fire and rescue services as outlined in Chap. 6. But such data also must be supplemented by data from other sources for the purpose of deeper analysis and contextual understanding. In the case of fire injuries or fatalities, information from databases in the health and forensic sectors, police, etc. (see Chap. 1) are needed. When evaluating fire safety interventions, such as fire safety education campaigns (Chap. 16) or cost-benefit analysis of "hard" fire safety measures (Chap. 13), the activities themselves have to be measured and data, including cost data, made available for analysis. In these latter areas, there is room for much improvement, as the evidence-based tradition within the fire safety community has been rather weak. GIS-based and geostatistical analysis, Chap. 18, where geo-coded fire data and census data are included in the models, is a powerful tool for investigating and visualizing the spatial and social distribution of fires, as well as for planning and prioritizing optimal areas for local fire safety activities.

Even if characteristics and risk factors are of vital importance for prevention, more is needed to develop a sound and evidence-based strategy for prevention. This need to be based on much richer data than the register data typically used in research today. The investigation of fatal fires needs to account for the full social and organizational environment around the victims to identify how the outcome could have been prevented. This requires additional scientific disciplines to be involved in the investigation, such as sociologists, political scientists, geriatrics, etc.

The investigation should probably also include non-scientific actors more familiar with the system, such as authorities at different levels and possibly companies in the field. To retain the interest of those actors, the generation of generalized scientific knowledge should be in tandem with local knowledge on actual events. One example of such process is the OLA-process regularly performed in the road sector in Sweden, where selected traffic accidents are reviewed by a group of selected actors, which has the capacity to implement measures to reduce the risk of similar accidents in the future.

Such a process is believed to result in the implementation of actual preventive measures in society in tandem with the long-term development of general scientific knowledge that may benefit actors outside the local context.

As previously mentioned, there is an enormous gap in knowledge regarding the fire risk of the great majority of people living outside the western countries. As described in Chap. 1, the most common source of residential death and injury data for many low-income countries is burn data, which often doesn't include the source of those burns (i.e. fire or another source). However, there is ample reason to assume that the bulk of fire fatalities in those countries also occurs in residential settings. Primitive stoves are a major cause of fires and burns in most developing countries, with women and children at particular risk.

In contrast to high-income countries, where an ageing population [8] will create challenges for residential fire safety, the situation in low-income countries is different, but probably even more problematic. On a global scale, more than one billion people live in informal settlements with little or no built-in fire safety. The urbanization is rapid; by 2050, two thirds of the world's total population will live in urban areas, and 1 billion dwellings will have to be built in such areas to accommodate this increase [9].

The fast population growth in, e.g., sub-Saharan Africa will create megacities with little means of providing its citizens with proper infrastructure or housing. One such example is Lagos, Nigeria, where the population in 2021 is estimated to be close to 15 million, a number that is expected to double by 2050 – making it the third largest city in the world [10]. It is evident that this development will create residential environments with serious possibilities of aggravating the burden of residential fire injuries and fatalities. Whether the residences will be in the shape of makeshift dwellings or substandard high-rise "slum" buildings, the risk for mass-causality catastrophic fires can be expected to be high.

It is not realistic to expect countries or cities under such a rapid expansion and lack of national education or capacity in fire safety engineering to be able to apply our western type of fire safety standards. There is a strong need now to begin fire safety "capacity building", including [11]:

- Enhanced fire loss data capture and analysis.
- Build-up of fire safety education and research capacity.
- Transfer of adapted technology and knowledge.
- Contextually appropriate adaptations of western codes and standards.

Fortunately, lessons learned in the western world can accelerate this capacity building – calling for a wide partnership with different stakeholders/resources.

In the ongoing work with the 2030 Agenda for sustainable development [12], fire is a topic, but most attention regarding fire in general seems directed towards wildfires coupled with climate change. However devasting those fires are, the potential for large-scale fire disasters involving mass casualities is probably higher in urban areas. There are, therefore, good reasons for emphasizing the risk for both small and large-scale fires in residential areas in the developing megacities. Such an emerging risk falls naturally, e.g. under the UN Sustainable Development Goal no 11.1 – "By 2030, ensure access for all to adequate, safe and affordable housing and basic services and upgrade slum.".

The International Association of Fire Safety Science (IAFSS) highlights the need for the fire safety community to be part of the solution to what can be called "Grand societal challenges" [13]. Two such challenges where fire safety has an important role to play were identified as (i) climate change, resiliency and sustainability, and (ii) population growth, urbanization, globalization and changing demography. In that context, it is evident that residential fire safety is a core fire issue in the 2030 Agenda.

6 Conclusions

This book provides a comprehensive overview of various aspects relating to fatal fires and their victims. Based on this, and the discussion above, several conclusions can be drawn including the ones mentioned below.

There is an increasing **need to focus on high-risk groups**, especially older adults and socio-economically marginalized groups, and this requires additional disciplines to be involved in fire prevention. It is not enough to have a focus on preventing the fire, instead fire safety promotion of tomorrow should also address the capabilities and limitations of the victims as well as the social and organizational context surrounding the individual. This has implications for the organization of fire safety practices, where it is hard to imagine successful fire prevention efforts without the involvement of social services as well as NGOs who are regularly in contact with the groups. It also has implications for the level of fire prevention in homes; given the limited amount of resources in society and the comparably low risk of fatal fires for the general public, it can hardly be motivated to invest in sophisticated fire protection technologies, such as detector-activated sprinklers, for all citizens. Rather, there is a need to improve our abilities to tailor the fire protection depending on the needs of the individuals. Finally, it has implications on fire investigation where not only cause and origin of the fire should be sought but also how different latent conditions contributed to the final outcome.

Most of the western countries have come a long way in reducing the number of fire fatalities, while the rates in many poorer countries are significantly higher. This calls for an increased **global perspective** on fire safety, e.g. in the spirit of 2030 Agenda goal 17 "Partnerships for the goals". This includes both research to understand the differences in the fire problems in these countries compared to the countries where most of the research has been performed. However, it also includes global cooperation and capacity building in countries with a high risk to not only understand, but also to reduce the risk.

For general fire safety in society, there is a need to **promote innovation**, and this can, at least partly, be addressed by appropriate incitement structures and an attempt to promote fire safety as an inherent quality of buildings and products. This can also help to address the limited adoption rate of available technologies beyond the smoke alarm, such as stove guards and residential sprinkler systems. A problem related to innovation for residential fires safety is the lack of resources and driving forces for a dedicated common effort; the system and its actors are simply too disparate and scattered compared to, for example, fire safety of underground structures. Most of the research and development within the area is founded by governmental agencies, with minimal contributions from the other system designers/actors.

There is also clearly a need for **increased knowledge** in several areas, not least about the situation in non-western countries with regard to fire safety. There is also a need for more knowledge about factors that promote and hinder effective prevention efforts and also the cost-benefit of available means for reduction of fire risk, both in general and for specific groups.

However, no change will occur without **political leadership**. Political goals should be set, strategies redesigned to meet these goals, and a sustainable governing system put in place to ensure their systematic implementation. The Vision Zero approach may serve as a model of inspiration. In addition to these national challenges, there is a need for strengthening global leadership as well, to reach improved international support, coordination, benchmarking and learning across nations. The residential fire problem can be seen as a core fire safety issue in relation to major challenges such as climate change, resiliency, sustainability, changing demographics and urbanization. Therefore, there are strong factual and strategic reasons to integrate the ongoing and future work on residential fire safety into major political initiatives such as the 2030 Agenda.

References

1. Larsson A-C, Patra A (2020) Studies on environmentally friendly flame retardants for cellulosebased materials
2. Almand K (2021) Fire safety innovation – a global view. FPE extra 2021 #67
3. Andersson P, Byström A, Fjellgaard Miklasen R, et al (2019) Innovativa elsystem i byggnader – konsekvenser för brandsäkerhet ["Innovative electrical systems in buildings – consequences for fire safety"; in Swedish]. Brandforsk report 2019:6
4. Lönnermark A (2018) Brandsäker energilagring – Sammanställning av risker och forskningsbehov ["Firesafe energy storage – summary of risks and research needs"; in Swedish]. RISE report 2018:42, Research Insitutes of Sweden (RISE)
5. NFPA (2020) NFPA FIRE & LIFE safety ecosystem. National Fire Protection Association
6. Efectis EU FireStat – Closing Data Gaps and Paving the Way for Pan-European Fire Safety Efforts. https://eufirestat-efectis.com/. Accessed 28 Oct 2021
7. ISO 17755-2: Fire safety — Statistical data collection — Part 2: Definition of terms
8. OECD (2019) Demographic trends. In: Organ. Econ. Coop. Dev. https://www.oecd-ilibrary.org//sites/c05578aa-en/index.html?itemId=/content/component/c05578aa-en#. Accessed 28 Oct 2021
9. UN (2019) World population prospects. In: Dep Enonomic Soc. Aff. United Nations. https://population.un.org/wpp/. Accessed 28 Oct 2021

10. World Population Review. https://worldpopulationreview.com/world-cities/lagos-population. Accessed 28 Oct 2021
11. Gell T, Almand K (2017) Fire safety without borders. Presentation at Nordic Fire & Safety Days 2017
12. UN The 17 Goals. In: Dep. Econ. Soc. Aff. United Nations. https://sdgs.un.org/goals. Accessed 28 Oct 2021
13. McNamee M, Meacham B, van Hees P et al (2019) IAFSS agenda 2030 for a fire safe world. Fire Saf J 110. https://doi.org/10.1016/j.firesaf.2019.102889

Dr. Marcus Runefors is a Lecturer at the Division of Fire Safety Engineering at Lund University in Sweden, where he also finished his PhD in the beginning of 2020. The topic of his PhD was fatal residential fires from both a prevention and response perspective, focusing on the effectiveness of different measures to prevent fatal fires for different groups in the population.

Prof. Ragnar Andersson is a Senior Professor of Risk Management affiliated to Karlstad University in Sweden where he served as full professor from 2001 until retirement in 2015. His educational background is in engineering and public health. After serving for the Swedish National Board of Occupational Safety and Health in the 1970s and 1980s, he took his PhD in Social Medicine at Karolinska Institutet, Sweden, in 1991 on occupational injury prevention. Dr. Andersson's research is focused on accident and injury analysis and prevention, injury surveillance, and macro-level determinants of risk in broad fields such as occupational, traffic, product, child, senior, and fire safety.

Mr. Mattias Delin holds a Bachelor of Science degree in Fire Safety Engineering from Lund University. For more than 20 years, starting 1998, he worked as a fire safety consultant focusing on fire safety in buildings, before he joined the Swedish Fire Protection Association and the Swedish Fire Research Foundation – Brandforsk as Research Director in 2019. Since 2021 Mattias is working full time with Brandforsk only. Mattias has also been member of the board and president for the Swedish chapter of SFPE, Society of Fire Protection Engineers.

Mr. Thomas Gell holds a Licentiate of engineering degree in Marine structural engineering from Chalmers University of Technology. For more than 25 years, he worked in various managerial positions with risk-related issues at the Swedish Rescue Services Agency and the Swedish Civil Contingencies Agency. In 2016–2019, he was Head of Research and Innovation at the Swedish Fire Protection Association and director of Brandforsk, the Swedish Fire Research Foundation. He has been particularly focused on research-related development, especially learning from events and systematic safety work. He currently works as an independent consultant. He is chairman of Karlstad University's Center for Research on Societal Risks and a US Fire Protection Research Foundation board member.

Index

A
Actors, 90, 107, 116, 117, 261–263, 265, 267, 268, 300, 309, 323, 364, 368–372, 374
Ageing, 71, 82, 83, 116, 295, 296, 366, 372
Alarm signal characteristics, 149
Alcohol, 10, 16–20, 22, 23, 34, 37, 47, 93, 112, 117, 129, 130, 134, 210, 244, 246, 310, 313, 314, 365, 366
At-risk groups, 37
Audibility, 127, 128, 149, 150, 156
Auditory arousal, 131

B
Benefits and costs, 222, 224, 227–228, 331, 332
Burn care, 59
Burn injuries, 61
Burns, 4, 5, 8, 10, 19, 20, 34–36, 47, 48, 51–54, 56–62, 93, 107, 112, 113, 117, 126, 151, 162, 164, 167, 168, 170, 172, 185, 210, 211, 253, 337, 372

C
Collaboration, 199, 267, 277, 278, 301, 322, 328, 330, 333, 335, 337, 339–341, 348, 356–358, 366
Community risk reduction, 275, 278, 301
Compartment fires, 148, 152, 154
Co-production, 328, 330, 339–341
Cost-benefit analysis (CBA), 104, 221–229, 232–238, 333, 371

D
Disabilities, 4, 22, 34, 61, 62, 68–70, 81, 107, 117, 129, 198, 200, 201, 207, 209, 212–214, 217, 310–314, 366

E
Economically efficient, 222, 228, 229, 238
Economic evaluations, 238, 335, 338
Effectiveness, 19, 32, 38, 90, 118, 123, 124, 132, 134, 135, 137, 184, 222, 225, 229, 244–248, 251–254, 281–288, 301, 369
Egress, 68–73, 76–78, 81–83, 137, 146, 148–151, 153–155, 162, 164
Emergency response, 91, 92, 328, 330, 339
Evacuation, 20, 22, 36, 68–83, 104, 105, 112, 115, 117, 128, 129, 135, 137, 199, 205, 263, 275, 298, 368

F
Fatal fires, 5, 6, 14–24, 32–34, 36–38, 92, 105, 118, 160, 163, 164, 172, 173, 214, 216, 244, 249, 303, 312, 314, 346, 355, 371, 373
Fire, 4–10, 14–24, 31–39, 46–48, 50–62, 68–76, 78–83, 90–108, 111–118, 124–131, 133–138, 144–149, 151–156, 159–174, 177–193, 198–217, 221–239, 244–247, 249, 251–254, 260–268, 271–288, 294–304, 308–323, 328–331, 333–342, 346–359, 364–374
Fire death definition, 102
Fire definition, 100–102

© The Editor(s) (if applicable) and The Author(s), under exclusive license to Springer Nature Switzerland AG 2023
M. Runefors et al. (eds.), *Residential Fire Safety*, The Society of Fire Protection Engineers Series, https://doi.org/10.1007/978-3-031-06325-1

Fire fatality, 14–24, 105, 129, 130, 134, 146, 163, 164, 170, 183, 198, 236, 244, 247, 251, 267, 294, 295, 297, 300, 301, 365, 371–373
Fire indicator, 202, 217, 319, 352
Fire mortality, 6, 18, 111, 127
Fire prevention, 5, 16, 23, 92, 117, 118, 161, 178, 221, 225, 236, 249, 272, 273, 275, 277, 294, 296–300, 303, 308, 313, 315, 321, 323, 346, 373
Fire risk, 90, 146, 160, 161, 184, 254, 266, 279, 297, 301, 308–313, 319, 322, 346, 372, 374
Fire safety, 5, 14, 31, 68, 90, 111, 124, 146, 159, 182, 199, 222, 244, 260, 271, 296, 308, 342, 347, 365
Fire safety strategy, 14, 16, 118, 244
Fire statistics, 8, 98, 99, 107, 163, 164, 173, 298, 317
Fire strategy, 76, 159–161, 322, 345–359
First response, 328–333, 335, 336, 338–340, 357, 359, 370
Functional limitations, 22, 23, 67–83, 246

G
Geographic information system (GIS), 308, 313, 316, 319, 332, 335
Geography, 315
Global burden of disease (GBD), 4
Global perspective, 373

H
Home safety, 263
Human response, 123–138
Human vulnerability, 112, 116

I
Ignition, 16, 19, 33, 49, 73, 94, 100, 105, 115–117, 125, 127, 129, 134, 154, 155, 160, 162–164, 166–173, 214, 253, 263, 295–297, 313, 367
Implementation, 74, 90, 107, 161, 162, 244, 260, 261, 277, 279, 281, 283–286, 298–300, 302–303, 308, 332, 347–354, 357, 366, 367, 372, 374
Income, 7, 8, 18, 19, 21–23, 35–38, 103, 249–252, 254, 281, 282, 300, 310–312, 316, 319
Individualised fire safety, 300, 302, 303
Inhalation injuries, 47–49, 51, 58–61

Injury pyramid, 15, 29–39
Innovation, 265, 355, 357, 366, 367, 373, 374
Intensive care, 58, 60, 61
Interior doors, 143–155, 215
Interior textiles, 165
International Classification of functioning, disability and health (ICF), 69, 70, 73, 76, 82, 295

K
Kitchen fires, 191–193, 323

L
Living conditions, 10, 52, 246, 294, 295, 308, 309, 313, 316–322

M
Management by objectives (MBO), 264, 267
Mattresses, 75, 133, 154, 161, 164–166, 170–173
Model for rescue operations, 201
Morbidity, 10, 46, 47, 58, 93
Mortality, 4–8, 10, 18, 20, 31–34, 36, 46, 47, 49, 58–60, 93, 111, 127, 365, 366, 368

N
Non-fatal fires, 15, 20, 21, 33, 37

O
Older adults, 5, 36, 79, 133, 253, 295, 296, 298, 300, 303, 373

P
Policies, 35, 70, 91, 95, 229, 260, 266, 272, 284, 294, 300, 308, 341, 351, 366, 370
Pressure effects, 146
Program evaluation, 284
Public education, 272, 277–279, 281, 282, 284, 285, 288

R
Residential fires, 14–24, 29–39, 47, 52, 54, 68, 70, 74, 91, 94–96, 98, 99, 101, 105, 106, 108, 112, 116, 118, 124–127, 129, 130, 132, 143, 144, 146–156, 161–164, 166, 167, 170, 184, 185, 192, 193, 198,

199, 202–204, 207, 208, 214–217, 222, 229, 232, 249–251, 268, 271, 285, 297, 308–323, 328–331, 333, 335, 337, 338, 340–342, 346–348, 355–358, 364, 367, 369, 370, 372–374
Residential sprinklers, 117, 177–179, 181–190, 192, 193, 374
Residential sprinkler systems, 177, 178, 186, 192, 374
Response time, 22, 104, 203, 217, 222, 224, 225, 227, 328, 331–335, 337, 339, 340, 357
Risk governance, 371–373
Risk groups, 10, 14–24, 32, 46, 52, 55, 80, 131, 225, 294–304, 314, 322, 355, 365

S

Semi-professionals, 328, 330, 332–337, 340, 341, 370
Smoke alarms, 15, 16, 18, 23, 32–34, 36, 38, 76, 90, 117, 123–138, 148–150, 166, 184, 192, 244, 245, 247–251, 253, 254, 287, 296, 300, 301, 310, 311, 366, 369, 374
Smoking, 10, 16–20, 22, 23, 112, 117, 129, 134, 146, 160, 163, 172, 173, 211, 246, 248, 249, 253, 281, 295, 297–299, 310, 313, 365, 366
Sociodemographic, 8, 9, 38, 52, 244–254
Sociodemographic factors, 18, 21, 22, 246
Socioeconomic factors, 112, 235, 310
Stove guards, 117, 160, 161, 167, 178, 190–193, 245–248, 254, 366, 367, 374

Strategies, 14, 16, 18, 38, 62, 68, 73–76, 79, 80, 82, 118, 159–161, 244, 267, 268, 279, 299, 322, 323, 341, 346–359, 369–371, 374
Surveillance, 90–108, 112, 264, 346, 366, 367
Sustainable residences, 358
Systems approach, 260, 262–264, 266, 298, 364

U

Unintentional fires, 4, 173, 340
Upholstered furniture, 126, 163, 164, 166, 168–173, 263, 367
Urban areas, 37, 321, 322, 334, 336–338, 340, 341, 372
Urgent rescues, 200, 202–207, 209, 212–217

V

Value of statistical life, 227, 238, 247
Vision zero, 260–268, 346, 368, 374
Volunteers, 281, 282, 300, 328, 330, 333, 336–341, 359, 370
Vulnerable, 5, 17, 20, 22, 46, 52–55, 82, 90, 104, 105, 116, 118, 131–133, 135, 138, 160, 161, 188, 190, 205–207, 213–217, 262–265, 286, 294, 295, 297–300, 317, 330, 338–342, 348, 358, 370

W

Water mist systems, 178, 185, 188–190

GPSR Compliance

The European Union's (EU) General Product Safety Regulation (GPSR) is a set of rules that requires consumer products to be safe and our obligations to ensure this.

If you have any concerns about our products, you can contact us on

ProductSafety@springernature.com

In case Publisher is established outside the EU, the EU authorized representative is:

Springer Nature Customer Service Center GmbH
Europaplatz 3
69115 Heidelberg, Germany

www.ingramcontent.com/pod-product-compliance
Ingram Content Group UK Ltd.
Pitfield, Milton Keynes, MK11 3LW, UK
UKHW021446190426
11946UKWH00022B/49